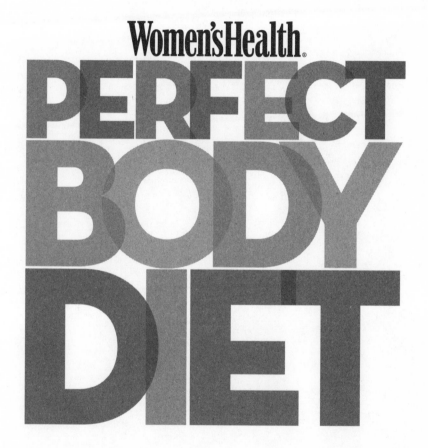

Women'sHealth

PERFECT
BODY
DIET

Foreword by **Kristina M. Johnson**, Editor-in-Chief of *Women's Health*

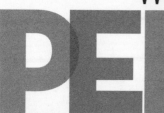

Women'sHealth®

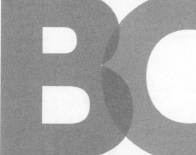

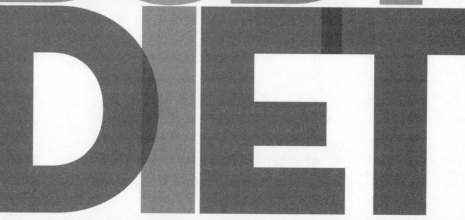

PERFECT
BODY
DIET

THE ULTIMATE WEIGHT LOSS AND WORKOUT PLAN
TO DROP STUBBORN POUNDS AND GET FIT FOR LIFE

CASSANDRA FORSYTHE, MS

RODALE®

PHOTOGRAPHS BY © TOM MACDONALD/RODALE IMAGES

BOOK DESIGN BY SUSAN EUGSTER

Library of Congress Cataloging-in-Publication Data

Forsythe, Cassandra E.
    Women's health perfect body diet : the ultimate weight loss and workout plan to drop stubborn pounds and get fit for life / Cassandra Forsythe ; foreword by Kristina M. Johnson.
        p.   cm.
    Includes index.
    ISBN-13 978–1–59486–791–0 direct-mail hardcover
    ISBN-10 1–59486–791–7 direct-mail hardcover
    1. Weight loss. 2. Physical fitness for women. 3. Women—Health and hygiene. I. Title.
    RM222.2.F6755 2008
    613.2'5—dc22   2007042968

2 4 6 8 10 9 7 5 3 1 direct-mail hardcover

womenshealthmag.com (♦

Here's to **every woman**
out there who's ever looked
in the **mirror**—and thought
better of it. We can't solve
those bad-hair days, but
perfection may be **closer**
than you think.

CONTENTS

ACKNOWLEDGMENTS

The editors of _Women's Health_ would like to give a shout out to several individuals who helped us create the _Perfect Body Diet_. Cassandra Forsythe provided the solid science that shaped the breakthrough concepts of the book, and Pam Liflander helped Cassandra bring her nutritional savvy to the page. Tom McGrath graced the text with his signature light touch and irreverent wit. And Jennifer Everett happily pitched in whenever we needed her expertise and flair. Amy Dixon, the face of _Women's Health_ on our DVDs and at womenshealthmag.com, shared her valuable insights on the book's fitness plan and posed for the photographs of the moves. Michelle Bower applied her talents to creating the workouts. Susan Eugster and her considerable design skills are responsible for the fresh look of the book, with Andy Carpenter and Andrea Dunham lending their artistry as well. Nancy Hancock, with the help of Kathryn LeSage, worked tirelessly to edit the book. And Robin Micheli made sure it all came together. To all of you, thanks. You rock.

FOREWORD

This book began as a conversation among the editors of *Women's Health*. The gist of it: Diets suck, to put it bluntly. We're sick of one-size-fits-all plans that are impossible to maintain. While we fully admit to trying them (crazy maple-syrup-and-cayenne concoction included), and we concede that they can help you drop a few pounds quickly, they're not a realistic or healthy game plan for losing weight and—here's the important part—keeping it off.

So we jotted down our diet wish list:

1. The *Women's Health Perfect Body Diet* should be custom-fit for every woman. After all, hormonally speaking, our bodies vary tremendously. I don't metabolize penne a la vodka at the same rate as, say, Eva Longoria or Jennifer Hudson. I want the best plan for *me*.

2. The *Women's Health Perfect Body Diet* should make me feel strong. Not weak. Not starving.

3. The *Women's Health Perfect Body Diet* should be easy to maintain as a permanent lifestyle change. Studies show that 95 percent of dieters gain back the weight they lose within 1 to 5 years. Thanks, but I'll pass. *Give me something I can stick to for life.*

Ambitious? Absolutely. But we at *Women's Health* wanted to provide you with a plan to change the way you eat and work out—a plan guaranteed to reveal your perfect body. We started out by consulting renowned nutritionists and fitness experts around the world. Each presented a potential plan, but nothing quite measured up. That is, not until we met nutritionist Cassandra Forsythe. Cassandra is a PhD candidate at the University of Connecticut (ranked the number one Doctoral Kinesiology program in the United States), and her name appears in the bylines of reams of research about diet and exercise. Her smart, realistic, science-based approach—not to mention her rock-solid body—syncs up with everything *Women's*

Health is about. Custom-fit? Check. Fills our tank? Check. Works with our busy-as-hell schedule? Check.

During our meetings with Cassandra, I emphasized that a deprivation diet is not an option—after all, if you're anything like me, that strategy ultimately sends you diving, face first, into a bag of Cool Ranch Doritos. Enough said. "Have you ever heard of glucomannan?" she asked. "Um, no," I admitted. "I don't read my nephew's comic books." She went on to explain that this multisyllabic mouthful is in fact an all-natural soluble fiber that, when added to your grub, slows digestion and makes you feel fuller, longer. And the grub that Cass had in mind is nothing less than great: She developed two complete diet plans (you'll find out which one best matches your body type and carb-sensitivity level by taking her simple breakfast tests), each with meal programs and recipes that'll keep you satisfied and on track. You just mix the plant-derived glucomannan powder into a few of your cinch-to-prepare meals each day, as though it's an everyday condiment. It's affordable, widely available, easy to incorporate, and, most important, tasteless.

But this book isn't just about what you put in your mouth. No *Women's Health* plan would be complete without energy-provoking, calorie-blasting workouts. The routines on these pages—each one designed to benefit your specific body type—will add muscle (minus the bulk) and make you feel stronger than ever.

So, dig in. After slurping down the Pumpkin Pie Smoothie on page 187, I know you'll feel the same way I do: This is the one diet that really rocks.

Kristina M. Johnson
Editor-in-Chief
Women's Health

INTRODUCTION:
YOUR PURSUIT OF PERFECTION

Okay, we know what you must be thinking when you pick up a book called *Women's Health Perfect Body Diet:* What exactly do we mean by "perfect"? Hollywood starlet perfect like, say, Natalie Portman? Superflexible yogalicious perfect like Christy Turlington? Oh-my-gosh-I-can't believe-she's-50 perfect like Kim Cattrall?

Yes. All of the above.

Or maybe none of the above. Because the truth is that having a "perfect" body means something different to every single woman on the planet. For some of us, it's getting a tummy so flat that we'll turn every head on the beach on our next bikini vacation. For others, it's simply slimming down our thighs so that pulling on our favorite jeans no longer feels like an Olympic event. When it comes to our bodies—just as when it comes to our lives—one size doesn't fit all. And it shouldn't. Our goals are as unique as we are.

Pardon us for patting ourselves on the back, but recognizing that fact is, we think, the genius of this book. When it comes to shaping up and slimming down, not every woman starts in the same place, and not every woman wants to end up in the same place. Just as important, the steps in between can end up being different, too. That's why we've crafted a plan with options, though they have one simple goal: to help *you* get *your* best body ever.

The *Women's Health Perfect Body Diet* Is as Unique as You Are

We don't need to tell you that there are a lot of weight-loss plans out there. In fact, these days it seems like the only thing more ubiquitous than new diet books are people who want to read them. Is it just supply keeping up with demand? Maybe. Or maybe it's the opposite: supply making the demand worse. Maybe we're gaining weight because we keep trying weight-loss plans that are fundamentally flawed.

Part of the problem is that diets are marketed as being effective for anyone, men and women alike. But we know that men aren't the same as women, and women aren't even the same as each other. We all metabolize food differently and have different energy needs. Some of us can tolerate all foods well, and some of us have problems digesting certain types of foods. So the promise of one diet that works for everyone is an empty promise.

Unfortunately, as smart as we are in many areas of our lives, a lot of us don't take our differences into account when we're trying to decide how to lose weight. We latch on to the latest fad or simply follow what our friends are doing. Word of mouth may be great for discovering a hot, young novelist or hilarious blogger, but trust us: It can be a disaster when it comes to dieting. Sure, the woman from your yoga class might have done well on a particular weight-loss plan—whether it was high-protein, high-carb, low-fat, all-chocolate, or "cleansing fast"—but you need to know why it worked for her before you try it yourself. When it comes to achieving your perfect size, one size doesn't fit all.

Perfect Body Principles

The *Women's Health Perfect Body Diet* makes it easy to lose the weight you want. Follow these simple guidelines.

» Calculate the right goal weight for *your* body.

» Determine which of the two diets is best for you.

» Always select from the vast array of good foods suggested in the *Perfect Body Diet*.

» Combine your food with the fiber supplement glucomannan to prevent you from eating foods that aren't good for you (like that giant slab of cake at your co-worker's birthday party).

» Eat five or six small meals a day, and don't let yourself get hungry.

» Choose the right exercise plan for your body shape. Exercise 6 days a week and be physically active for at least 30 minutes on the remaining day.

» Focus on the way your body feels and looks instead of worrying about a number on the scale.

The *Women's Health Perfect Body Diet* is unique because it offers options. It's an 8-week program based on two eating plans, both of which include balanced percentages of carbohydrates, protein, and fat. One plan is slightly higher in carbs, for women whose bodies react better to carbohydrates; the other is a bit lower, for those who do not metabolize carbohydrates as well.

Either of these plans will work for most women, but only one will be right for you. Once you determine which of the options suits your body best, you'll get immediate confirmation that it's the right regimen for you because it will fit into your lifestyle easily, and you'll find that you are satisfied, full, and functioning normally throughout the day. Best of all, you'll be able to stick with it for the long term, even after you've achieved your perfect body.

The *Perfect Body Diet* Keeps You Satisfied

If you feel like you're constantly restricting what you eat, you certainly aren't alone. Many women are "dieting" all the time. And that's exactly why most diets fail. We often restrict our calories to an extreme or follow a diet where the suggested foods are redundant or unpalatable. When feelings of boredom or starvation kick in, the diet gets kicked to the curb.

Most women think that in order to lose weight, they have to feel deprived all the time. But let's make this point loud and clear: You cannot restrict your food intake or food choices to the point where you're literally starving. You need to make sure that you are getting enough calories to function normally. If any diet restricts you to such small quantities of food that the diet book itself starts looking appetizing, then you know it's time to throw that diet out the window.

In Chapter 7, we'll help you figure out how many calories you need. You'll eat more frequently than you may be doing now, enjoying five or six small meals a day to evenly space out your caloric intake. And in Chapter 4, you'll learn about the *Perfect Body Diet*'s secret weapon, a revolutionary fiber supplement called glucomannan that will help control hunger by slowing the digestion and absorption of food, especially carbohydrates. Glucomannan will make you feel so satisfied that you won't even realize that you're on a diet. You'll learn how to incorporate 2 grams of this natural soluble fiber into at least three of your daily meals, so that you will be less hungry throughout the day and more satisfied with the foods you love to eat already. You'll not only stay full longer, you'll also boost your metabolic rate so that you burn body fat all day long.

The *Perfect Body Diet* Is Balanced

We can back up our theories on why some diets are better than others with reams of scientific papers. More important is this very scientific fact: There's no research that supports eliminating certain nutrients in one meal to attain a leaner, healthier body (such as separating carbohydrates from fat or eating fruit alone). What is most crucial is that you eat the right foods for your body, and for weight loss you'll need a slight caloric deficit. We'll show you how to calculate your proper calorie intake in Chapter 7.

You also need to take in the right balance of all the essential macronutrients. All women need lean proteins, complex carbs, and healthy fats at each meal. Together, these food groups replace and repair what you burn off and break down during a normal day, especially after exercise. They continuously supply your body with the right energy all day long, promoting weight loss and overall good health. We'll go over more about each of these types of nutrients in Chapter 6 and give you lists of foods to choose from each of these categories.

Remember those reams of scientific papers we mentioned? We won't bore you with all of them, but there are a couple of studies that really illustrate what balanced-macronutrient diets can do. Recently, researchers from Tufts University in Massachusetts published the first 1-year phase of a long-term dietary trial called the CALERIE study (that stands for Comprehensive Assessment of the Long-term Effects of Restricting Intake of Energy). This study divided overweight but otherwise healthy women and men into two dietary groups. One group ate a diet that, like the government-recommended diet, favored carbs, with 60 percent of calories from carbs, 20 percent from fat, and 20 percent from protein. The foods included carrots, chicken, rice, oatmeal, pizza, graham crackers, and yogurt with added fruit. The other group followed a diet in which the macronutrients were more evenly balanced, with 40 percent carbs, 30 percent fat, and 30 percent protein. The foods provided in this group included baked chicken, bulgur, beans, fruit, low-fat cottage cheese, nuts, steak, fat-free milk, and plain yogurt. Both diets were designed to help subjects adhere to a lower calorie level by including at least 25 grams of fiber each day, limited calories from liquids, and a large variety of low-energy-density foods (such as vegetables and berries).

After 3 months—the period when subjects were least likely to cheat and most likely to eat the food provided—the investigators looked at changes in self-reported hunger and satisfaction. They found that the subjects in the 60-percent-carb group had a significantly increased desire to consume nonstudy foods and a significant decrease in satisfaction with the type of food provided. In short, they were pretty miserable, meaning they were a lot less likely than the balanced-nutrient group to stick with the program.

Investigators took another measure after 6 months, this one looking at the difference in body fat loss between the higher-carb and the balanced-nutrient groups. The balanced group experienced a 23 percent reduction in body fat, compared with only a 17 percent reduction in the high-carb group. Although this wasn't statistically significant in the paper, it is clinically significant in that one group lost 5 percent more body fat.

This idea of balance is in direct opposition to the most popular diet types of the past few years. For instance, back in the days when Bill Clinton was president, most people were trying to lose weight by going the ultra-low-fat route—with only 10 to 15 percent of calories as fat (ironically, Bill himself was chowing down on Big Macs at the time). We've all seen where that particular diet fad left us: By the time George W. Bush took office, Americans were fatter and less healthy than ever—and the problem has continued to get worse. We now know that an ultra-low-fat diet is simply a bad choice. Here are a few reasons why.

Low-fat diets are bad for your health. Not to put too fine a point on it, but extreme low-fat dieting can increase your risk factors for cardiovascular disease. Heart disease is the second leading cause of death among women, and an ultra-low-fat diet can make your risk factors worse. For instance, when you follow a low-fat diet, you naturally increase your carbohydrate consumption, which in turn increases your levels of blood triglycerides—unhealthy fats that raise your risk for heart disease. It's true that reducing your fat intake may result in less LDL cholesterol—the so-called bad kind—but here's the kicker: Going too low on your fat intake can actually increase your number of "small" LDL cholesterol molecules, the ones that actually create plaque in your arteries.

Low-fat diets that are high in carbs also create swings in blood glucose and insulin that no woman really wants to deal with. In Chapter 3, we'll explain exactly how insulin and glucose prompt a hunger response. Low-fat diets are responsible for creating these swings because when you cut down fat and increase carbs, you increase the amount of glucose that enters your bloodstream, as well as the amount of insulin that your pancreas delivers to control glucose and bring it back into the normal range. If this glucose/insulin tug-of-war becomes a constant battle, your body can end up in a hypoglycemic (low blood glucose) state, and you'll find yourself on the road to constant hunger and, potentially, type 2 diabetes.

Low-fat diets can mess with your mood. In your body, insulin efficiently sweeps away excess glucose that is released into your bloodstream after you eat. When glucose is swept away too quickly, as happens when insulin has to work overtime in response to a low-fat, carbohydrate-rich meal, your blood sugar levels plummet and you become hungry and irritable.

UK researchers have shown that a low-fat diet (containing less than 55 grams of fat per day) increases feelings of anger, hostility, tension, and anxiety in normal, healthy young men and women, whereas a diet higher in fat (about 90 grams of fat) reduces these feelings.

Low-fat diets can actually make you fatter. Another low-fat strike against your body composition is that high insulin levels often make people eat more than they should. Studies of people with diabetes have shown that decreasing insulin secretion with drugs tends to spontaneously lower food intake. So, both the rise in insulin after a low-fat, high-carb meal followed by the drop in blood glucose will work together to foil your weight-loss plans because you'll want to eat more whether you really need to or not.

There's also this problem: When you eat large quantities of carbohydrates, your liver and muscles don't have the space to store the excess. This means the carbs are almost automatically converted to fat. As a result, low-fat, high-carb diets will just increase your body fat level unless you're using these carbs effectively throughout the day, as endurance athletes do.

Okay, so that's one diet fad down. What about the other, more recent diet phenomenon, low-carb eating plans? A typical very low-carbohydrate diet contains less than about 50 grams of carbohydrate per day, or about 10 percent of total calorie intake. It also contains a high amount of dietary fat, at about 140 grams of fat per day, and about 100 grams of protein per day. Such plans were originally designed to help people who were very overweight, had problems with blood glucose control, and had difficulties controlling hunger cravings (especially their carbohydrate joneses). And in fact, for the past several years, study after study has demonstrated that these characteristics are effectively managed with such plans, and the risk of disease is reduced.

However (and this is a very important "however"), when the media and food manufacturers glommed onto this diet, they touted it as one that *every* person could follow, no matter what his or her blood glucose control or body fat percentage. Many women who weren't obese were following this diet because they wanted to lose a couple of pounds fast. And it worked for some of them—but not for those who found the high percentage of fat and protein to be unpalatable (not eggs *again!*) or who found it difficult to severely limit their intake of healthy carbs such as fruit (an apple has 22 grams of carbs—nearly half your daily allowance on a very low-carb diet), low-fat yogurt (23 grams), and whole wheat bread (30 grams in the two slices you need for your sandwich).

Thankfully, those of us who are not extremely overweight or who don't have problems controlling carbohydrate cravings do not really need to restrict our carbs to very low levels. We can lose weight as long as our diets are lower in carbs than the 60 to 65 percent of total calories (270 to 300 grams of carbohydrate daily) recommended by the government. Remember, the more successful dieters in the CALERIE study ate 40 percent carbs.

The takeaway here is simple: Diets like the *Women's Health Perfect Body Diet* that contain a balanced ratio of calories from carbohydrates, protein, and fat help you retain more muscle mass and leave you less hungry. Donald Layman, PhD, and colleagues at the University of Illinois have published most of the convincing evidence. In several well-conducted studies, they clearly show that diets with carbohydrate intake under 150 grams per day and protein intake greater than 1.4 grams per kilogram of body weight result in increased weight loss, increased loss of body fat, less loss of lean muscle mass, improved blood glucose control, improved blood cholesterol profiles, and enhanced fullness.

Another recent study, published in 2007 by researchers at Purdue University in Indiana, compared weight loss, fat loss, muscle retention, mood, and hunger ratings among overweight and obese women on diets that were either 25 percent fat, 45 percent carbs, and 30 percent protein or 25 percent fat, 57 percent carbs, and 18 percent protein. After 12 weeks, the women in both groups lost about 18 pounds of body weight each, including 14.5 pounds of fat. However, the women in the first group, whose diet was more evenly balanced among the three macronutrients, lost less muscle—only 3 pounds, compared with 6 pounds in the other group. This shows that when calories are reduced, a more balanced intake of nutrients helps to preserve lean body mass, which is important for health and longevity. Lean mass (that is, muscle) is related to strength, and increased strength will protect you from injury. What's more, the women in the more balanced group felt fuller after eating than did the other women. Feelings of pleasure and satisfaction throughout the day were also higher for the more balanced group, and these same good feelings were decreased in the other group.

That's why the *Women's Health Perfect Body Diet* includes balanced amounts of both carbohydrates and healthy fats in its diet prescription. The plan provides less than 50 percent of daily calories from carbohydrates (fewer than 200 grams of carbs per day), so you get the benefits of carbohydrate restriction without feeling deprived of healthy carbohydrate foods. Likewise, your intake of healthy fat will fall between 25 and 40 percent of calories (55 to 70 grams daily), as opposed to the 10 to 15 percent common in low-fat diets.

The *Perfect Body Diet* Is Personalized

If you've tried other diets in the past, their one upside is that they may have helped you figure out which foods work best for you. For example, if you once tried to eliminate animal protein but ended up sick, unhappy, and fat, then you know that you shouldn't go out and try the newest vegetarian weight-loss plan. Every woman's body runs better on certain combinations of foods than on others, which may be one of the most important reasons you are not losing weight. In the *Perfect Body Diet,* we'll help you personalize your food choices so that your results will be the best possible.

That's why there are actually *two* eating plans in this book, each with a slightly different macronutrient balance to give you the most satisfaction, the greatest fat loss, and the fullest health benefits possible.

 One macronutrient mix, the **Greens and Berries Diet**, offers 20 to 30 percent of calories from carbs (90 to 125 grams of carbohydrate per day), 35 to 45 percent of calories from fat (60 to 70 grams), and 30 to 35 percent of calories from protein (120 to 140 grams).

 The other, the **Grains and Fruits Diet**, contains 35 to 45 percent of calories from carbs (150 to 185 grams), 25 to 35 percent of calories from fat (50 to 55 grams), and 25 to 30 percent of calories from protein (100 to 120 grams).

In both dietary plans, you will choose proteins from lean meats, fish, eggs, dairy, whey protein powder, nuts, beans, and, if you are vegetarian, soy. Your choices of healthy fat will come from cold-water fish (such as salmon and trout), nuts and seeds, egg yolks (yes, they're good for you, and we'll tell you more about that in Chapter 6), avocados, olive and canola oils, ground flaxseeds and their oil, and the fats found naturally in meat, dairy products, and soy. Carbohydrate choices will be those that are least processed and will depend on your diet plan. The Greens and Berries Diet, as you would expect, prescribes berries as the perfect fruit—and focuses primarily on green vegetables such as asparagus, broccoli, Brussels sprouts, green beans, collards, lettuces, and spinach because these are the choices that are highest in fiber. The Grains and Fruits Diet includes a wider variety of fruits, such as bananas, melons, and tropical fruits, and permits whole grains, such as brown rice, whole grain pastas, and sprouted grain breads.

The dietary mix that is best for *you* will depend on how well your body uses carbohydrates. Successful fat loss is dictated by your body's ability to process carbohydrates correctly. One of the best examples of this comes from research conducted by investigators at the University of Colorado. In their study, 21 obese women were randomly selected to follow either a calorically restricted diet that was higher in carbs and lower in fat or one that was lower in carbs and higher in fat. What they found was that the women who could metabolize carbohydrates well lost the most weight and body fat when they followed a diet that was higher in carbohydrates, whereas the women who could not metabolize carbohydrates very well lost the most weight when they followed a diet that was lower in carbohydrates. In Chapter 5, you'll use a simple breakfast test to determine your own carb tolerance.

How to Follow the *Women's Health Perfect Body Diet*

The *Perfect Body Diet* is literally different for every woman who follows it. You'll start by first identifying, in Chapter 1, what type of body shape you have. In Chapter 2, you'll figure out exactly what your body fat ratio should be for your perfect, healthy body—and how much weight you should realistically lose.

Chapter 4 will reveal the secret of glucomannan, the fiber supplement that will make it easy to stick to the *Perfect Body Diet*. Then, in Chapter 5, you'll determine which of the two diets is best for your body, based on a simple food investigation. This test will tell you more about your own digestion than you have ever known (or probably cared about). In Chapter 6, you'll learn about each of the macronutrients and the roles they play in your body and in the *Perfect Body Diet*.

Part 2 gives you the nitty-gritty information about exactly what you should eat. We'll give you an overview of the diet guidelines that hold true regardless of whether you follow the Greens and Berries Diet or the Grains and Fruits Diet—tips about meal timing, which supplements to take, what your best beverage choices are, and what to order when eating out. We'll also explain why you need to eat a higher number of calories at least 1 day every 2 weeks. This Perfect Body Break is just one of tons of great tips to keep you on the plan until you get to your perfect body weight.

Then you'll read either Chapter 8 or 9 to choose the right foods and meal plans for your diet: Greens and Berries, or Grains and Fruits. Among the delicious recipes you'll find in Chapter 10 are more than 80 dishes that incorporate glucomannan, so that you can make sure you are taking this vital fiber supplement with breakfast, lunch, dinner, and snacks.

In Part 3, we'll give you an exercise plan that is easy to follow and appropriate for your body shape. You'll learn how to weight train the right way, so that you build muscle where you want to and increase testosterone levels slightly, so fat loss is faster. Muscle development is key in boosting metabolism so that weight loss will come not just from eating less but also from the addition of calorie-burning muscle. You'll also learn which cardio activities are best for your body shape and how often you really need to do them in order to get the results you're after.

Finally, we'll show you how to maintain your weight loss once you've reached your perfect body goals. Because the *Women's Health Perfect Body Diet* isn't just the best weight-loss program you'll ever try—it's also the last program you'll ever need!

PART 1
PERFECT PLANNING

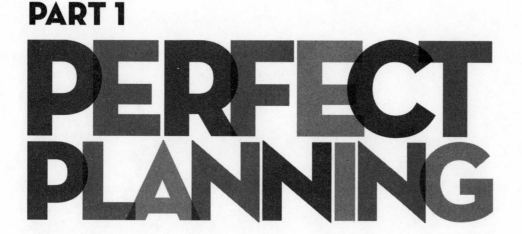

CHAPTER 1

Yes, Your Body Can Be Perfect

Quick quiz!

BODY FAT IS DISTRIBUTED DIFFERENTLY AMONG WOMEN BECAUSE OF . . .

a. Genetics

b. Dieting history

c. All of the above

d. I don't know . . . and I really hate quizzes

The correct answer is "c." (We will ignore those of you who chose "d.")

You only need to take a quick look around the gym to appreciate that women's bodies naturally come in many different shapes. Why? A woman's shape is dependent on where she stores her body fat—a phenomenon largely dependent on genetics. If your mother had big boobs and thick hips, you might be programmed the same way. If Grandma Rosalita was all paunch, a Buddha belly could be your natural tendency, too.

One relevant aspect of your genes is your ethnic background, which large population studies suggest plays a big role in body fat distribution. For instance, one study in the journal *Human Biology* found that women of Mexican American ethnicity tend to carry more abdominal fat, compared with women of European Caucasian heritage. So that's one explanation why your tall, leggy Minnesotan co-worker whose ancestors came from Sweden is likely to have a different body type than your friend whose South American roots make her shorter and more voluptuous.

Your hormonal profile is also linked to your genetic makeup, and it causes your body to keep fat rather than lose it. A 1995 University of Texas study has shown that high estrogen levels may be linked to bigger thighs, while an overabundance of either cortisol or insulin can cause weight gain around the stomach.

Warning! Hormonal differences may help explain why your body stores fat in a particular pattern, but we're certainly not recommending that you buy the latest "hormonal" fat-loss supplement targeted at reducing your estrogen or cortisol levels. There just isn't enough evidence yet that it's a good idea to manipulate your hormones to lose weight or influence where your body stores fat.

There's nothing you can do about genetic factors just yet (though we're rooting for you, Modern Science!), but you *can* manage what those genes have given you. You can control your body fat distribution naturally and safely by making wiser food choices and doing the right exercises for your body type. Here's where answer "b" comes in: You can modify how you live and what you eat. You can recognize what contributes to your fat storage areas. And you can learn to kick ass with what nature gave you. We're going to show you how to do that in this book.

The Obnoxious Party Guest: First to Arrive, Last to Leave

Where you store fat matters not just because of how it makes you look but also because it controls how you lose weight. The Golden Rule of Weight Loss: Where you put on fat first is where you will lose it last. So if you first started noticing a small bulge around your middle, don't expect to kiss that tummy good-bye in a week. Your arms and legs will probably slim down first, no matter how many crunches you do.

The point: There's no such thing as "spot reduction." Barring drastic interventions such as liposuction, you cannot choose where your body will lose fat first, regardless of how much you exercise a specific muscle group. All the leg lifts in the world can never transform J.Lo's curvaceous backside into Paris Hilton's skinny little booty. (Not that we hear Marc Anthony complaining.)

That said, your food and exercise choices have a big impact. For instance, if your tribe has been cursed by thunder thighs since the Paleolithic era, sitting at a desk all day is almost certainly going to make the situation worse. And if you binge on "low-fat" baked goods, you're kidding yourself. The extra calories will still increase your overall body fat, leaving you with a muffin top regardless of whether you were genetically meant to have one. Here's the truth: Exercising too little and eating too much—even if the food is "low fat" or "low carb"—will cause you to put on body fat.

Another theory suggests that body shape may be related to fluctuations in body weight. A yo-yo dieter whose weight dramatically shifts up and down may be inadvertently causing a redistribution of body fat to her upper body, regardless of her pre–yo-yo body shape. One Austrian study from the Medical University of Graz showed that yo-yo dieters have more fat in their upper bodies and thinner legs than women who haven't dieted as frequently.

A Few Words about Fruit (Though, Curiously, Not about Eating It)

You probably already know the most common way that body shapes are categorized: fruit. If most of your body fat is found below your hips and on your butt and thighs, for example, you're a "pear" because you are heavier on the bottom than on the top. A Pear often has cellulite on her lower abdominal region and legs, while her upper body is relatively slim. When a Pear gains 5 pounds, at least 4 of those are found below her waist.

An "apple," on the other hand, has a rounder appearance, with more fullness to the top. Most of her body fat can be found around her waist and midsection. An Apple usually has a wide torso with a fullness to her breasts, waist, and upper back. An apple-shaped woman likely has slim thighs and a flat bottom. When she gains 5 pounds, at least 4 of them go to her belly.

If your body doesn't look quite like either a Pear or an Apple type, you may be an "avocado." When you gain 5 pounds, they're distributed equally between your belly and your butt. Avocados may vary when it comes to the size of their thighs and breasts, but in general, they usually are capable of attaining the slim and trim "athletic body type." And when you get to that point, we'll start calling you a Banana.

Your basic body shape will dictate how you look even after you lose weight. An Apple can't turn into a Pear. Whatever your shape, though, the *Women's Health Perfect Body Diet* will definitely tighten up your body and reduce your overall body fat. This will reduce the areas of your body that make you resemble an Apple, Pear, or Avocado because your body will be in its leanest form, with proportions evened out to more closely resemble that Banana appeal. Apples will be able to look down and see their feet without a protruding bust and tummy blocking the view. Pears will slim their thighs. Avocados will melt off fat everywhere evenly.

What Kind of Fruit Are You?

Two easy ways to tell (and no quizzes!):

Step #1: Look in the mirror.

Step #2: Take your waist-to-hip ratio (WHR). Wrap a flexible measuring tape around your waist, right at your belly button. Then, measure around your hips at the largest part of your butt. Divide your waist measurement by your hip measurement. If this ratio is less than 0.80, you're a Pear. If it's above 0.85, you're an Apple. If it's in between, you're an Avocado.

Her Perfect Body

WHO: YVONNE B.

WHAT: THE *WOMEN'S HEALTH PERFECT BODY DIET* PUT AN END TO HER YO-YO DIETING

In the past 4 years, Yvonne B.'s weight has gone up and down like an elevator, from 138 to 98 pounds, from 115 to 103 pounds, from 125 to 109 pounds, from 120 to 115. "I believe that my yo-yo dieting has caused me to gain stubborn belly fat that I'm having a really hard time losing," she says. At 31 years old, she's been frustrated by her inability to whittle her middle back to the awesomeness she was able to achieve in her twenties. "I figure part of it is aging. Part of it is hormones—I had issues with missing my period for over a year. And, of course, part of it is stress and lifestyle—I am much more stressed and my life is much busier and less conducive to strict training/dieting. Whatever the excuse, it's friggin' frustrating!"

But the *Women's Health Perfect Body Diet* is teaching Yvonne about making good food choices for her body type. "I'm not crash dieting anymore or trying the newest fat-loss product that I see advertised." By eating better foods more often, she's finally seeing her weight and belly fat decreasing.

And a Banana's waist-hip ratio is also between 0.80 and 0.85, but total body fat and weight are much lower than an Avocado's.

Your Fruit, Your Strategy

On the *Women's Health Perfect Body Diet*, your natural body type helps determine what type of diet you follow and what kind of exercise you do. We'll get into details in later chapters, but here's a quick overview of what works best for each body shape.

APPLES

Overall strategy: Increase the musculature of your legs and buttocks while slimming down your midsection.

Diet: A 2006 study from the University Hospitals Coventry and Warwickshire, in Coventry, UK, shows that women with large waist-to-hip ratios, such as Apples, lose more weight and the most abdominal fat when their diets are low in carbohydrates and higher in protein and fat. As you'll learn in Chapter 5, high-fiber, low-carb foods such as green vegetables and certain fruits (including berries and, appropriately enough, apples) are usually the best carb choices for Apples because they are digested more slowly. Good fats and quality protein are also important so that the processing of carbs, and their subsequent conversion into blood glucose, is reduced to a slower pace, preventing the storage of body fat around your middle.

Apples who tend to have higher cortisol and insulin levels can control this by eating more frequent, smaller meals. As we mentioned earlier, cortisol can cause weight gain around the stomach, and this hormone is released in increased amounts when you go too long between meals. Don't worry about how long is too long—on the *Women's Health Perfect Body Diet*, you'll eat five or six times a day, so your next meal or snack is never too far off. Insulin is produced when you eat lots of simple carbohydrates (think big plates of pasta) or when you eat carbs without protein and fat (think pasta with fat-free tomato sauce and no meat or soy). A simple food challenge in Chapter 5 will help you determine whether you indeed have typical Apple hormone responses to carbs. Based upon the results of those tests, you will determine which of the book's two meal plans you should follow.

Exercise: A is for Apple—and also for aerobic exercise, such as biking and brisk walking, which you should do to build muscle in your lower body. Thirty minutes or more daily is the easiest way to lose fat. Also do resistance training to shape up leg muscles and create a higher, rounder butt. Chapter 13 features an exercise plan designed specifically for Apples.

PEARS

Overall strategy: Build the muscles in your upper body, creating the illusion that your bottom half is smaller.

Diet: A Pear generally stores less body fat when her diet is an even balance of protein, carbohydrates, and fats. Her lower-body fat cells will store dietary fat as it's consumed, making problem areas even worse. So eat lower-fat—but not fat-free—foods.

Hormonally, Pears may have relatively higher estrogen levels, compared with Apples, which means you have to be careful not to increase those levels even more with the choices you make. Birth control pills and foods containing phytoestrogens might be causing your estrogen levels to be higher than natural. Problem foods include soy and cruciferous vegetables such as broccoli, cabbage, and Brussels sprouts. Limit your intake of soy and crucifers to no more than three servings per week.

Pears, too, will take the food tests in Chapter 5 to ascertain which of the book's two meal plans is appropriate for them.

Exercise: Concentrate on resistance training that targets the upper body. Hill walking, running, and full-body pushups are also great for Pears to strengthen their bones and define their muscles, while creating the image of a smaller lower body. Cut down on weight-training exercises for the lower body, to prevent it from becoming any larger. In Chapter 14 you'll find an exercise program tailored to Pears.

AVOCADOS

Overall strategy: Increase your musculature and decrease fat in all areas.

Diet: When it comes to how the body responds to food, Avocados are less predictable than Pears and Apples. Some Avocados do better with a diet containing an even distribution of carbohydrates, fats, and proteins, while others lose more body fat if their meals contain fewer carbohydrates. To find out whether you need to keep your guacamole away from the chips, assess how well you tolerate carbs by performing the food challenge in Chapter 5. Then adjust your carbs up or down depending on your sensitivity.

Exercise: The best resistance training for you is an allover plan with full-body movements such as deadlifts, and the best cardio is higher-intensity interval training (running sprints on the treadmill or track) for the most fat burning possible. An Avocado-friendly workout program is the focus of Chapter 15.

Get Off the Diet Roller Coaster

We hear veteran dieters muttering under their breath: *It doesn't matter if I'm an apple, pear, avocado, or kumquat—I just can't seem to keep weight off once I lose it.*

There might be a physiological reason for that. A 2007 study in the journal *Appetite* shows that women who are overly concerned about their body image and food choices burn calories slower than women who have never dieted or been concerned about food choices. Constant dieting slows your metabolism over time. If your body is running fine on a low calorie level, it has learned to use calories slowly instead of burning them quickly, making it harder to lose weight, no matter how few calories you take in.

I'm Already a Banana

Really? Congratulations. Frankly, Bananas really shouldn't be dieting at all. Instead, you need to learn how to create balanced meals and eat them often to hold on to your athletic shape forever. When exercising, Bananas need to focus on resistance training to build muscle all over, while limiting the amount of cardio so that muscle gains won't be compromised by excess aerobic activity.

These strategies—conveniently part of the *Women's Health Perfect Body Diet!*—will help keep a Banana from turning into another type of fruit. For example, Tracy, a marketing consultant, looked like a Banana until several months ago, when she started to commute an hour to and from work each day. She started to develop what she called chair butt. In the past, if Tracy gained a few pounds, she would find a bit more fat around her belly. However, when her activity level decreased significantly because of her commute, her body fat started to accumulate on her butt, thighs, and hips. Her body had transformed into a Pear.

Then Tracy started the *Women's Health Perfect Body Diet* and returned to her normal Banana shape.

Depressed? Don't be. If you are a constant dieter, the *Women's Health Perfect Body Diet* will teach you how to eat *more* to weigh *less*.

A Final Word

Those are the basics of the *Women's Health Perfect Body Diet*. The next step is to determine what *your* perfect body will look like and what a realistic weight-loss goal should be. The next chapter will give you clear ideas on how much weight you need to drop and how that will affect the amounts and types of foods you can eat to achieve your perfect body.

CHAPTER 2

What's Your Perfect Weight?

Of all the numbers swimming around in your head—ATM card PIN, boyfriend's shirt size, precise number of calories in a scoop of Ben & Jerry's New York Super Fudge Chunk (310)—the digits that probably give you the most grief are your weight. And whatever your weight is now, you probably have a second number that plagues you nearly as much: what you *want* to weigh. Your mythical Perfect Body Weight.

Your ideal body might be inspired by a picture you saw on a magazine cover—or by your too-skinny friend who eats bowl after bowl of New York Super Fudge Chunk and never gains an ounce. But here's what you need to remember: Your body is unique, and you need to find a realistic number that is accessible for you. *Your* perfect body weight will take into account your height, bone structure, muscle mass, age, and breast size, as well as your father/mother's weight. Before we do anything else, we need to figure out exactly what number you should be aiming for.

Three Steps to Calculating Your Perfect Weight

To determine the body weight that's right for you, we're going to look at three different measures: baseline weight goal (or roughly what you should weigh, based on your height), bone structure, and overall body fat percentage. Here's how to figure out each one.

STEP #1: WHAT'S THE RIGHT WEIGHT FOR YOUR HEIGHT?

First, measure your height. Don't fall back on a number you kind of remember from the last time you went to the doctor or when your dad used to measure you in the laundry room doorway. Take off your shoes and socks, stand up straight next to a doorjamb, and use a pencil to mark off where your head is flattest. Then extend a tape measure from that mark to the floor.

» If you're over 5 feet, take the number of inches over and multiply that by 5. Add 100 to this number, and that will give you an idea of how much you should weigh.

» If you are 5 feet tall or shorter, use 100 pounds as your baseline.

*Her*PerfectBody

WHO: SUE F.

WHAT: SHE MET HER PERFECT BODY GOAL IN JUST 6 WEEKS!

Sue F. had tried tons of diets in the past, and she already made a habit of eating cleanly and rigorously exercising. She lived the "California lifestyle," spending lots of time outdoors with her two kids. Even so, Sue couldn't keep the weight off whenever she lost a few pounds. When she started the *Women's Health Perfect Body Diet*, she set a goal of getting—and staying—below 150.

In the first 2 weeks, Sue lost 8 pounds. After just 6 weeks, she had already lost 12 pounds and met her goal. "That was a major accomplishment," she says. "I feel really hopeful that this time I'll be able to keep those pounds off. I'm seeing such great results that I think I'm dieting for the last time." Sue says that she feels—and looks—fantastic. "My old jeans are fitting! It feels great not to be squishing into things. And I feel better about myself. I notice that I have more energy than ever before."

She really appreciated that the *Women's Health Perfect Body Diet* was easy to incorporate into her daily routine. "I liked how the diet was laid out very specifically at first, and then I was able to adapt it to my life," Sue says. "For me, the only big change was using the glucomannan, and it was so easy to add into the

Remember, this baseline is a rough estimate. But it does serve as a critical number for the other equations that come next.

YOUR BASELINE WEIGHT GOAL: _____

STEP #2: WHAT'S YOUR FRAME SIZE?

The idea of being "big boned" isn't just something your middle school PE teacher concocted to make certain kids in your class feel better. Your inner structure can run large or small, no matter how tall you are. Being big boned can add as much as 10 pounds to your baseline weight goal. And those are pounds that you will never be able to lose.

foods I already eat." Sue notes that even though she hasn't changed the quantity of food she's eating, the glucomannan makes that food seem even more satisfying. "The glucomannan made me feel gassy at first, but then I realized that I was using too much at one time," she admits. "When I dropped the dose to the correct level, the gassiness stopped." Sue was also happy to discover that the glucomannan wasn't a drain on her budget. "I was impressed by how inexpensive it is."

The recipes for the smoothies were Sue's favorites. "The smoothies are really easy to prepare at home, and I like knowing that I can control my ratio of proteins, carbs, and fats. I also notice that drinking smoothies throughout the day helps me stabilize my energy level."

Sue already had a serious fitness routine that focused on working one muscle group at a time. She would work her chest one day, move on to her legs the next, and so on. The total-body approach of the exercise program in the *Women's Health Perfect Body Diet* was a big change for her, and over time she recognized the benefit. "I realized that in order for workouts to be effective, you have to change them up every once in a while so that the body doesn't get complacent," she remarks. With the great results she's getting, Sue plans to stick with the whole eating and exercising program for good.

Figure out your frame size by measuring the circumference of your wrist with a flexible measuring tape, and then compare that number with the following chart.

HEIGHT	WRIST CIRCUMFERENCE	FRAME SIZE
Under 5'2"	Under 5.5"	Small
	Under 6"	Medium
	Under 6.25"	Large
5'2"–5'5"	5.5"–5.75"	Small
	6"–6.25"	Medium
	6.25"–6.5"	Large
Over 5'5"	Over 5.75"	Small
	Over 6.25"	Medium
	Over 6.5"	Large

If you have a large frame, add 10 pounds to your baseline. If you have a small frame, subtract 5 pounds. And if you have a medium frame size, don't adjust your weight calculation at all.

YOUR FRAME SIZE: _____

YOUR FRAME SIZE ADJUSTMENT: _____

STEP #3: HOW MUCH BODY FAT DO YOU HAVE?

Okay, this is a bit of a bait-and-switch. Your body fat percentage—the proportion of your bulk that's fat, compared with muscle and bone—won't help you figure out precisely how many pounds you ought to be. Still, it's one of the best indicators of whether you're at a healthy weight.

The National Institutes of Health recommends that women between 18 and 39 years old maintain a body fat percentage between 21 and 33 percent. However, since the high end of this range approaches the threshold for obesity, we recommend that you aim for 20 percent body fat, or somewhere between 16 and 26 percent, depending on your level of exercise and activity. This range is one that almost every woman should be able to achieve. Some women can look lean at 22 percent if they also have a lot of muscle, while others may not look so lean if they are shorter or work out infrequently. (To put this in perspective, professional gymnasts come in at around 10 percent, and swimmers are usually closer to 26 percent.)

Warning: Never allow your body fat to dip below 12 percent, or you will compromise body functions such as your ability to maintain a normal body temperature (you'll be too cold or hot all the time).

Again, you can't convert your body composition number into a goal of pounds to lose. But this number should just give you an idea of where you should be in terms of fat retention, regardless of your weight. For example, if you weigh 150 pounds and your body fat measures 20 percent, you're in good shape. But if you weigh 150 pounds and have 35 percent body fat, you'll want to reduce that percentage because, put another way, 53 pounds of you is fat. Periodically measuring your body fat is a great way to monitor your progress on the *Women's Health Perfect Body Diet*. Remember, less fat is better, and more muscle is better. It's more important to lose body fat than to lose actual pounds, so as you continue on the program, you will look forward to reducing your body fat percentage, and you won't care as much about "weight" or "scale" loss.

The best way to measure body fat is with a body composition assessment tool. Your doctor or even your gym might have one of these devices.

Bioelectrical impedance. This is a souped-up bathroom scale that you can purchase at a home goods store or pharmacy or find at your local gym. Though it can be less accurate than other methods, it's convenient and it indicates your current weight, as well as your body fat percentage. It does this by sending a mild electrical current into the soles of your feet (don't freak out—you won't even feel it) and measuring the time it takes the current to travel up through your body. Water and muscle conduct electricity more efficiently than fat does, so the more fat you have, the more slowly the current will travel.

To get the most accurate results, follow the machine's specific instructions. Make sure you're fully hydrated—that is, that you've been drinking enough fluids that your urine is odorless and a light yellow color. Don't exercise in the 12 to 24 hours before taking the test, and refrain from eating for 4 hours before. (The most convenient time to test is first thing in the morning after a day of relatively little activity.)

An alternative to the foot scale is a hand-held version. No matter which you choose, use the same model each time; different machines may give you different results, making it difficult to gauge true body composition changes.

Calipers. Your doctor or gym trainer can use these to perform the classic skin fold test, measuring your body in various places to determine the thickness of the fat under your skin. The results are only as good as the tester, so try to hook up with someone experienced or that's certified as a body composition tester. The measurements are plugged into an equation that's based on your age, ethnicity, and, of course, gender. To chart your progress, use the same tester and the same testing conditions (e.g., in the morning before breakfast).

DEXA scan. Probably the most accurate way to measure body fat is with dual-energy x-ray absorptiometry, or DEXA, which involves two different low-dose x-rays and a body scanner that reads bone and soft-tissue mass. This machine is most commonly used to test for osteoporosis by assessing bone mineral density. It requires a prescription and a hospital visit, although you might also be able to locate a DEXA machine at a specialized weight-loss center. The procedure lasts 6 to 10 minutes. But it might put you back as much as $250, so ask your doctor whether this is the best use of your money. Your insurance won't cover this exam unless you have bone density issues, which don't normally occur in younger women.

Your Magic Number

Okay, we've crunched all the numbers we need to crunch to determine your perfect weight. These assessments will give you the best understanding of how much weight loss is realistic for you and how much your body can change. Fill in the following chart to see where you are now and to help determine where you're headed:

》 Baseline weight goal: _____

》 Bone structure additions or subtractions: _____

》 **YOUR PERFECT BODY WEIGHT:** [_____]

That last number is your goal. Before we get to the specifics of the *Women's Health Perfect Body Diet* and exactly how you'll reach that target weight, we want to show you why the plan has been constructed the way it has—and why it's the best way to achieve your perfect body weight.

CHAPTER 3

Why You'll Never
Go Hungry Again

It's no secret what dooms most diets: hunger. Sure, you might be able to handle that famished feeling for a couple of days, weeks, even months, but eventually the need to feed always wins out.

Often, it's obvious why we feel like our diets are the starvation variety: We're not eating enough. When trying to drop a few pounds before, say, a friend's wedding, it's common to choose a diet so low in calories that it couldn't support the nutritional needs of an ant. As a result, we're racked with hunger, which also makes us tired and cranky. Now we're too hungry to exercise and too miserable to care. So we binge, which gets rid of the hunger but also ends our chances of looking great. Talk about a vicious cycle.

Thankfully, the situation isn't hopeless. In the next chapter, we'll share with you the *Women's Health Perfect Body Diet*'s secret weapon—a tool that will make you feel full, not famished, all day long, so that you can finally achieve your perfect body.

Before we get there, though, it's important to talk about what makes us feel hungry in the first place. It isn't necessarily what you think it might be—and there are a number of things that you can do to overcome hunger that *don't* require having a secret weapon.

How Our Brains Trick Us into Eating

Show of hands: Who thinks we eat because our bodies need nourishment?

It's a logical assumption, except we know from experience that it isn't always true. Many of us feel hungry all the time, even after we've just eaten. Or we continue to eat even after we've realized we're not hungry anymore. Or we eat because we're bored, depressed, or anxious.

What gives? Blame the way we've evolved—the way our bodies have learned to react to food. For most of history, food was extremely difficult to get. If you didn't eat when food was available, there was a very good chance that you might never eat again. So we developed the instinct to eat as much as we could, whenever we could.

Even though this learned response developed tens of thousands of years ago, it is still locked inside our brains today, when food is relatively fast, cheap, and easy. So it's hard to stop eating once we start because, technically, we're not supposed to. Instinctively, we automatically get hungry whenever we are around food.

Our busy modern lives have also contributed to our learned hunger. Many of us eat by the clock—when it says 12:00 noon, the fact that we've learned to consider this "lunchtime" leads us to feel hungry even if we've just eaten. Stress can also drive us toward food. This may be a biological function that has turned into a learned behavior. When you are stressed, whether by the ferocious German shepherd who's angry that you jogged past his yard or by the looming deadline that awaits you back at the office, your body rapidly depletes its energy stores and drains your blood glucose to prepare you to flee or fight. The brain responds by signaling for the stress hormone cortisol to be released in order to raise your blood glucose and provide more energy to help you escape the "threat." But increasing blood glucose, which increases insulin, also prompts your desire to eat. That sends you chasing after a quick fix: any sort of high-calorie, sugary mess. Your body knows that a chocolate bar will use all that insulin to shuttle the sugar through your body. Your mind just knows that the candy "satisfies" you by distracting you from the barking dog or snarling boss.

Memo to Mother Nature: Back Off!

To get your perfect body, you need to win the battle of learned behaviors. To put it another way, you need some willpower—the ability to "just say no" to the stimuli with which you associate food. It's not easy, particularly at first, but here's the good news: The longer you stick with it, the more your learned hunger will disappear.

Restraint is easier when you think about the big picture and how badly you want to get your perfect body. Bill Phillips, the creator of *Body-for-LIFE*, tells his audiences to repeat a mantra when they are faced with food challenges. His is: "I'm building my body for life." When food seems tempting, try whispering to yourself, "I can resist that. I am stronger than that cookie." Dorky? Maybe. But when it comes to willpower, you go with whatever works.

How Our Bodies Trick Us into Eating

When you can move past the psychological cues for hunger and learn to respond to the physical ones, you've taken the first step toward attaining your perfect body. But even physical cues can trick us into eating when we shouldn't. Understanding the physical stimuli behind hunger will give you better control over your appetite. Here are five physical factors that can make you hungry—and some advice on how to handle each of them.

The ghrelin response: Ghrelin is a protein secreted by your stomach and intestines. Your ghrelin levels rise when you haven't eaten in a while, which may contribute to that "feed me, feed me, feed me" feeling you get at certain points during the day.

Lack of sleep has also been shown to increase ghrelin levels. This would explain why some women experience strong hunger sensations after a wakeful night. To see whether ghrelin is affecting your hunger pangs, keep a food diary and a sleep diary for a week, noting what you eat before you go to bed and how many hours of sleep you get. You may think that your morning hunger is caused by the tiny dinner you had the evening before, when it may actually have been caused by the amount of sleep you had. The 2004 Wisconsin Sleep Cohort Study found higher ghrelin levels in people who got fewer than 8 hours of sleep per night.

Ghrelin can work against you when you want to lose weight. Research from Pennsylvania State University found that women who had lost significant body weight and fat had increased ghrelin levels that made them substantially hungrier than they'd felt before losing weight. This makes ghrelin one of the main obstacles to keeping off the weight you lose.

The good news is that time is on your side. If you can maintain your weight loss for at least 3 months, ghrelin will back off. In the meantime, keep ghrelin in check by eating five or six small meals spaced evenly throughout the day. Frequent eating prevents large increases in ghrelin, so you never get to the point where you will eat a rusty stop sign.

Protein and carbs have been shown to reduce ghrelin levels by increasing other hormones, such as glucagon, insulin, and cholecystokinin (CCK), that tell your body you have been fed. Fats alone are less effective in keeping ghrelin levels low, but they do slow the digestion of food so that your stomach feels fuller for a longer period of time. This is why the *Women's Health Perfect Body Diet* suggests that you consume protein, carbohydrates, and fat every time you eat: to suppress ghrelin and initiate fullness all the time.

The insulin response: Have you ever felt hungry 10 to 15 minutes after eating a rich piece of chocolate cake? Even though you just downed something that was supposed to "satisfy" your craving for sweets, you still felt like you needed to eat again. This is because insulin, the hormone released by your pancreas in response to a rapid rush of glucose to the blood, had to increase quickly to control all the carbohydrates that you just ingested. Experiments have shown that rapid elevations in insulin produce hasty feelings of increased hunger, heightened desire for more sweet foods, and greater food intake: in short, a downward spiral of sweets consumption.

For reasons that science does not yet entirely understand, not all women have this response to carbohydrate-rich foods, which is why sweets are less of a problem for some people. Women who are pear- or banana-shaped, for instance, are usually more tolerant of high-carbohydrate meals and have a lower insulin response. If that's you, consider yourself lucky. If you're apple-shaped, on the other hand, don't fret: You can control your insulin response by eating smaller, more frequent meals.

The glucose response: You may also get hungry when your blood glucose levels drop. Your body produces glucose on its own and also gets it from carbohydrate and protein foods. Your brain relies entirely on glucose for fuel, so your body always tries to maintain the minimal amount of blood glucose needed to keep your mind functioning properly, whether through hormonal responses or the initiation of food intake.

The normal range of blood glucose is slightly different for each woman, but in general, 80 to 120 milligrams of glucose per 100 milliliter (mg/ml) of blood is considered normal. Anything below 80 mg/ml is considered low blood glucose (known as hypoglycemia); anything above 120 mg/ml is considered high (known as hyperglycemia). Some women feel hungry and irritable as soon as their blood glucose drops below 80 milligrams. Others won't have this reaction until blood glucose has dropped much lower. As with the varying reactions to high-carb foods, we're not sure why different women respond in different ways. If you feel disoriented or very hungry in the morning or after a meal, your blood glucose levels might be dropping too much. Ask your doctor to check your blood glucose both in a fasting state and with a 5-hour glucose tolerance test, just to ensure that you are not at risk of any blood glucose–related disease, such as diabetes.

Your blood glucose levels usually start dropping approximately 3 hours after you've eaten a meal, as the supply of nutrients from food declines. Levels also drop rapidly after a carbohydrate-rich meal, due to the overzealous nature of insulin. Eating in response to low blood glucose is something your body must do, regardless of whether you are dieting. The best way to prevent low blood glucose and avoid getting to the point where you lose all control and eat anything in sight is, as we've said before, to eat every few hours. Each meal needs to contain all three macronutrients—proteins, fats, and the right carbohydrates for your body—to provide the most satisfaction and sustain glucose levels the longest.

The heat-production response: Body temperature can also have an effect on your appetite; when your temp falls, your hunger increases. This might be why we tend to eat more during winter—and also why restaurants keep their air conditioners cranked up, requiring you to cover that carefully selected date outfit with your emergency sweater.

In one study in the Netherlands, women were placed in a temperature-controlled metabolic chamber and monitored for energy expenditures and intakes at two different temperatures. When women were surrounded by an air temperature of 27°C (81°F), they had a significantly increased body temperature coupled with a significant reduction in hunger, compared with an air temperature of 22°C (72°F). At the warmer temperature, they ate less, moved less, and felt less hungry. The hotter women also chose foods that contained fewer calories and were less energy dense (fewer calories per weight of the food).

Does this mean that women who live in colder climates are destined to be constantly hungry forever? No. Your body gets accustomed to any particular temperature over time. It also prompts you to move more in order to make you feel warmer. This is why during winter months you might feel "cooped up" and need to get out and take a walk, even in the cold.

Brain chemical response: In his book *The Edge Effect,* Eric Braverman, MD, posits that the brain controls four important neurotransmitters, or biochemicals, that send signals to the rest of the body in order for it to function correctly. These are dopamine, acetylcholine, GABA, and serotonin. Each plays a role in digestion and weight control. When they are produced at the right levels, your body is able to run smoothly and efficiently on the energy it takes in through food. When the biochemicals are either too high to too low, your ability to control your weight and metabolize food is significantly affected.

Dopamine controls your ability to maintain an efficient metabolism as well as your self-control when it comes to food. When it is at the proper levels, you can quickly burn through the foods you eat and lose weight, and you can easily walk away from tempting foods like ice cream. When you are low in dopamine, your metabolism slows down, and the foods you eat start to form body fat. You are also less able to maintain self-control.

Acetylcholine helps determine brain speed and mental agility, and it provides the lubricants for your muscles, bones, and other internal systems. When your brain sends a low acetylcholine signal, you begin to crave fatty foods to provide extra lubrication. When you feel mentally slow, be vigilant about choosing good fats over bad fats.

GABA stands for gamma-aminobutyric acid, a biochemical that controls the way information is transmitted from your brain to the rest of your body. When you are low in GABA, you feel stressed and anxious. You can boost GABA by eating foods rich in vitamin B, the precursor to this biochemical. Good sources include nuts, beans, and pork.

Lastly, serotonin is a well-known neurotransmitter that is important for achieving restful sleep. Low levels of this critical biochemical can induce depression that often manifests in overeating. Antidepressant medications called SSRIs (selective serotonin reuptake inhibitors) are used to rebalance serotonin levels; however, some people who take them experience weight gain. If you are taking an SSRI, talk with your doctor about making adjustments to your drugs so that you do not experience this side effect. You can naturally boost serotonin by eating foods rich in its precursor, tryptophan. Poultry, fish, cottage cheese, eggs, avocados, and beans are among the best sources.

Big Stomachs, Big Appetites

There's one other physical factor that can affect hunger: the size of your stomach.

In 1988, Allan Geliebter, PhD, a researcher at the Obesity Research Center of St. Luke's–Roosevelt Hospital in New York City, found that the stomachs of lean people were significantly smaller than those of obese people. The leaner people could hold only about 1,100 milliliters in their stomachs, while the obese people could hold 1,900 milliliters.

In a study in 1996, Dr. Geliebter researched whether the stomach would shrink after someone lost weight. He measured the stomach size of eight obese subjects before and after they followed a very low-calorie diet for 4 weeks. He found that after following the diet and losing weight, the subjects' stomachs could only hold three-quarters of what they had held before. This indicated that the stomach adjusts to tolerate less food than it could previously hold.

However, this doesn't mean that the subjects' stomachs "shrank." What it does prove is that after receiving less food, your stomach adjusts its holding capacity and tells you that you're full when it's holding less. But just as quickly as it can reduce its holding size, your stomach can adapt to hold more. If you've eaten multiple large, heavy meals over several weeks, your body tells you to keep eating more just to get to that feeling of fullness. It has been shown that in women with binge eating disorders—those who eat extremely large volumes of food at one time—stomach capacity is even bigger than in women who are obese.

Why It's Good to Feel Full

Most women have been conditioned to think that feeling full is a sign of gluttony. If they're full, it means they ate too much.

But the truth is that fullness is something you should *want*, not something you should hate. Fullness should feel pleasant, not uncomfortable. Fullness should bring you back to a good mood instead of crankiness. Being full should make you smile because you know you've eaten the right amount of food for your perfect body. Fullness will help you stick to your weight-loss plan so you don't jump ship and swim to the nearest all-you-can-eat buffet.

How to achieve healthful fullness? First, there are different levels of fullness that you can achieve without unbuttoning your jeans under the table. Your brain is the organ that properly judges fullness. Food has to be at least partially digested before your brain gets the message to stop stuffing your face. Your brain also monitors your stomach contents, and once it recognizes that your stomach is full, it will tell you to stop eating.

There are about eight hormones in your stomach that are responsible for sending the signal to the brain that it's okay to stop eating. One of these is called cholecystokinin, or CCK, and as we've mentioned, it's one of the chemicals that counteracts hunger-producing ghrelin. It is secreted by cells in the intestine as well as by neurons in the brain, and it's launched when food begins to stretch the stomach walls. CCK then stimulates a special nerve—called the vagus nerve—that travels from the gut to the brain, to tell the brain that you're satisfied. It also stimulates your brain to produce another hormone called neuropeptide Y (NPY) that is integral in pushing yourself away from the table. These signals take 15 to 20 minutes to reach your brain, but once they get there, you immediately feel like you've eaten enough.

CCK stays in the blood for only 1 to 2 minutes before it stops working, and the amount of CCK released is in proportion to the volume of food in the stomach. So, when you eat a small meal and your stomach walls are barely stretched, less CCK is released. That's one of the reasons you don't feel very full after eating smaller meals and you feel fuller after eating larger ones. However, as we just explained, as you consistently eat smaller meals over time, your stomach will get used to holding less food, so it will "feel fuller" and its walls will stretch even if less CCK is released.

Even though your stomach can adjust to appreciate smaller meals more often, it still can't count calories: It doesn't know whether you've eaten 700 calories' worth of buffalo chicken wings or only 250 calories' worth of spinach-and-broccoli frittata. That's because these two meals take up about the same space in your stomach. Your stomach may feel full with either meal, but only one fits into your perfect body meal plan. Since your stomach can't read nutrition labels, we've designed both the diet plans in this book to help you monitor calories and macronutrients.

Fullness, then, depends partially on how much food your *stomach* "thinks" is enough for you to feel satisfied (a physiological process), but it also depends on what your *brain* perceives to be enough food (a psychological process). If you're used to eating a humongous bowl of pasta each night for dinner and you suddenly switch to eating a smaller plate of steamed green beans and salmon, you'll want to eat more food because your new meal

Hungry for More

Ever wonder why we keep eating even when we know we've had enough? First, remember the lag: It takes approximately 20 minutes for your stomach to send your brain the message that it's had its fair share, so you'll keep eating right up to the point where your brain finally gets the memo. By that time, you're really feeling stuffed. One good strategy to avoid this is to eat the food on your plate, and then wait the 20 minutes to see whether you are still hungry. If so, have a little more, then wait again.

Also, we often do not pay attention to what we're actually consuming, and we choose foods that are very easy to eat (for example, we scarf down an entire bag of crunchy corn chips). Or the food we're eating isn't all that filling because it is getting digested almost immediately: The classic Sunday breakfast of hotcakes and syrup literally leaves your stomach faster than it took to get there. When you follow the *Women's Health Perfect Body Diet* and choose the perfect foods that take longer to digest, you'll find that you won't have this problem.

Her Perfect Body

looks smaller and feels lighter to eat. To judge your true fullness, first give your brain time to recognize that you've just eaten; 15 to 20 minutes should be enough. Then, if you still feel empty, go ahead and eat something—but eat something you know won't counteract all your hard work. The secret ingredient we'll introduce you to in Chapter 4 will also prevent small-portion disappointment by making your lower-calorie meals much more tummy filling, hearty, and satisfying.

Another way to judge fullness is to keep in mind how many calories and what quantities of protein, carbs, and fats are in your food. If you know the value of the food you're putting into your body, you will be able to gauge whether it will fill you up for the long haul or for only an hour or two. For example, Tristan used to eat $\frac{1}{2}$ cup of raspberries and a stick of string cheese for her mid-afternoon snack at 3:00 p.m. She thought she was doing her body a favor because the snack only contained about 100 calories, 7 grams of protein, 7 grams of carbs, and 4 grams of fat. However, she felt incredibly hungry and empty by 5:00 p.m. In truth, her snack was not substantial enough to keep her full for more than 2 hours. A full cup of berries, a stick of regular-fat string cheese, and $1\frac{1}{2}$ ounces of nuts would better satisfy her because it has more calories, protein, carbs, and fat.

No matter what the underlying cause of your hunger, the solution to achieving your perfect body is to keep hunger from controlling you. You need to learn how to disregard the psychological and physiological cues and take back control over what you eat. That way, the nutrients you take in will be absorbed into your bloodstream at a steady rate, and you will no longer be a slave to hunger. Just switching to eating five or six small meals throughout the day will have a big impact. It will help you decide when to eat without relying on hunger as a cue, and at the same time, you'll always feel full. We'll go into the rules for spacing out your meals in Chapter 7, but for now keep in mind that proper meal spacing is a cornerstone of the *Women's Health Perfect Body Diet*.

CHAPTER 4

The *Perfect Body Diet's* Secret Weapon

Probably the easiest way to feel full—and, as a result, lose weight—is to get more fiber in your diet. Was that a groan we heard? Understandable. Getting a lot of fiber in your diet can be tough, and telling people you're on a high-fiber eating plan isn't exactly the sexiest conversation opener.

Luckily, the *Women's Health Perfect Body Diet* has the ideal way for you to get all the benefits of fiber without eating an uncomfortable amount of food or turning vegetarian. You will be using a special soluble fiber supplement that you can add directly to your foods. This extraordinary dietary fiber will help you avoid overeating while still making you feel full and satisfied. The secret weapon is called *glucomannan*. It makes your stomach full without adding any extra calories to your diet, and it's an indispensable tool for helping you stick to the *Perfect Body Diet*.

We'll provide more details on glucomannan in a minute. But first, let's look at why fiber is such a great weight-loss tool in general.

A Fiber Primer (Wait . . . Not as Boring as It Sounds!)

Fiber is at the forefront of the latest diet theories, and for good reason. Beyond keeping you regular, the bulking action of fiber slows down the emptying of food from your stomach and makes your blood glucose levels rise and fall more gently. This provides a steady supply of nutrients for your body to use, which translates into feeling fuller longer. And you guessed it: When you feel full, you won't overeat. In fact, when you eat a fiber-rich meal, you can actually consume less than you normally would, and you'll still feel satisfied. Less food means fewer calories, and fewer calories means less body fat. So by adding lots of fiber to your diet, you can easily reduce your calorie intake without feeling as if you haven't eaten your fill.

Better still, fiber is now thought to block calorie absorption by keeping the intestines from breaking down the caloric parts of food. A 1997 USDA study found that women who doubled their fiber intake from 12 grams to 24 grams per day absorbed 90 fewer calories—which over the course of a year can translate into *10 fewer pounds* on your body. In another study, this one from Penn State University, obese women who ate more fruits and vegetables to increase their fiber intake lost 33 percent more weight than women who simply limited portion size and cut back on fat.

Fiber actually stimulates your body to release more of the hormone cholecystokinin (CCK), which tells your brain you're full faster and for a longer time. This happens mostly because fiber expands in your stomach, stretching the stomach walls to stimulate CCK production, even when you've eaten a relatively small amount of food. So, fiber helps you feel full after eating a smaller quantity of calories. Fiber also slows the movement of food from your stomach to your gut, and when food moves more slowly, it allows more time for the intestine to keep producing CCK.

Soluble versus Insoluble Fiber (Also Not as Boring as It Sounds!)

"Fiber" is a type of carbohydrate found in fruits, vegetables, grains, and legumes. The term refers to the component of plant-based foods that is basically indigestible by the human body. There are two types of fiber: soluble and insoluble. When a specific food is said to contain fiber, that means that it contains some combination of the two types. When placed in water, soluble fiber dissolves and forms a thick gel. In the stomach, this gel slows the absorption of food particles (such as glucose from carbohydrates) from the gut into the bloodstream, so that you feel fuller longer.

The other type of fiber is called insoluble because it doesn't dissolve in water and doesn't expand in the stomach and intestines. Instead, insoluble fiber acts like a scrub brush, helping to push food and waste out of the body more quickly. This more efficient elimination prevents constipation, bloating, and digestive discomfort.

Insoluble fiber passes through your digestive tract without being broken down or absorbed,

*Her*PerfectBody

As a vice president of marketing for a consumer electronics firm, Sabrina D. could never find the time to stick to a diet. "I travel a lot for business. I've been eating hotel food every night, and I wasn't exercising at all. In 2 years, I had put on more than 30 pounds. But this diet is definitely a winner." After 4 weeks on the *Women's Health Perfect Body Diet*, Sabrina had already lost 9 pounds. "The first 2 weeks were slow, and now I'm taking off 2 pounds every week."

Sabrina's favorite part of the program has definitely been the glucomannan. "I can pass up food even when I like it, because I'm not hungry. I'm not tempted by anything."

Sabrina found success because she developed a strategy that worked for her.

"I keep a stash of glucomannan in my purse at all times, and I discreetly pour it into soup or chili. Not a single client has noticed or commented. I don't want to draw attention to my diet during a business meeting, so this worked really well for me."

At home, Sabrina uses the recipes in Chapter 10 and has even created some new ones of her own. "I love to cook, so when I can find the time I make a big batch, like three or four servings of tuna salad so that it's always in the fridge."

The biggest change in Sabrina's routine has been adopting the program's workout. "I had done lots of aerobics before. But this workout was entirely new, and I love it. And best for me, I'm able to do the program in hotel gyms. The workout is giving me great energy, and I feel more alert."

The proof is not just how she feels, but how she looks. "My waist got smaller, and there is much more definition around the sides of my stomach and upper arms," Sabrina says. "More than losing inches, there is more definition. My clothes are fitting much looser. I noticed even more of a change in the way my clothes fit than in what I've seen on the scale. I'm trying to get down to 133, which was my everyday weight about 2½ years ago. After 8 weeks, I'm less than 20 pounds away. I will keep up with this; I want to get back to my old self."

meaning that it basically provides zero calories to the body. Soluble fiber, on the other hand, provides about 2 calories per gram versus the typical 4 calories per gram from other carbohydrates. These 2 calories do not come from the fiber itself but instead from a metabolic by-product known as short-chain fatty acids. When soluble fiber reaches the large intestine, where your body houses most of its digestive bacteria, some of the bacteria can metabolize the fiber in a process called fermentation, producing short-chain fatty acids.

Bad for you? On the contrary—short-chain fatty acids totally rock. They can be used for energy by the cells of your intestines, and they help improve the strength and health of your intestinal lining, reducing inflammation and minimizing the opportunity for disease to flourish. Some of the short-chain fatty acids can also be absorbed into your bloodstream to give you a small energy boost. And they offer a whole host of other benefits, such as stabilization of blood glucose, stimulation of immune cell production, and reduction of unhealthy blood cholesterol.

There is, however, one not-so-wonderful aspect of fermentation: It may cause gas . . . a side effect coveted only by 11-year-old boys. But only certain types of soluble fiber, such as guar gum (an emulsifier used in many packaged baked goods, ice creams, salad dressings, and other foods), are fermented to the point of uncomfortable gas production.

Get Fibered Up: Seven Easy Tips

Adding fiber-rich foods to your diet will give you all of these great benefits. Each of us needs approximately 25 total grams of dietary fiber (consisting of both soluble and insoluble fiber) each day to help the food we eat pass through our systems quickly enough that it doesn't have a chance to be stored as body fat. But most of us take in only 7 to 10 grams of fiber, because it is often depleted from foods when they are processed. White bread, white pasta, and white rice contain zero grams of fiber. Also, most Americans don't eat enough fiber-rich fruits and vegetables, either because they can't (gas, remember?) or because they just don't want to (vegetables aren't always a girl's favorite foods). Another problem is that even the most fiber-rich foods contain only a few grams of fiber per serving.

As part of the *Women's Health Perfect Body Diet*, to decrease hunger and increase weight loss, you will increase your intake of both kinds of fiber from whole foods. Soluble fiber is less common than insoluble but is found in large quantities in foods such as oats and barley, apples, oranges, and lentils. Insoluble fiber is easier to get because it's the most prevalent type found in foods. It makes up most of the total fiber found in whole grains (such as brown rice and quinoa), cereal brans (such as wheat bran), beans, flaxseeds, vegetables, and nuts. Since vegetables and fruits contain so much water, they provide less total dietary fiber per ounce, making grains and cereals the most concentrated sources of total fiber. "Find a Reliable Source" is a cheat sheet to some of the most fiber-rich foods.

Use the following tips to get your fiber requirement from whole foods, which will be a mix of soluble and insoluble fibers. One note of caution: You'll still need to watch the quantities that you are taking in. To meet your fiber requirements, you are generally forced to eat more, which means that you might be consuming lots more calories to go along with all that extra fiber. (Hint: This is why glucomannan is such a key component of the *Women's Health Perfect Body Diet*.)

Find a Reliable Source

FOOD	TOTAL FIBER (G)
½ c pinto beans	11
1 c peas	9
½ c kidney beans	8
½ c Shredded Wheat cereal	5
1 apple, with skin	5
7 prunes	5
½ c chickpeas	4
1 pear	4
1 c blueberries	4
1 sweet potato	4
¼ c almonds	4
½ c Brussels sprouts	4
½ c corn	4
½ c lentils	4
¼ c sesame seeds	4
1 c oatmeal	4

1. Look for the word *whole*, as in "whole wheat" or "whole grain," on packaged breads, cereals, and snack foods (average of 3 grams fiber per ½ cup).

2. Eat fresh or frozen fruit (2 grams of fiber per piece or ½ cup), but avoid fruit juice, which is virtually fiber free.

3. Leave the skin on your vegetables (2 to 3 grams per ½ cup).

4. Have a bowl of fiber-rich cereal, such as Fiber One (14 grams per ½ cup) or All-Bran Bran Buds (12 grams per ⅓ cup).

5. Eat beans, such as black beans or kidney beans (15 grams per cup).

6. Add ground flaxseeds to your smoothies (8 grams per 2 tablespoons).

7. Read food labels carefully. Many food manufacturers have jumped on the fiber bandwagon and are adding fiber to foods you wouldn't think about, such as orange juice and yogurt.

And Now Back to Our Secret Weapon

We'll admit it: Getting the proper amount of fiber in your diet—even using the seven preceding tips—can be tough. Which is why we have our secret weapon—glucomannan.

Glucomannan is an ancient soluble fiber source that can help you lose weight, stay full, reduce your appetite, and improve your health more effectively than any other soluble fiber. It comes naturally from the root of the elephant yam, also known as konjac, a plant native to Asia. It's a very popular fiber product and is used to make various noodles and jellies. Also known as *moyu* or *juruo* in China and sold as *konnyaku* or *shirataki* noodles in Japan, konjac foods are popular in Asian markets.

If you're thinking that you've tried fiber supplements before and been disappointed with the results, we know exactly what you mean. In the past, using fiber supplements was never pleasant. Many had you feeling gassy and bloated—or even running for the bathroom.

Psyllium fiber, for example, acts like both a soluble and insoluble fiber because it forms a gel when mixed with water, and it causes your stool to move rapidly through your intestines. This makes it great for people with constipation, but it's not something you can use very often. If you were to add it to most of your meals, you'd be running for the nearest restroom every hour or so. Psyllium can also cause gas and bloating in a lot of women. Perhaps worst of all, it tastes a little like dirt.

Methylcellulose is a soluble fiber that produces less gassiness because it's said to be completely nonfermentable. Although it reduces constipation and helps people meet their daily fiber requirements, no study has ever shown that is able to help you lose weight or reduce food intake and hunger.

Wheat dextrin is another type of soluble fiber, but, as with methylcellulose, no one has shown that it can help people lose weight.

Glucomannan, on the other hand, will allow you to feel full, satisfied, and less hungry, without all the unpleasant side effects. When professors at Chicago's Rush University College of Nursing reviewed 12 glucomannan studies, they concluded that this fiber does help people lose body weight and body fat while decreasing food intake and increasing fullness.

Other fiber supplements introduced over the past 10 years, including guar gum and alginate, have also been thought to help with weight reduction, but studies have disproved these claims. In a recent Norwegian study of 176 women and men, these two fiber sources were tested along with glucomannan for their effects on body weight and fat loss. Three fiber combinations were given to the study participants. Each of the fiber supplements contained some glucomannan, but only one was a pure form; the remaining two also contained either guar gum or alginate. It was conclusively shown that glucomannan was the key ingredient for weight loss: The other two fibers did not promote any more weight loss, compared with glucomannan alone.

How Glucomannan Works

Glucomannan is the most soluble fiber found in nature. It has the densest dietary fiber known, and it has the highest water-holding capacity of any soluble fiber—it can expand to up to 100 times its own water weight. This swelling action has several beneficial effects for weight loss when you add glucomannan to the foods you already enjoy eating.

Several clinical investigations have shown that glucomannan can help people eat fewer calories, leading to a negative caloric balance. This is one of the principle ways in which you're going to lose weight and get rid of your unwanted fat forever. Glucomannan has the unique ability to instantly satisfy your hunger because it can be easily added to foods to make them thicker and heavier. You'll feel like you're eating more food because the food is bulkier and more satisfying.

Thickening your food with glucomannan forces you to take more time to eat your meal, allowing you to enjoy each meal just a little longer. Which, for instance, can you

Glucomannan to Hunger: Get Lost!

How our secret weapon reduces your appetite:

1. Glucomannan prevents glucose levels from dropping, thanks to the slower and sustained release of nutrients into the bloodstream.

2. At the same time, it neutralizes the insulin response so that insulin can't make you hungry after a meal.

3. It controls ghrelin, because the ghrelin responds to a disruption in glucose and insulin.

4. It may also increase the level of CCK in the gut, which is another way to control your appetite.

5. When your body is satisfied, your brain is satisfied, and your neurotransmitters will be balanced.

Glucomannan Delivers

» This superfiber supplement promotes a sense of fullness.

» It makes you feel more satisfied.

» It makes your food last longer.

» It allows you to reduce the total number of calories your body absorbs because you are excreting more efficiently.

» It lowers the energy density of the food you eat *without* increasing calories.

» It sustains the release of nutrients into your bloodstream for longer periods of time.

consume faster: chocolate milk or a thick chocolate milkshake? You know you'd have a far easier time slurping down the milk than the shake. Plus, it's much more satisfying to eat something that has substance rather than something that is thin and runny. Scientists have demonstrated that an increase in the time it takes your mouth and jaw to chew food can stimulate your digestive system's signals of fullness.

Thicker foods also make your stomach fuller, which increases those fullness signals, such as CCK, that tell your brain you've had enough. Even a slight stretching of your stomach walls after eating a bulky meal causes much more CCK to be released from the gut. By adding glucomannan to food, you'll feel the sense of fullness sooner after you begin to eat—in fact, you'll find that you begin to eat more slowly after just a few bites. And because the food is taking up more space in the gut, your brain will get the signal that you don't need to eat more.

Studies also show that the weight of food controls your appetite. Glucomannan fiber increases the food's weight without increasing calories. These denser foods also travel more slowly through your digestive system. Instead of a meal speeding down through your stomach to your intestines (and then out of you for good), it moves slowly, allowing you to experience a sense of fullness for hours afterward (instead of minutes), because CCK is released for a longer period of time.

As the food leaves your stomach and enters your small intestine, the nutrients are absorbed. When you add glucomannan to your foods, these nutrients will be taken up at a slower and steadier pace. Your body receives a constant supply of fuel. This is more desirable than receiving fuel in one large dose, because your body has more time to burn the fuel, rather than storing it as fat. More important for women, by slowing the rate of food absorption from the gut to the bloodstream, glucomannan reduces the amount of insulin produced after a meal, which we've already established as one way to control your appetite. (See Chapter 3 for more on insulin.)

Finally, because it is so viscous, glucomannan leaves your stomach and small intestine slowly. You'll pass more calories through your stool because glucomannan has soaked up all those calories and moved them out.

All these features point toward a significant new theory in weight loss that is well supported by scientific research. At least seven clinical trials of glucomannan have been conducted in overweight women and men. In all of these studies, glucomannan in doses of

Glucomannan Is Good for the Rest of You

Apart from the research into its role in weight reduction, glucomannan has been studied for its effects on constipation, blood cholesterol, blood glucose, insulin resistance syndrome, and blood pressure. Researchers have shown that glucomannan helps the body create and absorb less "bad" cholesterol. An 8-week study published in the *International Journal of Obesity* found that in obese subjects, serum cholesterol and LDL cholesterol were significantly reduced in the people who took glucomannan, compared with subjects who received placebos. These effects are beneficial for people at high risk of heart disease, but in healthy people, glucomannan won't negatively impact normal cholesterol balance.

By lowering blood glucose to a normal level, glucomannan has also helped many people who have an increased risk for diabetes or those who have diabetes already. A University of Toronto study of 11 people with type 2 diabetes found that glucomannan helped bring down high blood glucose levels by almost 6 percent in 3 weeks. When glucose levels are reduced from a high level, people become more insulin sensitive (and carbohydrate tolerant), which helps prevent the development of type 2 diabetes.

Let's look at a real-life example. A friend of ours, Lil, has used glucomannan and lost weight, but she is even more impressed by her increased energy levels. Lil was very hypoglycemic and had problems with blood glucose control before she began supplementing with glucomannan. When she added glucomannan to her foods, she found that the meals kept her blood sugars more stable, compared with the roller-coaster effect she experienced before using it. More stable blood glucose equals more stable energy.

2 to 4 grams per day significantly lowered body weight. In one study of obese women without dietary restriction, participants who received glucomannan at a dose of 3 grams per day for 8 weeks decreased their body weight by 5¹/₂ pounds. So, even *without* dietary change, glucomannan can help you lose weight. In the *Women's Health Perfect Body Diet,* you will cut back calories and utilize 6 grams of glucomannan per day, a one-two punch that will make it easy to meet your weight-loss goals.

Just Say No to Glucomannan Pills

Most people haven't heard of glucomannan before. And those who have heard of it haven't seen great weight-loss results for one simple reason: They don't know the secret to using glucomannan properly.

This dietary fiber is sometimes packaged as easy-to-swallow capsules. The packages suggest that you should take two or three capsules (providing a total of 2 grams of glucomannan fiber) 30 minutes before a meal so that the glucomannan can swell in your stomach and cause

A Word on Fat-Burner Supplements

What woman hasn't walked into a health food store or pharmacy and checked out the shelves of the latest weight-loss supplements? We're all a little curious to know whether they actually work.

Most weight-loss pills or "fat burners" are combinations of caffeine and other stimulants that claim to increase your metabolism and burn off fat. Due to their stimulating nature, they can make you so jittery and hyper that you forget about eating. However, losing body fat and weight is about eating better foods more often, not about passing up meals because your hand is shaking too hard to hold a fork.

Some fat burners have been banned because they contain ephedra, a potent stimulant that has been associated with increased heart rate and blood pressure, and even death. However, even some of the new ephedra-free herbal supplements may pose health risks. In a study published in the *American Journal of Medicine,* 10 healthy adults tried a single dose of one of two popular herbal weight-loss supplements. After the supplement had been metabolized, the subjects' heart rates increased by 11 to 16 beats per minute. One of the supplements also increased blood pressure by between 7 and 12 percent. These are the same kinds of issues that were found with ephedra, which the FDA banned in 2004. Your bottom line? It's best to just avoid these fat burners.

you to feel full. This fullness is supposed to help curb your appetite so you eat less at your next meal. However, we suspect that glucomannan may not work most efficiently when delivered in capsule form. When ingested in a capsule, the powder may not actually be completely released to expand in your stomach. Instead, gastric juices and acids break down the capsule walls slowly, and fluid from your stomach seeps in little by little. As the fluid comes into contact with the glucomannan, it causes the fiber to swell *inside* the partially intact capsule. You can see the way this happens if you try adding spoonfuls of cornstarch or wheat flour to a bowl of liquid: Unless you stir everything up to disperse the starch throughout the liquid, the outermost particles of starch will clump up, trapping the innermost particles so that they cannot dissolve. (Now you know why your grandma seemed to spend hours whisking the turkey gravy.) Likewise, partially encapsulated glucomannan becomes what glucomannan researcher Vladimir Vuksan, an associate professor in the nutritional sciences department at the University of Toronto, has called a fiber worm. Now, this isn't a parasite, it's simply the result of the expansion of glucomannan within the capsule to form a long, thin, worm-shaped gel. So, instead of swelling in your stomach to make you feel full, the fiber swells inside the capsule and passes through your digestive tract without performing its designated job.

The key to getting the desired effects from this superfiber is to remove it from its straitjacket (the sleeves of the capsule) and mix it directly into the food you're about to eat. This way, the glucomannan goes to work immediately. The food will be thicker, so you'll eat less. And the amount you do eat will be more slowly digested and absorbed in your stomach and intestines.

Since all of your food will get thicker and more satisfying with glucomannan, make sure to wash it down with plenty of water; drink at least 8 ounces of H_2O with every meal or snack. For the best taste and texture—clumps of glucomannan aren't exactly gourmet, and they could even get stuck in your throat—always mix the powder thoroughly into your grub and wait 2 to 3 minutes for it to soak up whatever sauce, broth, dressing, or other liquid is on your plate or in your bowl or glass. Sit back and watch your serving size expand without any extra calories. When used as we've directed here, glucomannan is an important part of the *Women's Health Perfect Body Diet*'s safe and effective weight-loss strategy. You'll find that it is easy to use and will help you enjoy the foods you already like to eat. You'll learn much more about incorporating it into your diet in Part 2. Chapter 7 will provide information on how to buy it and exactly how to use it, and Chapter 10 includes more than 80 recipes using glucomannan as an ingredient: 30 recipes you can use on the Greens and Berries Diet, 31 that work for the Grains and Fruits Diet, and 28 recipes that work for both.

CHAPTER 5

Which Plan Works Best for You?

Ready for a quick review? So far in the *Women's Health Perfect Body Diet*, we've done the following:

» Established that everybody's body can be perfect—
though not everyone will take exactly the same path to get there

» Crunched the numbers on what *your* perfect weight should be

» Given you a "secret weapon" for beating hunger

» Shown that a high-fiber, balanced diet works best—and explained
that the *Women's Health Perfect Body Diet* gives you a choice of two
different meal plans

The next step is figuring out which of those meal plans will be most effective for you. We're going to do it by testing your carbohydrate tolerance. Painful? Hardly. All you have to do is eat.

What's Carb Tolerance? (And, Um, Why Should I Care?)

Women generally know when they're lactose intolerant: They drink milk, and within a few minutes, they're gassy, bloated, and running for the nearest bathroom. It's an annoying problem that actually has a pretty simple solution: Stay away from milk.

But dairy products aren't the only foods that can cause physical discomfort (as well as physiological imbalances that can, in some cases, impede weight loss). If you've been trying to lose weight for long periods of time and have not had good results, the problem might not be your willpower, your exercise routine, or even your portion control. Instead, it might be that you don't process carbohydrates well—you're carbohydrate intolerant.

The American Dietetic Association has been telling us for decades that the perfect diet is based on a foundation of carbohydrates. Over the years, the USDA food pyramid has been improved to favor healthier, whole grains, yet we are still told that carbs should be the major component of our daily intake. So we've grown up eating a ton of carbs all day long: cereal for breakfast; a sandwich and chips for lunch; chicken, beef, or fish accompanied by a green vegetable and a starch—more carbs—for dinner. But while carbs are filling and relatively inexpensive, *too* many aren't good for you.

In fact, for some women—those who don't metabolize them well—carbohydrates are particularly detrimental. Carbs just might be the culprit behind your lack of weight loss and, even worse, your weight gain. Too many carbs actually slow down your fat-burning furnace so that your metabolism is not running as hot as possible. Remember, excess carbohydrate intake overstimulates insulin production, causing food to be stored as fat rather than used for energy. This deep-sixes your efforts to build a perfect body.

If you are cranky or forgetful after a high-carb meal, that could mean you don't process carbohydrates correctly and could be at high risk for diabetes. In a recent study, UK researchers had women eat a high-carb breakfast—the equivalent of two flapjacks or a large bagel—first thing in the morning. Then they monitored the women's memory and mood for the next 2 hours. Those who had the poorest recall and attitude also had the greatest fluctuations in blood sugar, an early warning sign for diabetes. If you can't metabolize carbs properly, your mood, ability to think clearly, and feeling of fullness will go downhill. You may not have realized that these issues are linked to what you eat, but they are.

Tests for Apples, Pears, and Avocados

The following tests will help you see how your body processes carbohydrates. If you process them well, you will feel satisfied for at least 2 hours after eating the high-carb meal in Test One, and you won't feel any change in your mood or ability to think and concentrate. But if you don't use carbs well, you'll feel hungry and irritable within 2 hours, and your mood and focus will diminish.

Women with apple-shaped bodies are more likely to be carb intolerant and will probably do best by following the lower-carb meal plan—the Greens and Berries Diet—in Chapter 8. Pears can usually tolerate carbs better, and the test will probably indicate that they should follow the relatively higher-carb plan—the Grains and Fruits Diet—in Chapter 9. Avocados can go either way; you can figure out which is best for you after taking the test. However, these are just generalizations. As we've pointed out again and again, every woman is different and individual, and *your* body may not be so easily categorized. That's the whole reason testing is necessary.

How to Do the Tests

These tests are best done in the morning, when your body will have the most pronounced response to a meal containing carbohydrates. At other times of the day, previous meals or your activity level can influence test results.

You are going to eat a different breakfast—one higher in carbs, one lower—on two different days. After each, you will assess your fullness, mood, hunger, and ability to focus. Repeat the tests in the reverse order to confirm the accuracy. So, for instance, take Test One on Monday and Test Two on Tuesday. Eat your normal breakfast on Wednesday. Then take Test Two again on Thursday and Test One on Friday. Test Two will help confirm the results of Test One, to ensure that you didn't get a false positive or false negative. It will also provide clarity if you scored somewhere in the middle on Test One. The cumulative results of testing four times total should tell you clearly which of the two eating plans is right for you.

Take the tests on mornings when you have few distractions or stresses—*not* on a day when you have an important morning meeting or a huge deadline that will distract you. Get a good night's sleep beforehand, so that your responses are not influenced by fatigue (a lack of sleep increases hunger and irritability). Eat each breakfast within 2 hours of waking. If you usually drink coffee or tea in the morning, do so. If you usually exercise in the morning, plan to work out at another time of day on the days when you take the tests. (Exercise improves overall carbohydrate metabolism, so it could alter the results.) After you eat breakfast, continue your day as usual, including normal eating and exercise.

Test One: The High-Carb Breakfast

1 large plain bagel, about 4 ounces

2 tablespoons no-sugar-added preserves or jam

Nutrition facts: 345 calories, 10 grams protein, 74 grams carbohydrates, 3 grams fiber, 1 gram fat

CHART YOUR RESULTS

After eating, complete the questionnaire on page 42 every 30 minutes for the next 3 hours, for a total of six assessments. At every 30-minute interval, check off the answer that most closely matches how you feel. Your answers may change as time goes by.

Test Two: The Low-Carb Breakfast

Scrambled Eggs with Feta Cheese and Salsa

1 medium apple (any variety), slightly smaller than the size of your fist

Nutrition facts: 307 calories, 22 grams protein, 30 grams carbohydrates, 7 grams fiber, 11 grams fat

test recipe

Scrambled Eggs with Feta Cheese and Salsa

   2 large eggs
   2 egg whites
   2 tablespoons crumbled full-fat feta cheese
      Salt and ground black pepper to taste
   ⅓ cup no-sugar-added salsa, such as Muir Glen Organic Salsa

1. Heat a nonstick skillet to medium-high. Coat with olive oil cooking spray.

2. In a medium bowl, mix together the eggs, egg whites, and feta cheese.

3. Add to the skillet and cook, stirring, for 3 to 4 minutes, or until firm.

4. Remove the eggs to a plate. Season with salt and pepper. Top with the salsa.

CHART YOUR RESULTS

After eating, complete the following questionnaire every 30 minutes for the next 3 hours, for a total of six assessments. At every 30-minute interval, check off the answer that most closely matches how you feel. Your answers may change as time goes by.

Your Carb Tolerance Questionnaire

Make photocopies of this questionnaire so that you can fill it out for each of your four tests (two Test Ones and two Test Twos). Score each test according to the instructions on pages 43 to 44, and compare your results for all four tests on page 45.

	30 MIN	1 HR	1½ HR	2 HR	2½ HR	3 HR
1. How satisfied are you?						
a. I am not satisfied at all						
b. I am somewhat satisfied						
c. I am comfortably satisfied						
d. I am very satisfied						
2. How hungry are you?						
a. I have never been more hungry						
b. I am more than slightly hungry						
c. I am slightly hungry						
d. I am not hungry at all						
3. How full are you?						
a. I am completely empty						
b. I am partially full						
c. I am full but not uncomfortable						
d. I am completely full						
4. How much food could you eat right now?						
a. I could eat a lot						
b. I could eat, and I do want to						
c. I could eat, but I don't want to						
d. I could not eat another bite						
5. How composed or anxious do you feel right now?						
a. I feel very composed						
b. I feel somewhat composed						
c. I feel somewhat anxious						
d. I feel very anxious						

	30 MIN	1 HR	1½ HR	2 HR	2½ HR	3 HR

6. How agreeable or disagreeable do you feel right now?

	30 MIN	1 HR	1½ HR	2 HR	2½ HR	3 HR
a. I feel very agreeable and pleasant						
b. I feel somewhat agreeable						
c. I feel somewhat disagreeable						
d. I feel very disagreeable and mean						

7. How happy or sad do you feel right now?

	30 MIN	1 HR	1½ HR	2 HR	2½ HR	3 HR
a. I feel very happy and elated						
b. I feel somewhat happy						
c. I feel somewhat sad						
d. I feel very sad and unhappy						

8. How energetic or tired do you feel right now?

	30 MIN	1 HR	1½ HR	2 HR	2½ HR	3 HR
a. I feel very energetic and spirited						
b. I feel somewhat energetic						
c. I feel somewhat tired						
d. I feel very tired and sluggish						

9. How clearheaded or foggy do you feel right now?

	30 MIN	1 HR	1½ HR	2 HR	2½ HR	3 HR
a. I feel very clearheaded						
b. I feel somewhat clearheaded						
c. I feel somewhat foggy						
d. I feel very foggy and confused						

10. How confident or unsure do you feel right now?

	30 MIN	1 HR	1½ HR	2 HR	2½ HR	3 HR
a. I feel very confident and sure						
b. I feel somewhat confident						
c. I feel somewhat unsure						
d. I feel very unconfident and unsure						

Scoring Your Tests

For each test, add up your total score for each half-hour increment using the following scale.

Calculate the following points for questions 1 to 4:

a = 1 point

b = 2 points

c = 3 points

d = 4 points

Calculate the following points for questions 5 to 10:

a = 4 points

b = 3 points

c = 2 points

d = 1 point

≫Your Perfect Body Diet Planner

Check off the appropriate response below to help chart your plan in the *Women's Health Perfect Body Diet*.

The results of the carbohydrate tolerance tests in this chapter reveal which of the two eating plans you should follow:

 ☐ **GREENS AND BERRIES DIET IN CHAPTER 8:** This is the lower-carb option of the two plans, offering 20 to 30 percent of calories from carbs (90 to 125 grams of carbohydrates per day), 35 to 45 percent of calories from fat (60 to 70 grams), and 30 to 35 percent of calories from protein (120 to 140 grams). The actual number of grams of each macronutrient that you take in each day will depend on your customized calorie counts, which you'll calculate in Chapter 7. You can further tailor this plan to your body by choosing your preferred foods from among the lists of sanctioned foods in Chapters 7 and 8.

 ☐ **GRAINS AND FRUITS DIET IN CHAPTER 9:** It allows you comparatively more carbohydrate-rich foods, providing 35 to 45 percent of calories from carbs (150 to 185 grams), 25 to 35 percent of calories from fat (50 to 55 grams), and 25 to 30 percent of calories from protein (100 to 125 grams). The actual number of grams of each macronutrient that you take in each day will depend on your customized calorie counts, which you'll calculate in Chapter 7. You can further tailor this plan to your body by choosing your preferred foods from among the lists of sanctioned foods in Chapters 7 and 9.

	FIRST TEST SEQUENCE		SECOND TEST SEQUENCE	
	Test One	Test Two	Test One	Test Two
30-Min Score				
1-Hr Score				
1½-Hr Score				
2-Hr Score				
2½-Hr Score				
3-Hr Score				

What Your Test-One Score Means

If your total score is below 20 for any of the half-hour time periods before the 2-hour mark, you have poor carbohydrate tolerance. You should follow the Greens and Berries Diet in Chapter 8 to reach your perfect body goal.

If your total score is above 20 for most of the time periods, you have very good carbohydrate tolerance and should follow the Grains and Fruits Diet in Chapter 9.

If your scores are above 20 until the 2-hour mark and then drop, you are in the middle. You can follow either diet, but we suggest you stick with the Grains and Fruits Diet, the relatively higher-carb plan. It allows a wider variety of foods, including brown rice and more fruit. You'll still lose weight.

What Your Test-Two Score Means

After eating the low-carbohydrate Test Two meal, most women should feel a bit more energetic (and less hungry) than they do after eating the high-carb Test One meal. But if your score is below 20 for most of the time periods, your body runs better with more carbohydrates. You should follow the Grains and Fruits Diet—the relatively higher-carb diet, which contains a little less fat and protein than the Greens and Berries Diet.

If your total score is above 20 for most of the periods (especially after 2 hours), you should eat according to the Greens and Berries Diet, the slightly lower-carbohydrate diet.

What Happens Once You Have the Results?

With the results of these tests, you now know which of the two diets you need to follow, based on which macronutrient ratio is best for your perfect body. In the next chapter, we'll tell you more about each of those macronutrients and how they're put to work.

CHAPTER 6

What to Eat:
Perfect Carbs, Fats, and Proteins

Now that you know which eating plan you'll follow, let's learn more about the basic nutrients and types of foods that you'll eat on the *Women's Health Perfect Body Diet*. (No tests, quizzes, or essay questions, we promise.)

This chapter covers the three main energy-providing nutrient categories: carbohydrates, fats, and proteins. You'll learn exactly what these nutrients are and where you can find them. Every food falls into at least one of these categories, and by having a better understanding of them, you'll be able to see why you react to specific foods and what you can do about it. That way, you'll be more successful on the *Women's Health Perfect Body Diet*, and it will be one you can follow for life.

First up: carbs.

Everything You Wanted to Know about Carbs (But May Have Been Too Bloated and Sleepy to Ask)

Let's play a little word association. When you hear the word *carbohydrate*, you think of . . .

Giant loaves of bread? Plates of pasta? Baskets of cookies? Well, you're right—all those things are carbs. But the classification *carbohydrate* also applies to fresh foods such as fruits, vegetables, beans, and legumes. Dairy products also contain some carbohydrates, though their makeup is higher in protein and fat (unless the fat has been removed).

Carbohydrates have a distinct molecular structure by which they can be further classified as a sugar, starch, or fiber. Common fibers are pectin (in apples) and cellulose (in many vegetables). Common starches are amylose and amylopectin (found in many grains and cereals). Common sugars include glucose (in most foods), fructose (found mostly in fruit), and galactose (the carb component of milk). Sugar alcohols, also known as sugar substitutes, create the taste of sweetness without adding extra calories. These are man-made and not naturally found in foods, so while they are considered carbohydrates, they are not digested the same way as other carbs.

When you eat foods that contain starch or sugar, your stomach and intestines break them down into individual sugar units. These single sugar molecules are easily absorbed through the intestinal wall into the bloodstream, where they can provide energy (in the form of blood glucose/sugar), if you need it. If you don't need the energy right away, or if you don't need all of it at that moment, then the sugars are stored in your muscles in a form called glycogen. However, since you have only a limited amount of muscle space in which to store glycogen, the liver will convert most excess sugar into body fat. That's what you're trying to get rid of.

Carbohydrate foods that contain more fiber than sugar and starch aren't broken down as easily and have less chance to affect your body fat levels. So the type of carbohydrate foods you eat is important because it influences how much body fat you have.

Sugars and starches are quick digesting and referred to as *simple carbohydrates*. Foods that contain simple carbs are mostly the man-made variety: high-sugar breakfast cereals, granola bars, and candy. Fruit juices also contain a lot of simple carbohydrates. Because simple carbs provide glucose in quantities too large to be used right away for energy, they are more likely to be stored as body fat.

Foods that are broken down slowly thanks to a high amount of fiber are called *complex carbohydrates*. These foods are less likely to be stored as body fat because they deliver a smaller, steadier influx of energy that your body will use as its provided. Examples of high-fiber foods are asparagus, beans, brown rice, sprouted grains, and glucomannan.

If you're not a big fan of high-fiber, good-for-you foods, another way to make even a simple carbohydrate food break down more slowly is to combine it with foods that contain proteins, fats, or dietary fiber (for instance, glucomannan). These other nutrients slow down the movement of food from your stomach into your intestines and, eventually, into your

Her Perfect Body

bloodstream. If you combine these foods with simpler carbs, your digestion time will be lengthened, and you'll receive your energy slowly and steadily, keeping you in control of your mood, stamina, and hunger. Otherwise, you'll receive your energy supply (blood glucose) too fast, causing your body to store it away quickly, leaving you slightly chubbier and yearning for more food.

THE PERFECT CARBS FOR YOUR BODY

What does all this mean in terms of what you should actually eat every day?

 Women with poorer carbohydrate tolerance, who are following the Greens and Berries Diet in Chapter 8, will choose from a list of carb foods that are slow digesting, usually high in fiber, and thus very satisfying. Shoot for 15 to 25 grams of carbohydrates every meal, or 90 to 125 daily grams of carbohydrates.

Women who can tolerate and use carbohydrates better and are following the Grains and Fruits Diet in Chapter 9 will choose from a list of carb foods that are digested a little faster but still make you feel full. You can have as much as 25 to 45 grams per meal, or approximately 150 to 185 daily grams of carbohydrates.

No matter which diet you follow, your intake of carbohydrates should be higher in your main meals and smaller in snacks. Remember, you'll be eating five or six times a day.

Followers of both diets should also remember this: The perfect carbohydrate-containing foods for women are those that come directly from natural sources: fruits, vegetables, beans, and whole grains. If you've tried low-carb diets, you may recall that on some diets, fruits and some vegetables were in the "bad carb" category, and you were instructed not to eat those. However, studies from the department of preventive medicine and public health at the University of Navarra in Pamplona, Spain, have shown that fruits and vegetables, as

Women, Carbohydrates, and Exercise

High-carbohydrate diets were all the rage when women starting working out in the mid-1960s. It was thought that the muscles needed additional glycogen (stored carbohydrate) for fuel during prolonged exercise and that carbs would provide energy to fight fatigue. So people ate large volumes of carbohydrates, such as giant pasta dinners, in an attempt to pump up muscle-glycogen levels as much as possible. This led to the development of eating strategies called glycogen loading (or carbohydrate loading) to supersaturate muscle glycogen levels, delay glycogen depletion, and prolong the onset of fatigue, thereby improving performance.

But that way of thinking is now almost 50 years old. Today, we know that high-carbohydrate diets may not be optimal for women, even female athletes. We now understand that women actually use significantly less carbohydrate during exercise than men, store less carbohydrate in their muscles, and store more as body fat. So while glycogen loading is a good strategy for your boyfriend, it's not the best strategy for you.

During exercise, women's bodies naturally prefer to use fat for energy rather than carbohydrates, so it's not smart to overdose on carbohydrate-rich foods. They won't help you exercise any harder or any better because they won't be used very well. And in some women, carbohydrate tolerance is so low that additional carbohydrate foods will just make their bodies hold on to more body fat.

well as fiber (that includes glucomannan for you), have an inverse relationship to weight gain. Simply put, the participants who included fruits and vegetables or fiber in their diets were more likely to lose weight than those who omitted them.

That's why on this diet you'll be eating lots of vegetables, fruits, and fruit smoothies (combined with glucomannan). All of these are body-friendly choices for the *Women's*

▶▶Your Perfect Body Diet Planner

THE GREENS AND BERRIES DIET IN CHAPTER 8: This is the lower-carb option of the two plans, offering 20 to 30 percent of daily calories from carbohydrates per day, or 90 to 125 daily grams of carbohydrates. The actual number of carb grams that you take in each day will depend on your customized calorie counts, which you'll calculate in Chapter 7. The best carbohydrates for you are those that are rich in fiber and digested slowly. Focus on green vegetables and berries (hence the diet's name), certain other fruits, and beans and legumes. We'll give you complete, detailed lists of the carb foods you should choose from, including their serving sizes, calorie counts, and carb and fiber grams, in Chapter 8. Your intake of carbs should be higher in your main meals and smaller in snacks. Remember, you'll be eating five or six times a day.

GRAINS AND FRUITS DIET IN CHAPTER 9: It allows you comparatively more carbohydrate foods, providing 35 to 45 percent of daily calories from carbs (150 to 185 grams). The actual number of carb grams that you take in each day will depend on your customized calorie counts, which you'll calculate in Chapter 7. Your body tolerates and uses carbohydrates better, so you can choose from a list of carbohydrate foods that are digested a little faster but still make you feel full. These foods include whole grains and a wide variety of fruit, as well as beans and legumes. Chapter 9 features your lists of prescribed carb foods, including their serving sizes, calorie counts, and carb and fiber grams. Your intake of carbohydrates should be higher in larger meals and smaller in snacks. You'll also be eating five or six times a day.

Health Perfect Body Diet. However, stay away from fruit juices—even those that are not artificially sweetened. They have significantly lower amounts of fiber, compared with fruits in their natural states.

FAR-FROM-PERFECT CARBS: JUST SAY NO

As you already know, there are lots of carbs that should just be shunned. Whenever you can, try to avoid processed foods, especially carbs that end up looking white: white flours, white rice, and white potatoes. If you avoid eating the foods on the following far-from-perfect carbohydrate lists, your perfect body will thank you.

Far-from-Perfect Breads

Savvy marketers have changed the lingo of the bakery aisle to the point that every product claims to be "whole" this or "multigrain" that. And if it hasn't been "stone ground," it's probably been "cracked." Some breads with healthy-sounding names are not so healthy, and some with ho-hum names are terrific. Here's how to separate the whole wheat from the chaff.

>> **Ignore the name.** They all sound compelling, and you'll only get confused. For example, a "light whole grain sourdough" sounds good. But it's probably made from mostly white flour. It may contain a little whole wheat flour, but if that's way down there on the ingredients list, right below the corn syrup and the yeast, don't bother. According to FDA regulations, all flour in bread that calls itself "whole wheat" has to be just that. There is no such rule for "whole grain."

>> **Know what you are looking for.** The first ingredient should be "whole wheat" flour, not "wheat" flour, "unbleached wheat" flour, or "unbleached enriched wheat" flour: All of these varieties have been stripped of their germ and their bran—and their fiber content. This applies to all flour-based products, including crackers, waffles, and pancakes.

>> **Be wary of enriched bread.** Many manufacturers "enrich" their denuded flour by adding back a few B vitamins and iron. Thanks, but no thanks. Instead of picking enriched bread, buy one that hasn't been robbed of vitamins and minerals in the first place. Whole wheat and sprouted grain breads are the best.

>> **Check the fiber content.** Two slices of most whole wheat breads contain 4 grams of fiber, so the minimum per slice you should look for is 2 grams. That's about three times as much as you'll get from the same amount of white bread. Just

Your Perfect Body Carb Caveats

1. Stay away from foods made with white flour, including white breads, crackers, cookies, muffins, pastas, and bagels. When you add water to white flour, it turns into wallpaper paste. That's exactly what happens with flour products as they lie around inside your body, so they slow down your metabolism and add useless calories. If you must eat flour products, make sure they are 100 percent whole wheat.

2. Get more of your calories from foods instead of drinks. Ditch the apple juice and eat the apple instead.

3. Eat vegetables—especially low-calorie, high-fiber vegetables—at most meals. This will keep you feeling more satisfied for a longer time after you eat.

remember: Refined flour plus a little fiber in the form of bran, whole grain, or guar gum doesn't pack the same vitamin and mineral punch as a whole grain alternative.

》》 **Never buy . . .** potato bread; white bagels, muffins, waffles, or pancakes; white bread; or light bread.

Far-from-Perfect Snacks and Cereals

Most packaged snack foods and breakfast cereals are loaded with sugar. Read the ingredients and walk away if you see the words listed below, because they are all synonyms for sugar.

》》 Cane juice

》》 Corn syrup

》》 Dextrose

》》 Fructose

》》 Glucose

》》 High fructose corn syrup

》》 Lactose

》》 Maltodextrin

》》 Rice syrup

》》 Sucrose

Also stay away from "100-calorie snack packs." Just because they are prepackaged to contain a predetermined number of calories doesn't mean that they are good for your body. So, even if it's sold in small portions, stay away from:

- Candy
- Chips
- Chocolate bars
- Chocolate-covered pretzels
- Cookies, cakes, and most commercial pies
- Granola bars
- Nachos
- Popcorn, buttered, microwaved
- Soda (regular)
- White flour crackers

Far-from-Perfect Vegetables

You really can't go wrong eating vegetables—unless you ruin a good thing by coating them in deep-fried flour or dipping them in a dressing that's high fat or packed with soybean oil (check the ingredients list). Here are a few to avoid.

- Deep-fried breaded onion
- Tempura vegetables
- Wasabi peas

Far-from-Perfect Fruits

Make sure that your favorite frozen berries and fruits have no added sugars, and stay away from dried fruits with extra "sweetness." Even if the package says that it has no additives or preservatives, read the ingredients label to ensure that the only thing in the package is the fruit. Here are a few that might trip you up.

- Dried cranberries with added sugar (Craisins is the best-known brand)
- Dried pineapple or mango rings (often contain extra sugar)
- Unsulphured papaya (processed and coated with honey)

The Perfect Fats for Shedding Body Fat

It was only a few years ago that the phrase "perfect fats" would have been considered an oxymoron. Fat was evil, fat was a villain, fat was to be avoided.

Today, it's clear that eating the right kind of fat is not only *not* bad for you, it's essential for good health. What's more, dietary fat can be an incredible tool for helping you get rid of body fat. Here are a few of the benefits of putting the right kinds of fat in your diet.

>> Fats found naturally in foods help protect against heart disease and cancer.

>> Fats crank up your metabolic rate and increase the amount of body fat you burn off. Research has shown that when you replace carbohydrates with good sources of fat, your body increases the enzymes that help turn fat into an energy source.

>> Fat supplies the fat-soluble vitamins A, D, E and K, and it helps your body produce estrogen and progesterone.

>> The right fats make your skin soft and supple instead of dry, wrinkled, and flaky. Without fat you'd have sandpapery skin, brittle nails, and dull, lifeless hair.

>> Adding fat to meals and snacks, especially those that contain fiber, helps you feel more satisfied and keeps you feeling full longer. Good fats help slow your digestive rate, so that food leaves your stomach slowly and enters your bloodstream at a steadier rate. When there is some fat in your meals, your body produces more cholecystokinin, or CCK—the hormone that makes you feel satisfied after eating. A little dietary fat also reduces the amount of ghrelin in your body, thereby suppressing your desire to eat.

A BIG FAT LESSON

So what fat-centric foods should you be eating? We'll recommend some in a minute, but first let's get a better understanding of what we're talking about. Fats and their liquid form—oils—are classified as being saturated, monounsaturated, or polyunsaturated. Actually, every fat or oil is a mixture of all three of these, but one type will predominate in any given fat-based food. For example, if you cooked exclusively with olive oil, a rich source of monounsaturated fat, and ate everything else completely fat free, you'd still obtain some saturated and polyunsaturated fats because small amounts are also found in olive oil.

Let's look in more detail at the different types of fats.

Saturated fatty acids are solid and stiff at room temperature. Butter and other dairy products are examples, as is coconut oil. These are the ones that some dietetic associations have told us to limit in our diets to avoid raising blood cholesterol to dangerous levels. But the latest research shows that these fats may not have the detrimental effect we've been warned about. A 2004 review in the *American Journal of Clinical Nutrition* concluded that there has not been sufficient research on the way saturated fats affect coronary artery disease and other health issues to justify the recommendation that all people limit their saturated fat intake.

This doesn't mean you should eat buckets of butter; it just means that the saturated fatty acids found naturally in foods have not been proven to be dangerous in moderate amounts, such as 2 cups of 2% milk a day, 2 tablespoons of cream cheese with your lox, or 1 tablespoon of butter on your whole grain bread. It also means you don't have to drink only fat-free milk or avoid red meat if you don't want to. A moderate amount of saturated fat may not be unhealthy or fattening as long as it's part of a diet that also contains healthy amounts of monounsaturated and polyunsaturated fats. So eat your butter, but also have some almonds, which are rich in monos, to balance it out.

Monounsaturated fatty acids are liquid or soft at room temperature and are found in the highest quantities in foods such as olives, avocados, nuts, seeds, and egg yolks. They are also the most prevalent form of fat in meats; for example, the fat in beef is 50 percent monounsaturated and 35 to 40 percent saturated. Monounsaturates are the type of fat our bodies prefer to use as energy. And Wisconsin researchers have shown that exercise increases the metabolism of monounsaturated fat more than saturated fat in women. This means that more fat can be burned for fuel during and after exercise when you eat foods rich in monounsaturated fat.

Polyunsaturated fatty acids are found in many foods from both plant and animal sources. Most polyunsaturated fatty acids can't be made by your body, so you have to obtain them through your diet. These food-dependent types of polyunsaturates are called essential. There are two categories of essential polyunsaturated fats: omega-3s and omega-6s.

Omega-3 fats, especially those from fish, have gotten a lot of good press in recent years, and for good reason: They're pivotal in maintaining good health. Increased quantities of omega-3 fatty acids have been associated in clinical trials with lower rates of cancer, depression, mental illness, adverse pregnancy outcomes, infectious disease, osteoporosis, lung disease, menstrual pain, cognitive decline, eye damage, rheumatoid arthritis, kidney disease, menstrual problems, ulcerative colitis, Crohn's disease, and cystic fibrosis.

Eat in the Moment

A University of Illinois study found that people who consumed monounsaturated fats from olive oil, avocados, and nuts before a meal ate 25 percent fewer calories than those who didn't. Treat yourself to a tablespoon of natural peanut butter or a handful of nuts right before going out, and you'll feel a little less hungry before you eat and more satisfied during dinner.

Perhaps most important to the *Women's Health Perfect Body Diet*, they can also help control body fat and increase fat burning.

The three omega-3 polyunsaturated fatty acids commonly found in our diets are alpha-linoleic acid (ALA), eicosapentaenoic acid (EPA), and docosahexaenoic acid (DHA). These are found only in specially raised eggs, a few plant foods (such as walnuts, flax, and canola oil), and a few fish (such as salmon, trout, and sardines). (Fish oil has gotten so much attention because it is rich in both EPA and DHA.)

Omega-6s, the most common of which is linoleic acid (LNA), are healthy when they're consumed in an almost equal ratio with omega-3s. Overconsuming omega-6s, on the other hand, sets up our bodies for increased inflammation, which is a risk factor for many diseases. Omega-6s are found in the highest quantities in vegetable oils such as corn oil, soybean oil, and safflower oil. They also make up the majority of the polyunsaturated fat found in meats such as chicken, beef, and pork. Because corn and soybean oil are added to many food products (such as salad dressings, corn chips, baked goods, and even fruit snacks) and because many of us eat meat products often, our ratio of omega-6s to omega-3s weighs heavily toward the omega-6s. To balance out the two types of polyunsaturated fats, watch out for these added oils; eat lots of fish, ground flaxseeds, and walnuts; and use canola, olive, or flaxseed oil for salad dressings and when cooking.

Here's a list of foods that contain omega-3s and omega-6s. This list gives the values for 100 grams of food, unless otherwise indicated. Although you'll probably never eat 100

Why Fish Is Better Than Flax

All omega-3s are not all created equal. Even though both flaxseeds and fish such as salmon are rich sources of dietary omega-3 fats, they contain different *types* of omega-3s. The bottom line is that the omega-3s found in fish are easier for your body to use than those found in flax. The type of omega-3 in flaxseed oil, called ALA, must first be converted in the body to EPA and DHA before the fat-burning and health-promoting effects can be experienced. The rate at which flax omega-3 is converted to EPA and DHA is quite low—about 5 to 15 percent of the total amount you eat. It probably wouldn't hurt to use flaxseed oil in your salads or smoothies, but don't assume that this will give you all the omega-3 you need. You still must include fish in your diet, and if you absolutely hate fish, take six 1-gram fish oil capsules per day.

grams of flaxseeds, you might well eat 100 grams of fish. For best results, choose foods with more omega-3s than omega-6s.

FOOD	OMEGA-3s (G)	OMEGA-6s (G)
Flaxseed oil	55.3	13.4
Flaxseeds, ground	18.2	4.3
Canola oil	9.3	20.3
Walnuts, chopped	9.0	38.1
Hemp seeds	7.0	21.0
Salmon, Atlantic	2.3	0.6
Herring, canned	2.1	0.3
Soybeans, roasted	1.4	10.7
Sardines, canned	1.4	3.5
Butter	1.4	2.2
Trout, farmed	1.2	0.9
Olive oil, extra-virgin	0.7	8.0
Wheat germ, toasted	0.7	5.5
Omega-3 egg, 1 large	0.4	0.7
Pumpkin seeds	0.1	20.7
Sunflower seeds	0	30.7
Almonds	0	9.2
Olives	0	1.6
Egg, 1 large	0	0.7

THE NEW FAT-LOSS FATS

Research has shown that certain special fats, like the Enova brand oil that is derived from canola and olive oils, can help you lose weight. You may have noticed this new cooking oil on your supermarket shelves. Several clinical studies show that compared with other cooking oils, less Enova oil is stored as body fat, which means it can help you reach your perfect body more quickly. Enova oil doesn't taste any different than other cooking oils, and it doesn't have any nasty side effects (such as diarrhea or fat-soluble-vitamin depletion).

Enova oil is dramatically different from other oils in its basic chemical composition. Saturated, monounsaturated, and polyunsaturated fats are *triglycerides,* consisting of a molecule of glycerol with three arms of fatty acids composed of carbon, hydrogen, and oxygen. Enova oil molecules, in contrast, have only two fatty acid arms and therefore are called *diglycerides*. Your body does not process diglycerides the same way it treats triglycerides; instead, it stores less of the Enova oil and burns more of it for energy.

An important study in the *American Journal of Clinical Nutrition* found that Enova oil, the only brand of diglyceride oil available in North America, promoted weight loss and body fat reduction. It may help you both burn more calories and eat less food.

Since this oil is new to the market and its long-term effects are not completely known, it's a good idea to rotate its use with olive oil or canola oil to ensure that you don't miss out on the health benefits of these other oils.

Another special fatty acid that is associated with body fat reduction and weight control is gamma-linolenic acid (GLA). Gamma-linolenic acid is a special type of omega-6 poly-

Trans Fats: The New Villain

Although they occur naturally in some foods, such as dairy products, trans fats have been added to other foods by a very unnatural process called hydrogenation. Food chemists took polyunsaturated fats rich in omega-6 fat and bombarded them with extra hydrogen molecules to create solid trans fatty acids. These new fats were supposed to replace the demonized saturated fats as a solid fat source that was very shelf stable. But it turns out that trans fats increase blood cholesterol and increase disease risk more than saturated fats have ever been shown to do.

To avoid trans fats, check all food labels for the words *hydrogenated* or even *partially hydrogenated* before the name of a particular oil, such as soybean oil. Even if the food label says that it contains zero grams of trans fats, that only means the food contains no more than 0.5 gram of trans fats, which is still bad for your body.

In response to the backlash against trans fats, the food industry has come up with another winner: *interesterified fats.* These are created by blending highly saturated hard fats such as palm oil or fully hydrogenated vegetable oils with other liquid oils. However, interesterified fats have a similar negative dietary impact, particularly in terms of blood cholesterol levels and blood glucose control.

unsaturated fatty acid found in the highest quantities in evening primrose oil (from the seeds of the evening primrose plant) and borage oil (from the seeds of the borage plant). Research at UCLA and the University of California, Berkeley, showed that GLA helped prevent fat regain after weight loss in overweight and obese people. The subjects were given either 860 milligrams of GLA from 5 grams of borage oil per day or 5 grams of olive oil, while losing weight with diet and exercise. After 1 year of weight loss, the participants continued the same supplementation for another 2 years without any dietary guidance. After the first year without dietary help, the participants taking the GLA from borage oil did not gain back any weight, while the ones taking olive oil gained back about 5 pounds. After the second year, there was an even greater difference between the groups: The people taking borage oil gained back only about 4 pounds of weight, while the ones taking olive oil gained back 17. The investigators hypothesized that borage oil (GLA) supplementation prevented weight regain by improving blood glucose handling, depressing fat production, and increasing fat burning.

Since we can't get borage oil from a food source (unless you want to eat borage seeds, which we doubt anyone would want to do), you must supplement with borage oil or evening primrose oil capsules to get GLA. The recommended dose is 3 to 5 grams of GLA (providing 520 to 860 mg of GLA) per day.

WHY CHOLESTEROL ISN'T AS BAD AS YOU THINK

Dietary cholesterol has gotten a bad reputation for all the wrong reasons. Many years ago, scientists assumed that the cholesterol found naturally in foods such as eggs and other animal products increased the cholesterol in our blood and thereby raised our risk for heart disease. So we were told to avoid it at all costs. Thousands of egg yolks were washed down the drain, and labels on food packages bragged that foods were low in cholesterol or, better yet, cholesterol free.

For the past 10 to 20 years, scientific evidence has proved again and again that dietary cholesterol has little or no impact on blood cholesterol levels in most people. A 2006 study in the journal *Current Opinion in Clinical Nutrition and Metabolic Care* concluded that 70 percent of people experience little to no increase in blood cholesterol in response to high amounts of dietary cholesterol (such as three eggs a day for 30 days). The only people who should watch the amount of cholesterol they eat are those who have already suffered a heart attack. And even these folks are never instructed to completely eliminate cholesterol from their diets. So start enjoying your eggs again, and stop buying foods just because they're cholesterol free. Dietary cholesterol is a normal component of healthy cell membranes, and your body also uses it to help produce hormones such as estrogen, progesterone, and testosterone. It's found naturally in many of the recommended foods in the *Women's Health Perfect Body Diet*, including salmon, poultry, and dairy products.

JUST THE FACTS, MA'AM
Speaking of foods recommended by this diet, there's also a lot of confusion about the fat in other specific foods that we'll be telling you to eat. Here are the facts about other healthy sources of fat.

Nuts Won't Make You Fat
Recent studies have shown that nuts have many health benefits, including protection against heart disease, high blood pressure, and adult-onset diabetes. Yet many women shy away from eating nuts for the same reasons they buy fat-free foods: They're afraid of high fat content.

When people think of fatty foods, they often think of nuts, and for good reason. It's true that all nuts (except chestnuts) are high in fat. By weight, the total fat content of nuts ranges from 45 to 75 percent, but this fat is largely the healthful monounsaturated and polyunsaturated kinds. For example, almonds and pistachios are well known for being high in mono-

Five Ways to Eat More Nuts

» Toss a handful of sunflower seeds into hot or cold high-fiber cereal.

» Sauté walnuts in a nonstick pan over low heat. Add the toasted nuts to salads and whole wheat pasta.

» Sprinkle chopped pecans over a casserole, cooked vegetables, or stir-fry.

» Add almond slivers to an omelette.

» For a savory popcorn alternative, spray a handful of almonds with nonstick cooking spray and bake at 400°F for 5 to 10 minutes. Take them out of the oven, then sprinkle with a mixture of salt, ground red pepper, and thyme.

Go Nuts!

Here is a short list of the benefits of some of your favorite nuts. A typical serving of nuts is about 1 ounce, but enjoy up to 3 ounces per day as long as you're accounting for the additional calories by subtracting other foods. You'll be eating lots of nuts (2 to 3 ounces per day) by following the meal plan.

Almonds: Packed with protein, fiber, calcium, and iron, almonds are also one of the best sources of vitamin E, which protects against stroke and cancer.

Hazelnuts: Along with one of the highest ratios of good fat to bad, hazelnuts are packed with folate, a vitamin that protects against birth defects.

Peanuts: These legumes (they're actually not nuts at all) are a good choice for keeping cholesterol levels at bay. They provide more protein (7 grams per serving) than tree nuts.

Pecans: These help fight high cholesterol because of their high monounsaturated fat content.

Pistachios: They're a great source of potassium that may lower your LDL cholesterol.

Walnuts: Walnuts have an abundance of polyunsaturated fat, which may protect against adult-onset diabetes.

One note about storing nuts: With their high fat content, nuts turn rancid quickly unless stored in tightly sealed containers in a cool, dark place, such as your freezer. Proper storage will let you enjoy them for at least 3 weeks. Or buy 'em and eat 'em right away.

unsaturated fat, containing 53 to 64 percent monounsaturates for the total amount of fat. Walnuts are another unique nut because they're loaded with the same heart-healthy omega-3 polyunsaturated fatty acids found in flaxseeds.

Of course, nuts and seeds are also a concentrated source of calories. When you look at the nutritional information for a 1-ounce serving of walnuts, you'll see that they supply a hefty 190 calories. Considering that 1 ounce is about $^1/_4$ cup, or just enough nuts to fit into the palm of your hand, this seems like too many calories for such a small serving. However, because nuts contain fiber, not all of the calories they provide are absorbed by the body. Even better, researchers now speculate that, rather than expanding your waistline, eating nuts may actually help you keep off the pounds. A 2007 Purdue University study of 20 women found that 2.2 ounces of almonds eaten daily was associated with a decrease in calorie intake from other foods. So while eating pounds and pounds of nuts each day would probably make you gain weight, a daily 2-to-3-ounce serving, as recommended by the *Women's Health Perfect Body Diet,* won't expand your waistline.

In Mediterranean countries, where the consumption of nuts is almost double that of the United States, the rate of obesity is significantly lower. In the famous Nurses' Health Study, which looked at body weight and body mass index in a group of 86,000 women, the women who ate at least 1.5 ounces of nuts per day weighed much less than women who did not eat nuts at all. And in few controlled feeding studies where women were given nuts daily, body weight actually declined when they regularly ate between 1 and 3 ounces ($^1/_4$ to $^3/_4$ cup) of walnuts, pecans, and almonds per day.

Nuts also contain protein and at least 3 to 5 grams of fiber per serving. This causes them to be digested very slowly, which makes them very satisfying and helps to reduce hunger. The fat found in nuts also helps your body use more fat as fuel and increases your metabolic rate. In this way, your body has to expend energy to digest nuts, which lowers the number of calories they may add to your body.

Finally, and most important, nuts are not fully digested. Since the surface of the nut is hard and dense, your digestive enzymes can't always break nuts completely apart. A research study with peanuts actually found that 17 percent of the fat in nuts was eliminated in stools, indicating that fat absorption was impaired. Since all of the fat cannot be absorbed into your body, you obviously do not receive all of the calories and the fat listed on the Nutrition Facts label. So go ahead and enjoy nuts. A couple of handfuls—equating to 1 to 3 ounces, or $^1/_4$ to $^3/_4$ cup—is a good daily amount.

The Real Deal with Dairy Fat

All the hype about dairy makes it hard to know whether it's on the yes or no list in terms of dieting. In the past 3 years, researchers such as Michael Zemel, PhD, of the University of Tennessee, have published more than 60 studies connecting dairy and body weight reduction, many of which support the idea that dairy might be a key to increased weight loss. However, other experts, including Pamela Peeke, MD, a clinical assistant professor of medicine at the University of Maryland School of Medicine and the author of *Body-for-LIFE for Women,* caution that there is no overwhelming consensus yet and that the data are still new.

Some research suggests that dairy-fueled weight loss leads to a more toned physique.

"On dairy-rich diets, more of the weight you lose is fat and less is muscle," says Dr. Zemel. Other scientists have recognized that people who eat dairy often weigh less than those who don't. One reason may be that high levels of calcium appear to help release fat-burning hormones and enzymes. And when your body receives too little dietary calcium, it releases chemicals that leach calcium from your bones and teeth—and that slows down fat burning. "On a low-calcium diet you're breaking down less fat, and you're making more fat," Dr. Zemel says. The best weight-loss results were with people who initially consumed only one serving of dairy a day (such as a 1-ounce slice of cheese) and then tripled their intake, which happens to be the US government's recommended daily allowance.

Popping a handful of calcium-fortified Tums or other calcium supplements may not do the trick. In order to enhance weight loss, the calcium must react with the proteins in dairy products. You're best off adding dairy to your daily food intake and trimming your calories somewhere else.

Can you simply trim the calories from dairy and get the best of both? Unfortunately, it's not that easy. Low-fat yogurt is one of the best sources of calcium (1 cup provides almost half your daily recommended intake of calcium), and the fat that it contains helps your body absorb more of the calcium and use more of the protein; it also will keep you satisfied longer. Fat-free yogurt won't have the same effect. Not all fat-containing dairy products are also high in calcium—full-fat cream cheese, sour cream, and ice cream are actually poor sources—but if you omit all the fat from your favorite dairy products, you won't reduce the hunger hormones that make you want to overeat.

In addition to being more satisfying, the fat in dairy helps control how quickly the yogurt, cheese, or milk is digested and will help you reach your goals for fat intake. Plus, dairy products such as yogurt, ricotta, and cottage cheese are great foods in which to mix glucomannan, the fiber supplement that will also slow your digestion and keep you fuller longer.

You can limit full-fat dairy products, such as high-fat cheeses, because the fat in dairy is rich in saturated fatty acids. Some saturated fat is good in your diet, but too much may not be very healthy. So the bottom line is to make sure your daily diet incorporates a minimal amount of dairy fat, such as a 6-ounce container of low-fat yogurt and one or more 4-ounce glasses of 2% milk.

If you are lactose intolerant, you may still be able to eat yogurt because the lactose content is quite low; or look for dairy products with added lactase, such as Lactaid brand milk and cottage cheese, which contain the enzyme your body needs to break down the lactose molecule.

Choosing Cooking Oils

When some fats are heated at very high temperatures, such as in a deep fryer, the heat can bump off a hydrogen molecule, leaving an unpaired electron. This is known as oxidation, and it allows the unpaired electron to steal hydrogen molecules from your body. The theft can damage your DNA and cell membranes, causing illness and faster aging. A 2003 review of animal studies, published in the journal *Current Opinion in Clinical Nutrition and Metabolic Care,* concluded that oxidized fat promotes atherosclerosis (hardening of the arteries). A 2002 study in the *Journal of Nutritional Biochemistry* linked oxidized fats to compromised immune function and reduced bone growth in dogs. (Our take is that if it's no good for Fido, it's probably not good for you either.)

This is one of the reasons why you should rarely eat deep-fried foods such as french fries and hot wings. If you use oil for sautéing, pan frying, or baking, the temperature does not get hot enough to make the fat unstable.

Oils that are more susceptible to oxidation are those that are highly unsaturated (such as polyunsaturated oils, including safflower oil and corn oil) rather than less unsaturated (such as monounsaturated fat from olive oil or canola oil or saturated fat from butter). For this reason, if you do occasionally fry foods, choose monounsaturated-rich oils such as olive oil, because they are less polyunsaturated than other common cooking oils. Or use butter, which is even less polyunsaturated. Olive oil and butter also contain high amounts of antioxidant vitamins E, D, and A, which helps protect the oil against heat damage.

To sum up, the best oils for cooking are:

➤➤ Extra-virgin olive oil

➤➤ Canola oil

➤➤ Enova oil (made from olive and canola oil)

➤➤ Butter

THE PERFECT FAT RATIOS

Experts recommend that you take in equal amounts of fat calories from polyunsaturated and monounsaturated fat, with slightly fewer calories from saturated fat. Then, among the polyunsaturates, you need to eat a balance of omega-6s and omega-3s. In order for you to get this ideal balance, try to incorporate the following oil-based fats into your diet equally throughout the week. These will complement the other fats you take in naturally from foods, so that your ratio of saturates to polyunsaturates to monounsaturates is perfect.

➤➤ Your Perfect Body Diet Planner

GREENS AND BERRIES DIET IN CHAPTER 8: With this plan, you get 35 to 45 percent of your daily calories from fat (60 to 70 grams). The actual number of fat grams that you take in each day will depend on your customized calorie counts, which you'll calculate in Chapter 7. In Chapter 8, we'll give you complete, detailed lists of the foods that you should choose from, including their serving sizes, calorie counts, and grams of total fat, as well as saturated, monounsaturated, and polyunsaturated fat content. You can tailor this plan to your body and tastes by choosing your preferred foods from among those lists.

GRAINS AND FRUITS DIET IN CHAPTER 9: You'll get 25 to 35 percent of daily calories from fat (50 to 55 grams) following this plan. The actual number of fat grams that you take in each day will depend on your customized calorie counts, which you'll calculate in Chapter 7. Chapter 9 features your lists of prescribed fat-containing foods, including their serving sizes, calorie counts, and grams of total fat, as well as saturated, monounsaturated, and polyunsaturated fat content. You, too, can tailor this plan to your body by choosing your preferred foods from among those lists.

➤➤ Canola oil and olive oil (rich sources of monounsaturated fatty acids and omega-6 polyunsaturated fatty acids)

➤➤ Fish oil capsules (a rich source of the omega-3 polyunsaturated fatty acids EPA and DHA)

➤➤ Flaxseed oil (a rich source of the omega-3 polyunsaturated fatty acid ALA)

➤➤ Butter (a rich source of saturated fatty acids— but use it in smaller amounts)

➤➤ Natural nut butters, no sweeteners added (rich sources of monounsaturated fatty acids)

FAR-FROM-PERFECT FATS

The following list outlines fats that every woman should try to avoid completely because they can greatly exacerbate your risk for disease.

» Bacon, chicken wings, T-bone steak, poultry skin

» Hydrogenated or partially hydrogenated oils

» Interesterified oils

» Soybean oil

» Vegetable oil and shortening

FATS ARE YOUR FRIENDS

Remember, the right fats in the right quantities are not going to instantly put flab on your frame. By following your personalized diet and including good fats in most meals, you will get the health and weight loss benefits without feeling guilty. The creamy texture that fats often add to your meals will make them more enjoyable. So go ahead and have some fun with fats!

The Pros of Protein

Whether you're following the Greens and Berries Diet or the Grains and Fruits Diet, you'll be eating high-protein foods such as lean meats, fish, eggs, dairy, whey protein powder, nuts, beans, and—if you are vegetarian—soy at every meal and snack. Frankly, it's a nutritional no-brainer: Protein-rich foods help reduce food intake, prevent the return of hunger, and preserve precious muscle when you're dieting so that the weight you lose is primarily fat. In short, high-protein foods are essential for helping you achieve your perfect body quickly.

HOW PROTEIN HELPS

Let's take a closer look at the ways protein aids weight loss.

For starters, protein stimulates the production of a hormone called *glucagon*, which helps your body use stored fat for energy. Protein foods are also more costly to digest, compared with carbohydrates and fats. Basically, when you eat, it "costs" your body energy to turn any food into a usable energy source. This cost is called the *thermic effect of food*, or TEF, and protein foods have the highest TEF. Protein helps increase your metabolism so that you burn body fat more quickly.

It also helps you stick to your diet because protein foods are very satisfying. They help maintain normal blood glucose levels and blood amino acid concentrations, which have a satiating effect. A 2000 study in the journal *Appetite* found that a meal containing at least 24 grams of protein, compared with a meal containing only 9 grams of protein, led women to eat 17 percent fewer calories at the next meal. So, eating high-protein foods will help prevent you from overeating later in the day.

Given all that, it's no shock that additional studies have shown that the most effective weight-loss diets are those that, like the *Women's Health Perfect Body Diet,* include a high quantity of protein. For instance, several dietary trials have found that calorie-reduced diets result in substantially more weight loss when protein accounts for at least 25 percent of total calories. And a study at the University of Illinois, Urbana, showed that women who exercised and followed a diet with 30 percent of calories from protein lost more body fat and less muscle than women who ate a diet with only 15 percent of calories from protein. On the *Women's Health Perfect Body Diet,* you'll get between 25 and 35 percent of calories from protein (100 to 140 grams), and you'll do one of the body-type-specific workout plans laid out in Part 3. Exercise and a high-protein meal plan: a perfect combination.

PERFECT PROTEIN SOURCES

So what are the best ways to get protein into your diet? Some types of proteins may be better than others for staving off hunger. Overall, the best sources are animal products, including chicken, turkey, fish, beef, eggs, and cheese. They supply all nine of the essential amino acids (building blocks of protein) that your body cannot produce on its own. Research from the University of Toronto suggests that white fish such as snapper, orange roughy, cod, and tilapia are more satisfying than beef or chicken; however, the type of protein that will most satisfy *you* likely depends on your own personal preferences.

Animal protein also provides a wide variety of healthy fats. For instance, half the fat found in a steak is the good-for-you monounsaturated fat oleic acid. Salmon and trout are protein foods that will also give you two of the essential omega-3 fats (EPA and DHA).

If you're not so keen on meat, poultry, and fish, or you don't have time to cook them, you might want to try adding whey protein powder—a concentrated protein source that comes from milk—to your daily diet. Investigators have shown that, like animal protein, whey protein helps to decrease food intake at a later meal. You'll find several recipes in Chapter 10 that use whey protein powder. It works perfectly in smoothies and can be added to yogurt for an extra protein boost or mixed in water and poured over your cereal for a milk-free, high-protein breakfast option. You can buy it in health food shops and some grocery stores. Most brands taste great, but you'll have to shop around for the one that best suits your tastebuds. The ones we particularly recommend are Dymatize Elite Whey, which contains a special enzyme blend that makes it tolerable for even the most lactose-intolerant woman; Designer Whey Protein; Metabolic Drive by Biotest; and Optimum Nutrition Whey.

THE PROBLEM WITH TOO MUCH SOY

Unless you are a vegetarian who doesn't eat dairy or eggs, we don't recommend adding lots of soy to your diet plan. Soy can be beneficial or detrimental for health, depending on its source. In its pure form, including soybeans (edamame), or its fermented form (tofu, tempeh, and miso), it is a rich source of fiber and contains a variety of vitamins and minerals. Second-generation soy foods such as soy milk, cheeses, ice cream, hot dogs, and burgers are not the best choices, due to all the additives that are used to make them taste like "real" food.

More important, a joint study by Cornell and Yale found that when powdered soy protein isolate and soy protein burgers were substituted for meat protein, calcium was not absorbed as well in the body. This could lead to more fragile bones.

If you really dislike milk, don't replace it with regular soy milk, which is packed with several different types of simple sugars. Instead, find a soy milk with no added sugars (though sweeteners such as Splenda are okay). Or mix vanilla whey protein powder or rice protein powder with water and use that as a milk substitute.

Another reason soy products are popular with women is because they are rich in estrogen-like compounds called *isoflavones*. These phytoestrogens are thought to protect women against cancer, reduce the severity of menopause, and lower risk for heart disease. But again, the truth depends on the type of soy food you are eating. Pure soy foods provide 30 to 40 milligrams of isoflavones per serving, whereas the isoflavone concentrations of second-generation soy foods range from 0.04 milligram per gram in soy sausage to 0.10 milligram per gram in soy milk. So, depending on your sources of soy, you might not be reaping the benefits you thought.

Furthermore, the effect of isoflavones on cancer risk and other health issues may not be substantiated. A recent review of 41 studies in the journal *Circulation* found that neither soy nor its component isoflavones helped to prevent breast or uterine cancers, reduce hot flashes, or significantly lower cholesterol.

Soy was also thought to help with weight loss. However, in a study conducted by the New York Obesity Research Center at St. Luke's–Roosevelt Hospital, this notion didn't hold up.

Groups of overweight women were counseled to decrease their caloric intake by 500 calories a day for 12 weeks; in addition, a soy protein–rich group was counseled to consume 15 grams of soy protein per 1,000 calories daily. The study showed no advantage to eating soy. Both groups lost a similar amount of weight, and there was no difference in body fat percentage or waist circumference.

"But I Don't Eat Meat. . . ."

Marni is an accomplished endurance athlete. She doesn't eat any meats or poultry, so she drinks smoothies made with whey protein powder or pasteurized egg whites, and she always includes cheeses like ricotta and cottage cheese in her diet. She also enjoys plant-based proteins such as beans, hummus, tahini, nuts, and seeds. With this variety of foods, she's ensuring that she gets enough protein to satisfy her appetite and help prevent her muscle from breaking down.

If you, like Marni, are a vegetarian, you needn't miss out on protein. Complete proteins (those that contain all nine of the amino acids that your body can't produce on its own) are available in plant sources such as soy protein (in soybeans/edamame, roasted soy nuts, tofu, and soy protein powder), rice protein powder, and hemp seed protein (in hemp seeds and hemp seed protein powder).

The remaining plant sources of protein, termed *partial proteins* in the *Women's Health Perfect Body Diet*, are incomplete because they are lacking or low in one or more of the essential amino acids. Essential amino acids that are missing or in short supply are termed *limiting amino acids*. To ensure that you take in enough of all of the essential amino acids, combine foods that complement each other's limiting amino acids. Plant food combinations that non–meat eaters should include in their diets are:

- » Rice with beans
- » Corn with beans
- » Corn tortillas with beans
- » Whole wheat pasta with beans
- » Nuts and seeds with beans
- » Nut butters with whole wheat breads
- » Tahini (sesame seed paste) and hummus (a chickpea spread or dip)

HOW PROTEIN POWERS YOUR WORKOUT

In the *Women's Health Perfect Body Diet*, you'll be physically active every day, with 3 days of resistance training each week, 3 days of aerobics and abdominal exercise, and 1 day with at least 30 minutes of general physical activity. Because of your high activity level, your protein needs are going to be higher than those of women who are permanently affixed to their sofas. One of the world's experts on protein metabolism for athletes, Stuart Phillips, PhD, of McMaster University in Hamilton, Ontario, suggests that people who exercise regularly should consume 0.6 to 0.8 gram of protein per pound of total body weight. This means that if you weigh 140 pounds, you should consume at least 85 grams of protein a day. However, for those who are exercising and following a calorically restricted diet, increased protein intake—up to 1 gram per pound of body weight—will help preserve muscle tissue and prevent the accumulation of body fat better than lower amounts of protein. In the *Women's Health Perfect Body Diet*, your diet will provide at least the minimum amount of protein for your body weight so that your daily protein needs are always met.

Eating some protein before working out will help you burn more body fat during your exercise session. Two hours prior to your workout is ideal, though that can be tough if you exercise first thing in the morning. In that case, we recommend eating a small amount of food containing at least a little bit of protein as soon as you wake up. Something light and fresh, such as half a cup of low-fat plain yogurt with some mixed fresh berries, is an excellent choice for both the Greens and Berries Diet and the Grains and Fruits Diet.

Within an hour after a good workout, it's crucial to eat a meal containing protein. Eating at least 10 grams from full protein sources (more on that below) combined with some carbohydrates will help you repair muscle damage that occurs after exercise. It will also ensure that you build more muscle and replenish the glycogen stores you used to work out. A perfect postworkout snack is an apple plus 2 ounces of low-fat (not fat-free) cheese for the women following the Grains and Fruits Diet, or a whey or rice protein smoothie made with berries and a teaspoon of natural peanut butter or flaxseed oil for the women following the Greens and Berries Diet. Either of these snacks guarantees that you'll get all three nutrients together.

LET'S TALK ABOUT WHAT PROTEIN FOODS TO EAT

Regardless of which of the two eating plans you use, you're going to differentiate between foods that we'll call *full proteins* and ones that we'll refer to as *partial proteins*. Full proteins are complete proteins, meaning that they contain all the essential amino acids in fairly equal quantities. Partial proteins are missing or limited in one or more of the essential amino acids.

On both diets, you should aim to eat at least three of your meals from the *full* protein list and three of your meals from the *partial* protein list. You need to have one or the other form of protein every time you eat, and if you have both in one meal, that's perfect, too. Always try to incorporate full proteins into your three main meals (breakfast, lunch, and dinner). Choose partial proteins for your two or three daily snacks between your main meals. If you are vegetarian, have partial proteins even more often.

A typical portion of full protein such as meat, chicken, or fish is 3 to 4 ounces (an amount roughly equal to the size of your palm). A typical serving of cheese is 1 to 2 ounces (1 ounce being about the size of your thumb). A typical serving of eggs is two; a typical serving of pasteurized liquid egg substitute is about ²/₃ cup. Among partial proteins, a typical serving of beans is ¹/₂ cup. A typical serving of tofu or edamame (soybeans) is ¹/₂ cup or

➤➤Your Perfect Body Diet Planner

GREENS AND BERRIES DIET IN CHAPTER 8: With this plan, you'll get 30 to 35 percent of your calories from protein (120 to 140 grams). The actual number of grams that you take in each day will depend on your customized calorie counts, which you'll calculate in Chapter 7, but aim for the higher end of the spectrum (140 grams). In Chapter 8, we'll give you complete, detailed lists of the foods you should choose from, including their serving sizes, calorie counts, and grams of protein. You can further tailor this plan to your body by choosing your preferred protein sources from among those lists.

GRAINS AND FRUITS DIET IN CHAPTER 9: Following this program, you'll take in 25 to 30 percent of your daily calories from protein (100 to 120 grams). The actual number of grams of protein that you take in each day will depend on your customized calorie counts, which you'll calculate in Chapter 7, but shoot for the lower end of the range (100 grams). You'll find lists of the protein foods we recommend in Chapter 9. Customize your plan by picking your favorites from among those sanctioned foods.

4 ounces. A typical serving of rice protein is 1 to 2 tablespoons. Chapters 8 and 9 include lists of the *Women's Health Perfect Body Diet*'s recommended full and partial protein foods for the Greens and Berries Diet and the Grains and Fruits Diet, respectively.

Think of protein as the centerpiece of your plate. You'll craft each meal and snack by building around your protein choice, adding in carbs and good fats. Always eat a wide variety of proteins, regardless of which diet you are following. Variety will make it even easier to stick with the *Women's Health Perfect Body Diet* because you won't get bored. Thanks to a full complement of protein options to mix and match, with a little imagination, you won't eat the same meal twice during the entire 8 weeks.

Get It Together, Girl

Now that you understand all the nutritional underpinnings of the *Women's Health Perfect Body Diet*, we're ready to show you how to put the plan into action. That's what Part 2 is all about.

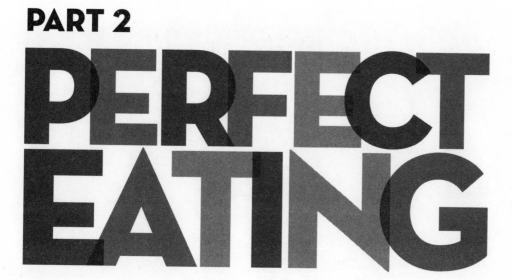

PART 2
PERFECT EATING

CHAPTER 7

Putting It All Together

You've got the whole picture now: You're ready to shed fat, lose weight, and gain lean, attractive muscle in just 8 weeks. You'll be eating five or six satisfying meals a day to evenly space out your caloric intake. You'll use 2 grams of the super-fiber glucomannan in at least three of those meals. This dietary plan will not only help you stay full longer, it will also boost your metabolic rate so that all day long, you'll burn calories—calories that have taken up residence on your body in places where they don't belong.

This program is about eating, and shifting to new ways of doing it. You'll eat a generous mix of proteins, carbs, and fats, so you won't be cutting out many of your favorite foods. You won't feel hungry because the glucomannan will slow down the delivery of nutrients from the good, healthy choices you are making, stretching out your feelings of satiety instead of your stomach. You'll be enjoying your food—just as you should.

Customizing the Meal Plans

In the next two chapters, you'll find day-by-day meal plans for both the Greens and Berries Diet and the Grains and Fruits Diet. Each plan is based on consuming 1,600 calories per day—about what it takes for the average exercising woman to lose weight without feeling famished.

You can follow the meal plans to the letter and you should reach your goal. But you'll probably achieve your best results by customizing the plans to fit your specific calorie needs. The formula on the opposite page helps you figure out exactly how many calories your body needs each day, as well as how many you should add or subtract from the standard meal plans to create your own calorie count.

For the first 2 weeks, the meal plans tell you precisely what to eat and when to eat it. Follow these as closely as you can, substituting only when you run across some that you really never want to see again—or that don't seem to like you, no matter how much you like them. If broccoli gives you gas or you get heartburn when you eat tomatoes, just ignore them when they show up on the meal plans. Listening to your body will help you function better and lose more body fat.

You can make exchanges by referring to the lists of your perfect foods and how many carbs, fats, and protein they contain. Just substitute one food in the same macronutrient group for another, based on their concentrations of carbohydrates, fat, and protein.

For Weeks 3 to 8, you can repeat the first 2 weeks over again. Or choose the recipes that really rocked to create your own sets of meals within your calorie count.

Women's Health Perfect Body Diet Commandments

1. Eat vegetables—best source of carbohydrates.

2. Eat dairy—supports bone health and weight loss.

3. Eat beans—best natural source of dietary fiber.

4. Eat berries—highest-fiber fruit, rich in antioxidants.

5. Eat nuts—healthy dietary fats.

6. Shun added sugars—to control insulin.

7. Choose full-fat or low-fat foods—ignore the "fat free" hype.

8. Take fish oil supplements—for omega-3 essential fatty acids.

9. Use glucomannan—to keep you full without taking in more calories.

Customize Your Calorie Count in Three Simple Steps

Your metabolic rate—how fast your body is currently burning the foods you are eating—will determine how many calories you should be consuming in any one day to achieve weight loss. To determine exactly what your target caloric intake should be, complete the equation below.

STEP #1: Calculate your resting energy expenditure (REE). This tells you the absolute minimum number of calories your body needs just to keep your heart beating and your brain thinking properly. To figure it out:

» Multiply your body weight in pounds by 7.18.   _____ **x 7.18 =** _____

» Divide that number by 2.2.   **÷ 2.2 =** _____

» Add 795.   **+ 795 =** _____

                                            REE = _____

STEP #2: Now factor in your physical activity level (PAL).

PAL calculates the additional calories needed for your body to perform daily tasks, such as walking around the office or exercising at the gym.

» Under 35 years old and less than 30 pounds over your ideal weight, use 1.5 for your PAL.

» Under 35 and more than 30 pounds over your ideal weight, use 1.4 for your PAL.

» 35 years and over and less than 30 pounds over your ideal weight, use 1.4 for your PAL.

» 35 years and over and more than 30 pounds over your ideal weight, use 1.2 for your PAL.

    REE (from step 1) x PAL = _____

This is your total energy expenditure, or the number of calories you need to eat each day to *maintain* your current weight.

STEP #3: Figure out the number of calories you should eat per day *to lose weight*.

On days you exercise:

    » Your total energy expenditure – 300 calories = _____

On days you don't exercise or exercise less intensely:

    » Your total energy expenditure – 500 calories = _____

These are your daily calorie goals. Adjust the meal plans in the next two chapters to hit those goals.

Why It Pays to Plan

Diets are like chess games, as geeky as that might sound—they work best when you approach them strategically. If you figure out what you're going to eat at the beginning of each day—before you take your first bite—you won't be scrambling to find the right foods when your stomach starts sending out SOS signals later on. If you plan ahead, you'll be able to take the right foods with you to work or resist the ravioli when you go out to lunch because you know just what to order. Hey, you may even save some bucks. Having perfect meals and snacks with you all the time means you won't be stopping to fork out for expensive food on the run.

Remember, you'll be spacing your five or six meals evenly throughout the day. That means you're eating every 2 to 3 hours, depending on what time you wake up and what time you generally go to sleep. Your first meal should begin no later than 2 hours after you wake up. A typical day might look like this.

7:00 a.m.: wake up

8:00 a.m.: breakfast

10:30 a.m.: snack

1:00 p.m.: lunch

3:30 p.m.: snack

6:00 p.m.: dinner

8:30 p.m.: snack/dessert

Why do you have to eat so often? It's a great way to keep hunger from getting pushy during the day. And going too many hours between feedings lets your metabolism run down. Eating at frequent intervals helps you speed it up. One of the first scientific studies that explored this concept was back in the mid-1980s. For a period of 2 weeks, researchers from the University of Toronto asked their subjects to eat either three meals a day (at 8:00 a.m., 1:00 p.m., and 7:00 p.m.) or 17 "mini-meals" every hour. The people who nibbled throughout the day had a metabolic advantage, compared with those who gorged on three meals. The nibblers had much lower insulin levels and more stable blood sugar levels than did the three-squares group, whose bodies would go into little starvation panics between meals and overstimulate their fat-storing hormone, insulin. The all-day eaters used more of the food they ate for energy. By stoking their digestive fires, they turned themselves into fat-burning machines. In support of this, a recent investigation conducted in healthy women

Your 100-Calorie Cheat Sheet

Need to subtract 100 calories from the meal plan to reach your perfect calorie count? Or add more calories without doubling up on portions? Use the following lists to find 100-calorie portions of foods.

If you're on the Greens and Berries Diet and need to drop 100 calories, choose carbohydrate foods only. Adding calories? Go for fat and protein.

If you're on the Grains and Fruits Diet, subtract excess calories from the fat foods only. Additions should come from either carbohydrate or protein foods.

100-CALORIE PERFECT CARBOHYDRATE FOODS

- ½ c cooked pearled barley, brown rice, bulgur, rolled oats, or whole wheat pasta
- ⅔ c cooked whole wheat couscous or wild rice
- 1¼ slices sprouted grain bread
- 1 whole wheat tortilla (6")
- 6 reduced-fat Triscuit crackers
- ⅔ c shredded wheat
- ½ c Fiber One cereal
- 3 c air-popped popcorn with 1 tsp butter
- 1 ear corn on the cob, with 1 tsp butter
- ⅔ c cooked corn or peas
- ½ c mashed sweet potato, no butter or milk added
- 1 small baked sweet potato, no butter or sour cream
- 1 large apple, banana, pear, or peach

100-CALORIE PERFECT FAT FOODS

- ⅓ Hass avocado
- 1 Tbsp butter or oil, such as flaxseed, olive, or canola
- 3 Tbsp unsweetened shredded coconut
- ⅓ c full-fat soft crumbled feta cheese
- ⅓ c part-skim ricotta cheese
- ½ c full-fat cottage cheese
- 1 slice (1 oz) full-fat hard cheese, such as Cheddar or Colby
- ⅔ c whole milk
- 1 large egg, plus 2 egg whites
- ¼ c hummus, made with olive oil or canola oil
- ⅛ c nuts of any type, including almonds, brazil nuts, cashews, and sunflower seeds
- 2 Tbsp shelled hemp seed kernels, such as Manitoba Harvest Hemp Seeds
- 2 Tbsp natural nut butters, such as almond, peanut, etc.

100-CALORIE PERFECT PROTEIN FOODS

- 3 oz canned light tuna in water
- 1 c liquid egg whites or egg substitute
- 6 large egg whites
- ⅔ c 1% fat cottage cheese
- 2 slices (2 oz) low-fat hard cheese
- 1 scoop whey protein powder in water
- ⅔ c low-fat plain yogurt
- 2 oz skinless chicken or turkey
- 2 oz lean steak: eye of round, top round, or top sirloin
- 2 oz lean fish: tilapia, cod, halibut, snapper, or fresh tuna
- 3 oz seafood and shellfish: shrimp or scallops
- ½ c firm tofu
- 2 Tbsp rice protein powder mixed with water

ages 18 to 42 showed that when they ate six regularly spaced meals per day, the energy burned per meal (the thermic effect of food) was higher than when they ate either three or nine meals per day. Irregular eating can lower the amount of energy your body can expend after eating a meal, while regular eating keeps it high. Further, several scientific review papers show that eating more than three small meals per day (nibbling, not gorging) is associated with a lower risk of weight gain and obesity.

We're not suggesting that you eat 17 times a day—who has time for that, anyway? But eating every 2 to 3 hours, five or six times a day, will help you reach your fat-loss goals.

A Perfect Day of Eating

Let's take a look at how you should approach those meals and snacks during the day.

BREAKFAST

First point: Don't skip it. Women who eat breakfast tend to be better at keeping their weight in line. Members of the National Weight Control Registry, a study of an elite group of adults who have maintained a loss of at least 30 pounds for a year or more, report that they eat breakfast regularly.

Coffee might be one of the first things you reach for when you get out of bed. This is fine, as long as you don't use it as a replacement for real food. Although the caffeine may wake you up, it's a short-lived energy fix. Your body needs a complete meal within 2 hours of waking to crank up your metabolism and help you eat less throughout the day.

If you're one of those people who have a hard time getting out of the house fully dressed and into work on time, breakfast may seem like an impossible dream. But you can do it. Start by deciding on one thing you'll eat every day. It really doesn't hurt to eat the same breakfast all the time, because your snacks, lunch, and dinner will provide nutritional variety to keep you healthy and satisfied. And you'll never be left guessing what to have, how to make it, or where to get it. Pick something you love to eat, and it will be easy to maintain the habit.

Breakfast doesn't have to be hard or time-consuming. It takes only a few minutes to blend one of the smoothies we've created for you in Chapter 10. It's also easy to make a meal at night, store it, and eat it while you're commuting or when you've arrived at work. When you look through the meal plans, you'll find that all of the breakfasts include gluco-mannan. It makes smoothies thick and filling, but it can also easily be added to many other common breakfast foods, such as yogurt or oatmeal. The Gluco-Granola recipe on page 181 combines oatmeal with whey protein and a small handful of nuts to provide protein and good fats. You can also add glucomannan to scrambled eggs.

LUNCH

Lunch can be as effortless as throwing together whatever you find in your fridge, using leftovers from your previous night's dinner or foods you cooked in large batches on the weekend. Salads are ideal as long as you add the right amounts of protein and healthy fats and mix glucomannan into the dressing. (Glucomannan will make the dressing thick and creamy, so if you're used to eating vinaigrette, you can thin out the mixture with a little bit

What *Not* to Eat for Breakfast

The old standby breakfast of white toast and jam with coffee (or worse, pancakes and syrup) is just not good for your body at all. Although it has a relatively low calorie count, it can throw some people into a glucose/insulin loop, all but guaranteeing zero weight loss for the day. Your body has a harder time using sugar and carbs you eat at breakfast than it does at other times of the day (such as after your workouts), so it's better to feed your morning hunger with a healthy high-fiber, protein- and fat-containing breakfast than with a toaster special. A study presented at the 2006 annual meeting of the European Association for the Study of Diabetes found that simple, fast-digesting carbs at breakfast result in a higher blood sugar swing than occurs at any other time of the day. This was the case even in people without diabetes. This is why the *Women's Health Perfect Body Diet* meal plans in Chapters 8 and 9 prescribe balanced breakfasts, such as high-fiber cereal with 2% milk and almonds, to keep you satisfied longer and help you lose the weight you want.

Aside from sugar, coffee on top of carbs only makes things worse for some people. Researchers at the Yale University School of Medicine have shown that people who drink moderate amounts of caffeine can develop hypoglycemic symptoms, such as shakiness, irritability, and hunger soon after eating, at a blood glucose level that is not usually considered low. This is similar to your body's response to a large, carbohydrate-rich meal. It will affect any woman who eats only simple carbs with coffee, but it will be even worse for women who are carb intolerant.

So, if you eat cereal, make sure that it's high in fiber and accompanied by a protein source (1% or 2% milk) and some fat (nuts or nut butter), and ease up on the coffee to automatically improve your glucose control.

of water.) Soup and salad can be a substantial meal: Mix glucomannan into a soup such as low-fat clam chowder or vegetable barley, then build a green salad topped with chicken or shrimp and an olive-oil-and-vinegar dressing.

When eating out or getting takeout for lunch, you can still choose foods that fit into the *Perfect Body Diet*. When choosing a restaurant, don't pick a place that will sabotage your diet—for instance, if you're a Greens and Berries girl and can't eat pasta, don't submit yourself to the temptation of the Tuscan Villa's fettuccine primavera. As always, salads and soups present easy ways to include your glucomannan—just keep capsules in your purse and add them to your salad dressing or soup.

🍐 If you're on the Grains and Fruits Diet and have the option of choosing a sandwich, make sure it contains protein and a vehicle for mixing in the glucomannan. For example, crack open two capsules to mix 2 grams of glucomannan into the mustard, hummus, or pesto within the sandwich.

🍇 If you're following the Greens and Berries Diet, order a vegetable-and-protein dish such as a chicken and veggie stir-fry, hold the rice; mix the glucomannan into the sauce and voilà—you've got a thick and satisfying lunch that won't put you over your calorie goals or upend your macronutrient ratios. The prescribed food lists in Chapters 8 and 9 will make it easy to identify the right restaurant meals for the *Women's Health Perfect Body Diet*—just make sure that the dish's ingredients are included on your lists.

If you happen to find yourself in an eatery that does not offer meals that fit your plan, make the best choice possible, and get back on track with your subsequent snacks and meals.

▶ Lose Weight with Smoothies

The smoothies we've created in Chapter 10 offer an excellent way for you to get a nutritious, quick, and easy breakfast, midday snack, or even late-night low-cal dessert. With the addition of glucomannan, the smoothie will be thick and satisfying to help you eat less and feel in control of your appetite the next time you have a meal. The smoothies are all rich in all the major macronutrients. Choose the one that is right for your body type.

Many of these smoothies contain protein- and calcium-rich yogurt. The live acidophilus cultures in yogurt can help prevent constipation and diarrhea, and they will prevent the bacterial imbalances that are quite common in women.

DINNER

Many women eat so little during the day that come dinnertime, it's tempting to have whatever the cat's eating. It's hard not to start nibbling on whatever's close at hand or end up eating a meal of epic proportions that completely busts the calorie meter. But dinner doesn't have to be desperate. On the *Women's Health Perfect Body Diet,* you'll be eating continuously throughout the day, so your appetite won't have a chance to grow into Godzilla. Your dinner will be about the same size as all your other meals, and you can cook it fresh most of the time, following the recipes we'll give you in Chapter 10. If you know that some nights you'll be too whipped to even consider mixing it up in the kitchen, try doubling the recipes (if they don't already serve more than one) so that you have a second meal to freeze. Or consider spending one evening making all your dinners for the week. Eat one, refrigerate one for tomorrow, and freeze the rest.

All of your dinners should contain glucomannan. This will help you avoid multiple return trips to the kitchen after dinner and prevent late-night sugar cravings. It will also promote better sleep by helping you feel satisfied all night long.

DAYTIME SNACKS

Snacking every 2 to 3 hours is a core concept of the *Women's Health Perfect Body Diet.* Your first snack of the day will be 2 to 3 hours after breakfast. Make sure it contains perfect carbohydrates, fats, and proteins from the lists in Chapters 8 and 9.

If you're following the Greens and Berries Diet, your snacks will contain a little less carbohydrate and a little more fat and protein. A good snack for Greens and Berries Diet women is 1½ servings of Bodacious Spinach and Bean Dip (page 182) with celery sticks.

On the Grains and Fruits Diet, your snacks will contain a little less fat, with a little more carbohydrate and protein—you can have one serving of the Bodacious Spinach and Bean Dip (page 182), but with four wheat crackers.

Try to include glucomannan in your snacks as often as possible, but don't stress out if you can't. The right combination of carbs, fats, and proteins will go a long way toward keeping your hunger at bay and your metabolism high. Avoiding high-sugar snacks also makes you less likely to eat more food (especially more sugar) later in the day. Australian scientists compared one snack food that was high in carbohydrates but also contained 10 grams of protein and 4 grams of fiber with another that had little protein and fiber but the same number of calories, mostly from sugar. The result: When people snacked on protein and fiber, they consumed 16 percent less sugar the next time they ate. When the afternoon munchies strike, instead of picking up a low-fat blueberry muffin, eat one of our home-made Pumpkin Protein Fiber Muffins (page 191), which includes healthy fats.

EVENING SNACKS

You've probably heard about people who lost weight by never eating after 6:00 p.m. You've probably read advice never to eat before bedtime because then "everything will be stored as fat!" And it may simply seem like common sense. But the truth is, your body won't turn late-night calories straight into fat.

Researchers from Oregon Health and Science University who monitored 16 female rhesus monkeys on a high-fat diet for a year found that while all the primates gained weight, those who munched most of their food after 5:00 p.m. did not gain any more weight than the ones who gobbled most of their grub earlier in the day. Your body is still metabolically active when you sleep, so it will use midnight-snack calories for energy just as it would at any other time of the day.

So it's true, we're telling you: Go ahead and snack before bed. The key is keeping to the *Perfect Body Diet* schedule and not deviating from your plan of eating every 2 to 3 hours. You can eat your last snack an hour before bed or even right before bed if you want to. If you eat dinner at 6:30 p.m. but don't go to sleep until 11:30, plan on having a snack at around 9:30—3 hours after your previous meal.

You can think of the last snack of the day as your dessert, and choose something that you really enjoy but haven't had all day long. Fresh fruit with nuts is an excellent after-dinner snack. And if you make sure that you have glucomannan with dinner, you don't have to have it with this nosh.

Eat to Support Your Workouts

When you're scheduling your six small meals, consider your workouts and what time you do them. Never do weight training or another workout for longer than 15 to 20 minutes on an empty stomach. Without access to energy from a recent meal, your body will pull calories from your muscle mass, depleting the precious muscle you've worked so hard to develop. Plus, this won't do much to aid your fat-loss goals, because later in the day, your body will revolt against its earlier starvation, causing you to crave more calories. We want you to eat at least 2 hours before an exercise session longer than 20 minutes in duration, so that you have enough energy to work out.

After you exercise, your fat cells release fatty acids into your bloodstream to be transported to your muscles for energy, so it's advised that you wait about 30 minutes to eat after working out. If you immediately consume food, you slow the amount of fat that can reach your muscles and be used as fuel because your body will use the food as fuel rather than the fat. However, if you wait *too* long to eat after exercise, you'll dive into a state of low blood sugar, so you'll feel worse for the remainder of the day—and you'll have a hard time convincing yourself to go back to the gym for your next workout. Eat within 30 minutes to 1 hour after your workout for the most fat burning without sacrificing your hunger control.

Your postworkout meal should contain a full-protein source and one of the perfect carbohydrate choices for your diet plan. Your body needs the energy of a full meal combined with the complete spectrum of amino acids found in a full protein in order to properly repair the damage caused to your muscles during your workout. If your meal plan has you scheduled for a snack, make sure it contains a full protein.

One other thing to keep in mind: Your workouts will be the lightest on the last day of each week. Remember to cut back your food intake on those days by an additional 200 calories (to the 500-calorie reduction level), which you can easily subtract from your meal plan lists. The meal plans in Chapters 8 and 9 take this into account for you.

Are Convenience Foods Okay?

Sometimes. When you are too busy to cook or absentmindedly leave your carefully prepared lunch sitting on the kitchen counter at home, something less than perfect is better than nothing. But less than perfect doesn't mean total crap. Many prepackaged and prepared foods contain a lot of preservatives and extra ingredients that don't support your perfect body goals. These things include Far-from-Perfect fats (such as interesterified and partially hydrogenated oils) and added sugars.

One advantage of low-calorie frozen meals and meal-replacement shakes is that many of them can easily accommodate glucomannan. Food manufacturers chill frozen foods with added water, so you can even mix the glucomannan into solid frozen foods such as broccoli or rice. To choose frozen meals that most closely adhere to your eating plan, carefully read the Nutrition Facts and ingredient labels. Compare them with the food lists in Chapters 8 and 9 so you can choose the right instant meal for your body. The varieties of frozen meals that we recommend are Weight Watchers Smart Ones and Lean Cuisine Spa Cuisine Classics.

   If you're following the Grains and Fruits Diet, your meal can contain rice or pasta.

On the Greens and Berries Diet, choose a meal that is made mostly with vegetables to meet your lower carbohydrate needs.

No matter which diet you're following, make sure that the meal includes a protein—preferably a full-protein choice such as chicken.

Grains and Fruits Diet adherents should choose a lower-fat option (less than 10 grams).

Those on the Greens and Berries Diet can have a little more fat.

Meal-replacement drinks that contain all the macronutrients (such as Myoplex Lite Ready to Drink) can stand in for solid food as long as they meet the following requirements.

For the Greens and Berries Diet: Drinks should contain no more than 10 grams of carbohydrates.

For the Grains and Fruits Diet: Drinks should contain 10 to 40 grams of carbs.

Watch out for simple sugars (anything like glucose, fructose, brown rice syrup, dextrose, cane sugar, etc.) and bad fats (anything hydrogenated or interesterified). Add 2 grams of glucomannan to the drink to make it thicker and more satisfying.

Meal-replacement bars are another handy option.

For the Greens and Berries Diet, choose from among Atkins Advantage High Protein, Worldwide Sport Nutrition Pure Protein, EAS AdvantEdge Carb Control, EAS Myoplex Carb Control, Balance Bar Carb Well, and Revival Smart-Carb soy protein bars.

On the Grains and Fruits Diet, look for Genisoy Soy Protein Bars, Kashi Go Lean Crunchy! bars, Promax protein bars, Balance Bar Gold, and Greens Plus Protein Food Bars.

Fast Food Lite

You didn't have time to pack a lunch, you can't get to a supermarket for a frozen meal, and you're ready to eat your car. Crisis? No. Head to the nearest fast-food joint. You'll be able to find something to eat that matches the *Women's Health Perfect Body Diet*. It just takes a little ingenuity.

AT THE BAGEL SHOP

If you're on the Greens and Berries Diet, walk on by to the build-your-own salad buffet at the other end of the shopping center. If there's no salad bar, order some tuna salad or soup and skip the bagel.

For those following the Grains and Fruits Diet: Combine carbs, proteins, and fat with a whole grain bagel, lox, and cream cheese. But eat only half a bagel—whole wheat or pumpernickel—and have just a thin coating of regular or low-cal vegetable cream cheese. Mix your glucomannan into the cream cheese and you'll be full!

AT THE SANDWICH/SUB SHOP

For the Greens and Berries gatherers, a salad or low-carb wrap with chicken, turkey, tuna, or roast beef will meet your protein, fat, and carb goals. Don't forget to add glucomannan to the dressing or condiments.

Grains and Fruits girls can order a 6-inch whole grain roll with turkey, mustard (for the glucomannan), olives, and veggies.

AT THE DRIVE-THRU WINDOW

On the Greens and Berries plan, have a salad with cheese, with low-cal dressing (to mix in your glucomannan) and grilled (not fried) chicken.

A Sneaky Tip for Portion Control

Pay close attention to portion control while you're following the *Women's Health Perfect Body Diet*, especially when you're snacking. A natural way to limit yourself is to make sure you never eat from a bag or a box. It's easy to scarf a whole bag of popcorn when it's making a direct trip from the container to your mouth. You usually have no idea how much you've eaten.

This is called ghost eating because there is no visual cue that reminds you to stop eating. Researchers at Cornell University, led by Brian Wansink, PhD, demonstrated how important visual cues are in controlling food intake. They served a free soup lunch to 54 adults, half of whom ate from normal 18-ounce soup bowls, while the other half ate from identical bowls that, unbeknownst to the participants, were slowly refilled through tubing connected to the bowls. In just 20 minutes, those who ate out of the refilling bowls consumed 73 percent more soup than did participants who ate from the normal soup bowls! The "endless soup" subjects averaged 113 more calories than the others, yet rated themselves as being no more full, leading Dr. Wansink to conclude that we count calories with our eyes and not our stomachs.

Before you find yourself with a bottomless stomach, learn to portion out the amount of food you should eat into a small bowl or into small plastic bags for when you're on the go.

Get your Grains and Fruits with a yogurt-and-fruit parfait with extra fruit and no granola. The yogurt alone accounts for your protein, fat, and carbs, so you're all set.

Restaurant Rules

Just because you're changing your eating habits doesn't mean that you can never go out to eat again. Generally, friends don't say, "Wanna go for a hike to celebrate your new job?" It's more like, "Congrats on your new position! Let me treat you to dinner!" You should never stop enjoying yourself, your friends, or nights out on the *Women's Health Perfect Body Diet.* You just need to remember what to pick from the menu so it fits your strategy.

Choose a mix of carbs, proteins, and fats based on the lists of perfect foods that fit into your plan.

An ideal selection for the Greens and Berries Diet is steamed salmon with creamed cauliflower, to which you can add glucomannan.

Grains and Fruits dieters might choose grilled pork tenderloin with glucomannan-friendly sautéed zucchini.

Choose an entrée featuring your perfect foods and eat half of it. Take the other half home for tomorrow's lunch. You can also skip the appetizer, unless it's a salad with light, glucomannan-laced dressing. And forgo dessert, unless you can get fresh fruit.

Don't miss an opportunity to add glucomannan to your food. Look for a dish or condiment that mixes well with the fiber. For example, order a salad or steamed fish with sauce on the side. You can also mix glucomannan into a hearty soup, such as clam chowder, to make it even thicker and more filling.

Please Use a Condiment

Little extras can add a lot when you're working to achieve your perfect body. Not only are spicy sauces and other enhancements useful for mixing with glucomannan, they can really amp up the flavor of your food. We encourage you to use fresh herbs and spices in your cooking, but think of accessorizing your dishes with other ingredients.

Beware of some add-ons that are high in sugar. Regular ketchup, for example, is loaded with high fructose corn syrup, and a single tablespoon contains 4 grams of sugar.

On the opposite page, we've listed condiments that are low in sugar and bad fats to help you stick with your plan.

FOOD	SERVING SIZE	CALORIES
Barbecue sauce, low-sugar, such as Walden Farms Calorie Free Original BBQ Sauce	2 Tbsp	0
Capers	1 Tbsp	2
Curry paste, no sugar added	1 Tbsp	4
Glorious Gluco-Mayo (page 189)	1 Tbsp	100
Sun-Dried Tomato Pesto (page 190)	2 Tbsp	140
Horseradish	1 tsp	2
Hot-pepper sauce, such as Tabasco	1 tsp	1
Hot-pepper sauce, mild, such as Frank's RedHot	1 tsp	1
Jam or preserves, no-sugar-added, such as Polaner Sugar Free Preserves	1 Tbsp	10
Ketchup, low-sugar, such as Heinz One Carb Ketchup	1 Tbsp	4
Liquid smoke	1 tsp	0
Mayonnaise made with olive or canola oil, such as Cains All Natural Mayonnaise with Omega-3	1 Tbsp	100
Mustard, yellow, Dijon, or spicy	1 Tbsp	10
Salsa, no-sugar-added or low-sugar, such as La Mexicana Fresh Salsa	2 Tbsp	10
Soy sauce, preferably low-sodium	1 tsp	10
Tomato/pasta sauce, no-sugar-added or low-sugar, such as Ragú Light No Sugar Added Tomato & Basil pasta sauce	½ c	60
Wasabi	1 tsp	15
Worcestershire sauce, in moderation	1 tsp	0

Your Glucomannan Guidelines

All of the research on using glucomannan for weight loss has focused on getting at least 6 grams per day. On the *Women's Health Perfect Body Diet,* you'll use at least 2 grams of glucomannan at least three times a day, for a total of 6 to 8 grams daily. This will greatly improve your hunger management.

LET'S GO SHOPPING!

Glucomannan is often available at health food stores, including the Vitamin Shoppe chain, which has its own house brand. But if you can't find this superfiber at your local strip mall, try online distributors. Here are several products we recommend.

» Your Perfect Mannan from www.yourperfectmannan.com comes in convenient 1-gram packets like the ones in which artificial sweeteners are packaged, so it eliminates the need to break open capsules.

» NSI Glucomannan capsules from www.vitacost.com ($9.99 for 180 capsules) is the brand that was used in the *Women's Health Perfect Body Diet* pilot program.

» SlimStyles PGX capsules or granules are available from www.slimstyles.com.

If you can't find any glucomannan supplements, look for "konjac root" or "konjac mannan," which are exactly the same as glucomannan. You might want to compare prices among traditional retailers and online distributors: The price of glucomannan can vary and does not necessarily reflect quality.

We also recommend products from NexGen Foods. Their muffins, in flavors such as wild blueberry and banana walnut, have our favorite fiber baked right in. You can order these goodies at www.nexgenfoods.com.

NOW YOU'RE COOKING—WITH GLUCOMANNAN

Glucomannan won't work if you just sprinkle it on food, like tossing croutons on top of a salad. You must break open the capsule (if there is one) and mix the powder into something with a soft consistency, such as mustard, mayonnaise, salsa, gravy, or salad dressing. It works like cornstarch, thickening sauces, gravies, soups, stews, casseroles, puddings, and pie fillings without affecting taste. It also makes muffins moister and fruit crumbles thicker. Yet, unlike cornstarch, glucomannan does not contain starch and sugar, so it's calorie free. It is also gluten free, making it the perfect substitute in cooking and baking when flour and other glutinous starches must be avoided (such as when you are following the *Women's Health Perfect Body Diet*). The ideal dose of powder is 2 grams per serving. So, if the meal is for one, add 2 grams of powder. If it's for more, increase the amount proportionally, so each serving delivers 2 grams. The recipes in Chapter 10 are scaled to provide the right amount per serving.

When adding glucomannan to a dish, always mix it with a small amount of room temperature or cold liquid (water, stock, soy sauce, wine, etc.) until you get a smooth paste, then add this mixture to your food or recipe ingredients. If you add glucomannan directly to hot food, it may lump up on you because the heat activates the fiber too quickly. Mixing glucomannan with something cool allows it to absorb the liquids slowly so that it's easily and fully dissolved.

Since all of your food will get thicker and more satisfying with glucomannan, make sure to wash it down with plenty of water; drink at least 8 ounces of H_2O with every meal or snack. For the best taste and texture—clumps of glucomannan aren't exactly gourmet, and they could even get stuck in your throat—always mix the powder thoroughly into your grub and wait 2 to 3 minutes for it to soak up whatever sauce, broth, dressing, or other liquid is on your plate or in your bowl or glass. Sit back and watch your serving size expand without any extra calories.

The following foods all work great with glucomannan. For more ideas of foods and recipes to make with glucomannan, see Chapter 10.

» Applesauce, unsweetened

» Barbecue sauce, low-sugar, such as KC Masterpiece Low Calorie Classic Blend

» Cottage or ricotta cheese

» Creamed vegetables

» Eggs: salad, scrambled, omelette-style, or quiches

» Gravy

» Ground meats such as turkey, salmon, or beef

» Hot whole grain cereals: oatmeal, oat bran, or cream of wheat (for the Grains and Fruits Diet only)

» Hummus made with olive oil or canola oil, such as Tribe of Two Sheiks

» Ketchup, low-sugar, such as Heinz One Carb

» Mayonnaise made with canola oil or olive oil

» Mustard: yellow, Dijon, or spicy

» Nut butters, like almond, peanut, or tahini

» Pesto

» Salad dressings made with olive oil or canola oil

» Salsa, no-sugar-added or low in sugar, such as La Mexicana Salsa

» Smoothies

» Soups

» Soy sauce, preferably low-sodium

» Tomato/pasta sauce, no-sugar-added or low-sugar, such as Ragú Light No Sugar Added Tomato and Basil Pasta Sauce

» Tuna or chicken salad

» Vegetable dips made with yogurt or low-fat sour cream

» Yogurt

It's easy to just mix glucomannan into the creamier foods you eat throughout the day. Get creative. We love to eat cooked vegetables like peas and green beans. Since glucomannan can't be added to vegetables alone, we create a ratatouille version, adding the superfiber to $\frac{1}{4}$ cup of salsa or a no-sugar pasta sauce and then mixing in the cooked veggies.

While you'll add glucomannan to most of your meals, you needn't include it every time you eat. Among the snacks recommended in the Greens and Berries Diet and the Grains and Fruits Diet are measured servings of berries, raisins, nuts, seeds, and cucumbers; it's not possible or necessary to add glucomannan to these foods.

We also don't recommend adding glucomannan to beverages. Because the fiber has a thickening effect, it would turn a regular glass of water, milk, sugar-free beverage, or other liquid into a smooth gel that you probably wouldn't find appetizing—or thirst quenching.

GLUCOMANNAN AND YOUR GUT

Glucomannan supplementation will increase stool frequency slightly so that you become more regular. Your stools won't be loose, but they'll be much easier to pass. Some people do get gassy initially. After a few days, you'll likely find that your extra gas significantly reduces or disappears completely. Women who experience diarrhea-predominant irritable bowel syndrome (IBS) may find that glucomannan exacerbates their symptoms.

If you have IBS or initial gassiness that does not resolve on its own, there are a couple of easy solutions. You can simply halve your glucomannan dose—take just 1 gram, instead of 2, three times a day. Or take one of two additional supplements: an enzyme to digest fiber (such as Beano) or a complete spectrum supplement with carbohydrate enzymes (look for the following ingredients: amylase or alpha-amylase, hemicellulase, cellulase, lactase, maltase, glucoamylase, or alpha galactosidase). Take either of these about a half hour before you eat food with glucomannan. Follow the package instructions for the proper dosage.

Other Important Supplements for Your Perfect Body

While glucomannan is the most important supplemental nutrient for the *Women's Health Perfect Body Diet,* you also need a steady supply of other nutrients, many of which you can't get in ideal quantities from food. The *Women's Health Perfect Body Diet* is full of a wide variety of nutritious and satisfying foods that should meet most of your dietary vitamin and mineral requirements. However, some women may have dietary preferences that cause them to fall short. For example, if you are lactose intolerant and avoid most dairy products, you will have to add calcium, magnesium, and vitamin D to your diet.

For this reason, you may want to take a daily multivitamin. In most research settings involving reduced-calorie weight-loss diets, participants are required to take a daily multivitamin to ensure that all nutrient needs are met.

The best multi for you is one that meets or comes very close to meeting all the DRIs (Dietary Reference Intakes), the intakes recommended by the US government. Compare labels of different brands to see which ones come close. *Women's Health*'s pick for the best: One-A-Day Women's. This classic brand's formulation adheres to the DRIs more closely than most other multis.

You should also take fish oil supplements. Fish oil is the best source of omega-3 essential fatty acids, fats that can help reduce the storage of body fat and help burn more body fat during exercise. This compound is incredibly important to supplement because your body cannot produce it and must obtain it from food. Unless you eat salmon three to five times a week, you should supplement to ensure that your body gets what it needs.

It's important to buy a pure and potent fish oil product. Most brands are screened for their potential content of mercury or PCBs, toxic chemicals that can accumulate in fish. Log on to www.ConsumerLab.com and other Web sites that rate different brands of fish oil. Look for a brand that provides at least 0.18 gram of EPA and 0.12 gram of DHA per capsule, for a total of at least 0.30 gram of omega-3 fats per 1-gram capsule. Take at least three 1-gram capsules daily to reach the dose that's been shown to provide health benefits.

What to Drink: Perfect Body Beverages

We've covered what to eat. How about what to drink? Our bodies don't always know what to make of liquid calories. Some beverages quench our thirst, while others go the extra mile and satisfy our hunger, too. The right beverage at the right time can be another secret weapon in helping you drop pounds. Here's how to deploy that weapon for maximum effect. These guidelines apply to both the Greens and Berries Diet and the Grains and Fruits Diet.

GOT WATER?

When you're trying to lose weight—or even just trying to stay healthy—drinking water is crucial because it flushes toxins out of your system and carries away unused sugars from your body. That said, the once sacred "drink eight full 8-ounce glasses daily" guideline is not necessarily the golden rule anymore, since your body may be getting the liquid it needs from other sources, including foods such as fruits and vegetables. One study conducted by researchers at the University of Nebraska found that hydration could be maintained simply with juices, diet beverages, and milk. Overall, choosing water or choosing to pass is really about knowing what your body needs.

Rather than focusing on *how much* liquid you need, focus instead on drinking fluids

What About Sweets?

Sugar substitutes are one tool for helping you get over a bad sweet craving. They can make foods more palatable without adding extra calories or causing a spike in blood sugar. For example, you may switch your normal morning glass of orange juice for sugar-free Crystal Light Sunrise. Or, you might buy a low-carb meal-replacement drink with an artificial sweetener. Both of these will cut out the excess sugars that cause fat gain and will help you save calories.

Sugar substitutes are safe to eat and have been available for decades. So are these additives really good for you? Despite a handful of scary studies back in the 1970s that linked saccharin to increased rates of cancer in rats, there's little evidence that artificial sweeteners cause problems in humans. As a precaution, the FDA has established maximum intakes for sugar substitutes. The rules: A 150-pound adult can ingest 8½ packets of Sweet'N Low, 87 packets of Equal or NutraSweet, or 25 packets of Splenda every 24 hours with no adverse effects.

Here's a caveat: A 2001 study from the journal *Headache* found that aspartame can trigger headaches. Some experts believe that phenylalanine, one of the amino acids used to make aspartame, has a negative impact on brain neurotransmitters. If you're prone to headaches (especially skull-splitting migraines), avoid foods with aspartame or phenylalanine in their ingredients lists.

If you want to stay away from artificial sweeteners, use a small amount of honey and maple syrup instead. Although they contain the same quantity of carbohydrates as sugar (about 15 grams per tablespoon), both natural sweeteners contain additional vitamins, minerals, and antioxidants that may benefit your health. Also, honey and maple syrup are sweeter than sugar due to differences in the type of sugar they contain (fructose versus just glucose), so you can use less and still get the sweetness you want.

Stevia is another natural sugar substitute. Known in South America as the "sweet herb," stevia comes from the leaves of the plant *Stevia rebaudiana* Bertoni, which is native to Brazil and Paraguay. It's 200 to 300 times sweeter than sugar, so just a small amount will sweeten even a strong cup of tea. It's naturally low in carbohydrates and contains zero calories. Stevia can be used exactly as you'd use sugar, including for baking. In fact, you'll notice that it's called for in many of the recipes in Chapter 10.

Due to a lack of studies, stevia has been approved by the FDA as a dietary supplement but not as a food additive. So you can buy stevia only in health food stores or over the Internet. The type of stevia that works best in baking and beverages is one that also contains the natural dietary fiber inulin. The brand we like most is Wisdom Natural Sweetleaf SteviaPlus powder.

consistently throughout the day. Dehydration can lead to fatigue, irritability, and decreased performance, both mentally and physically. Even a small drop in your body's water levels can hurt you. A recent study from Tufts University found that mild dehydration—a loss of just 1 to 2 percent of body weight as water—was enough to impair thinking. Also, when you're suddenly feeling hungry even though you've just eaten, it may be that your body is actually feeling slightly dehydrated and craving fluids. So if you haven't been drinking recently, reach for a tall, cold glass of water and see whether it makes those thoughts of food go away.

A WORD ABOUT CAFFEINE

Coffee may keep you going during the day, but when you're trying to lose weight, it's smart to be a little wary of it. Some women—interestingly, they're often the same ones who are carbohydrate intolerant—do not react well to caffeine. It makes them irritable and shaky and can lead to increased hunger. Researchers have shown that caffeine causes the brain to demand more blood sugar, while at the same time it decreases the amount of blood sugar that can actually be delivered to the brain. So if you have a problem keeping your blood sugar levels regular, caffeine may exacerbate the feeling and make you yearn for more food to bring blood sugar back up. If this sounds like you, avoid caffeinated drinks entirely.

WHY WATER IS BETTER THAN SPORTS DRINKS

Unless you're exercising for more than 90 minutes at a high intensity—say, training for a half-marathon or triathlon—all you need to drink when working out is 8 ounces of water. Sports drinks contain sugar that your body opts for use for fuel, rather than burning your your fat stores.

If you're strength training or doing cardio in a warm environment, be sure to drink about 20 ounces of H_2O an hour before your workout and another 20 ounces during exercise.

Following your workout, your best bet is to stick with a meal or smoothie that fulfills your

> ## Wake Up Your Sex Life with Coffee

Coffee is a liquid aphrodisiac. It wakes up the nervous system almost immediately and increases bloodflow to your genitals, making sensitive nerve endings more easily accessed and stimulated, says Lynn Fischer, author of *The Better Sex Diet.* But take it black, she cautions: Milk, like most dairy products, contains the sleep-inducing amino acid tryptophan.

protein, carbohydrate, and fat ratios for your particular diet, be it the Greens and Berries Diet or the Grains and Fruits Diet. You can err on the side of eating a few more calories and macronutrients than in your other daily meals because, after you work out, your body is craving the calories and will burn them off for energy instead of storing them as fat. If you work out in the morning, eat or drink a little something, such as a piece of string cheese or a Pumpkin Protein Fiber Muffin (see page 191), beforehand, then follow your workout with a breakfast such as the Super Fiber Breakfast Bowl (page 201 or 220). If you work out before dinner, choose one of the dinner options from the meal plans in your respective diet chapter. Or choose one of the filling and yummy protein-rich smoothies for a no-hassle option.

Your Perfect Body Beverage Lists

Both Greens and Berries Diet and Grains and Fruits Diet followers can drink these beverages. Listed first are those that contain no calories, with the ones containing caffeine marked with a star.

NO-CALORIE BEVERAGES

>> All herbal teas

>> Coffee, decaf or regular, black*

>> Diet sodas, caffeine-free
   or with caffeine*

>> Diet tonic water

>> Earl Grey, English breakfast,
   and orange pekoe teas*

>> Fruit waters, with no calories

>> Green, oolong, and white tea*

>> Sparkling mineral water

>> Sugar-free hot chocolate

>> Unsweetened iced tea,
   decaf or regular*

>> Water, with a wedge of lemon

BEVERAGES WITH CALORIES

The following beverages contain calories. That doesn't mean you can't drink them, but you need to make sure you account for them when totaling up your daily calorie intake. Women who are less carbohydrate tolerant may want to stay away from alcohol because it can cause fluctuations in blood sugar levels that are just as bad as eating a handful of candy. If you do like alcohol, keep your intake moderate: no more than one or two drinks a day of wine or clear spirits.

>> Cow's or goat's milk, 1%: 1 cup = 118 calories, 14 grams carbs, 10 grams protein,
   3 grams fat

>> Cow's or goat's milk, 2%: 1 cup = 122 calories, 11 grams carbs, 8 grams protein,
   5 grams fat

» Smoothies made with proteins and fruits (see recipes in Chapter 10)

» V8 juice, preferably low-sodium: 4 ounces = 25 calories, 5 grams carbs, 1 gram protein, 0 grams fat

» Light beer, 12 ounces = 95 calories, 4 grams carbs, 0 grams protein, 0 grams fat

» Wine or clear spirits in moderation

Wine, red, 5 ounces = 125 calories, 4 grams carbs, 0 grams protein, 0 grams fat

Wine, white, 5 ounces = 122 calories, 4 grams carbs, 0 grams protein, 0 grams fat

Gin, 80 proof, 1.5 ounces = 97 calories, 0 grams carbs, 0 grams protein, 0 grams fat

Vodka, 80 proof, 1.5 ounces = 97 calories, 0 grams carbs, 0 grams protein, 0 grams fat

FAR-FROM-PERFECT BEVERAGES

These beverages should be avoided. The calories, carbohydrates, and sometimes, alcohol that they contain will set you back from achieving your perfect body goal.

» Alcoholic drinks containing sugar or mixers

» Beer, regular

» Chocolate milk

» Fruit juice

» Regular sodas

» Rice milk

» Smoothies made with only fruit juice

» Soy milk

» Sports drinks, like Gatorade, made with only sugar

» Sweetened iced tea

» Tonic water, not diet, made with sugar

Take a Perfect Body Break

So you've made it for 2 weeks on the *Women's Health Perfect Body Diet*. Break time! Now, and after every consecutive 2 weeks, you can feel free to splurge with one meal that's forbidden on your meal plan. Craving a couple slices of pizza or a big slice of apple pie à la mode? Go for it. Just don't overdo it—no gorging yourself at a buffet. Your goal is to cheat in moderation by eating a meal that adds about an extra 300 to 500 calories to your total calorie count (one slice of pizza is about 300 calories).

The purpose of the Perfect Body Break is both noble and practical: to make sure you don't go out of your friggin' mind! We want you to burn calories, not burn out. If you think you may never set eyes on a molten chocolate cake again—much less let it melt in your mouth—you may lack the will to go on.

This little bonus also may have physiological implications. Scientific research has shown

Clear Thinking on Alcohol

Every calorie counts when you're counting, and alcohol ratchets up the total pretty fast. The best rule of thumb: "The blander the drink, the fewer the calories," says George Delgado, a New York beverage consultant. That means sticking with clear spirits such as vodka or gin—both of which have 80 to 90 calories per shot—and zero-cal mixers like club soda or diet tonic water.

that short-term overfeeding, such as an increase of 500 calories over your most recent caloric intake, can help increase your metabolic rate. As we've mentioned, when you reduce your caloric intake for weight-loss purposes, your metabolic rate sometimes declines, and that can be the reason your weight loss stalls. Eating extra calories every 14 days can help prevent this decline and keep your weight continuing to drop. In a 2000 investigation, Swiss researchers showed that when healthy women ate extra calories from carbohydrates for 3 days, their 24-hour metabolic rate increased by 7 percent. When they overate fat alone, their metabolic rate did not increase significantly.

In another 2000 investigation, UK researchers showed that metabolic rate increased by 8 percent in women who for 1 day ate 50 percent more carbohydrates or fat calories than they needed to maintain their body weight. Overall, this means that giving yourself a Perfect Body Break every 2 weeks can help you prevent weight-loss plateaus by counteracting the decrease in metabolism that occurs with chronic dieting. Since studies give conflicting evidence about which macronutrients should be increased to best boost metabolism, we recommend choosing a mixture in the form of a special dessert or comfort food that you've been craving.

What If I Blow It?

Don't even go there. You won't blow it, because if you eat too much of something on the meal plan one day or sneak in a food that's Far-from-Perfect, all is not lost: You can just make up for it by working out harder that same day. Add another set or two to your body-type-specific workout program, or ramp up the intensity of your cardio with a few more intervals. And whatever you do, don't think of it as punishment. You're simply putting to good use the extra energy you gave your body when you provided it with a higher-than-usual number of calories. Why not use those extra calories rather than store them as fat? It's a win-win! Then tomorrow, you can just go back to the *Perfect Body Diet* as if nothing ever happened—no biggie.

CHAPTER 8

The Greens and Berries Diet

Get ready: Here's the part where we tell you what to eat if the test in Chapter 5 indicated that you should follow the Greens and Berries version of the *Women's Health Perfect Body Diet*. First we'll give you lists of your prescribed foods in each of the macronutrient groups. Starting on page 111, we'll give you 14 days' worth of sample meal plans. You can follow these as presented, making adjustments only as needed to hit your customized calorie count. Or you can use the prescribed foods lists (which include serving sizes, calorie counts, and grams of carbs, protein, and fat, as relevant) to build your own meals. Because after all, that's the beauty of the *Perfect Body Diet*: It helps you eat in the way that works best for *you*.

Your Perfect Carbs

You should shoot for 20 to 30 percent of calories from carbohydrates, or about 90 to 125 daily grams of carbohydrates. (See "Your Perfect Body Diet Planner" on page 100 if you'd like to calculate a daily intake total based on your customized calorie count.) The best carbohydrate foods for the Greens and Berries Diet are those that are digested slowly, low in total carbohydrates, and rich in fiber, such as green (and other colored) vegetables and berries. Use the name of your diet to help you remember which types of carbohydrate foods you should eat. Please refer to the following lists

▶▶Your Perfect Body Diet Planner

You can use the following calculations to personalize your daily balance of the three macronutrients based on the calorie count you determined in "Customize Your Calorie Count in Three Simple Steps" on page 77.

FOR CARBOHYDRATES

Your ideal daily carb intake is 20 to 30 percent of calories. Multiply your customized calorie count by 0.20. Then divide the result by 4, since a gram of carbohydrate provides 4 calories. For example:

$$1,500 \text{ daily calories} \times 0.20 = 300$$

$$300 \div 4 = 75$$

On a 1,500-calorie diet, the minimum daily carb intake is 75 grams.

To find the upper limit of your range, multiply your customized calorie count by 0.30. Then divide the result by 4. For example:

$$1,500 \text{ daily calories} \times 0.30 = 450$$

$$450 \div 4 = 112.5$$

So the maximum daily carb intake is about 113 grams.

FOR FATS

Your ideal daily fat intake is 35 to 45 percent of calories. Multiply your customized calorie count by 0.35. Then divide the result by 9, since a gram of fat provides 9 calories. For example:

to choose carbohydrate foods that are perfect for you. If a food you are craving is not on the lists, try to avoid it or at least eat it infrequently. Your best bet for this diet is to focus your carbohydrate choices on vegetables, berries, certain other fruits, and beans and legumes.

VEGETABLES

Not surprisingly, given the name, on the Greens and Berries Diet you can eat the vegetables below any time of day. They have few calories, contain a lot of fiber, and provide a lot of water, so you can eat lots of them and not gain weight or add body fat. Eat them with most of your

$$1{,}500 \text{ daily calories} \times 0.35 = 525$$

$$525 \div 9 = 58.33$$

On a 1,500-calorie diet, the minimum daily fat intake is about 58 grams.

To find the upper limit of your range, multiply your customized calorie count by 0.45. Then divide the result by 9. For example:

$$1{,}500 \text{ daily calories} \times 0.45 = 675$$

$$675 \div 9 = 75$$

So the maximum daily fat intake is 75 grams.

FOR PROTEIN

Your ideal daily protein intake is 30 to 35 percent of calories. Multiply your customized calorie count by 0.30. Then divide the result by 4, since a gram of protein provides 4 calories. For example:

$$1{,}500 \text{ daily calories} \times 0.30 = 450$$

$$450 \div 4 = 112.5$$

On a 1,500-calorie diet, the minimum daily protein intake is about 113 grams.

To find the upper limit of your range, multiply your customized calorie count by 0.35. Then divide the result by 4. For example:

$$1{,}500 \text{ daily calories} \times 0.35 = 525$$

$$525 \div 4 = 131.25$$

So the maximum daily protein intake is about 131 grams.

meals so that you fill up your stomach without filling out your waistline. Indulge in these as much as you want, as long as you stay within your daily calorie count and carb limit.

VEGETABLE	SERVING SIZE	CALORIES	CARBS (G)	FIBER (G)
Artichoke	1 each, heart	60	9	4
Asparagus	12 spears	43	7	3
Bamboo shoots	½ c	12	2	1
Bean sprouts (adzuki, lentil, mung, etc.)	1 c raw	31	6	2

(continued)

VEGETABLE	SERVING SIZE	CALORIES	CARBS (G)	FIBER (G)
Bell peppers (red, green, yellow)	1 medium, raw	32	7	2
Bok choy	1 c cooked	22	3	2
Broccoli	1 c cooked	44	8	4
Brussels sprouts	½ c cooked	32	13	4
Green beans	1 c cooked	27	6	2
Cabbage	1 c raw	22	4	2
Cauliflower	1 c cooked	28	5	3
Celery	3 medium stalks	30	7	3
Cherry tomatoes	10 each	35	7	2
Collards	1 c cooked	50	9	5
Cucumber	1 medium, peeled	24	5	1
Eggplant	1 c cooked	27	6	2
Endive	1 c raw	8	1	1
Garlic	1 clove	4	1	0
Kale	1 c cooked	36	7	3
Kohlrabi	1 c cooked	47	11	2
Leeks	1 c cooked	32	7	1
Lettuces (red, iceberg, romaine, radicchio, green leaf)	2 c raw	10	2	1
Mushrooms	10 raw	30	4	0
Okra	1 c cooked	51	11	4
Onions	½ c cooked	39	9	2
Radishes	1 c raw	15	3	1
Spaghetti squash	1 c cooked	41	10	2
Spinach	1 c cooked	41	6	4
Tomatoes	1 medium, raw	25	5	1
Zucchini and summer squash	1 c cooked	25	5	2

FRUITS

Berries, the other namesake of the Greens and Berries Diet, are Mother Nature's perfect fruits. They contain a very small amount of carbohydrates per serving and are loaded with fiber and antioxidants. The darker the berry, the more vitamins it contains. For all fruits, always choose fresh, not dried, varieties; and stick with whole fruit, not fruit juice, whenever possible. Don't add sugar or artificial sweetener to your fruit either; these foods are sweet enough on their own.

FRUIT	SERVING SIZE	CALORIES	CARBS (G)	FIBER (G)
Apples	1 medium	80	22	5
Apricots	1 medium	16	4	1
Blackberries	½ c	37	9	4
Blueberries	½ c	40	10	2
Cherries	1 c, with pits	84	19	3
Cranberries, unsweetened	¼ c	23	11	2
Grapefruit	½ medium	45	11	2
Peaches	1 medium	42	10	2
Pears	1 medium	97	25	4
Plums	1 medium	36	9	1
Raspberries	½ c	30	7	4
Strawberries	½ c	22	5	2

BEANS AND LEGUMES

Beans and legumes have an extremely high fiber content, so they are perfect slow-digesting carbs for the Greens and Berries Diet. The following nutritional information is for a ½-cup serving of cooked beans (either canned or fresh).

BEAN/LEGUME	CALORIES	CARBS (G)	FIBER (G)
Adzuki	147	28	8
Black	113	20	7
Black-eyed peas	100	17	6
Chickpeas	134	22	6
Fava/broadbeans	93	16	5
Great Northern	104	19	8
Kidney	110	19	9
Lentils	114	19	8
Lima	94	18	7
Navy	129	24	6
Pink	125	23	4
Pinto	117	21	7
Refried, canned, no added fats	100	18	6
Soy (edamame)	126	10	4
Split peas	115	21	8
White	127	23	9

WHOLE GRAIN BREAKFAST CEREALS

The following cereals are options on the Greens and Berries Diet because they are quite high in fiber and very slowly digested.

FOOD	SERVING SIZE	CALORIES	CARBS (G)	FIBER (G)
All-Bran Bran Buds	⅓ c	75	24	13
Fiber One	½ c	61	25	14

SNACKS

Stay away from common carbohydrate snacks such as pretzels or crackers. If you're hungry, eat more of the perfect carbohydrate choices in the previous lists, or choose foods from the protein or fat lists throughout the rest of this chapter.

Your Perfect Fats

This diet requires 35 to 45 percent of calories from fat. This comes out to 60 to 70 grams of fat per day. (See "Your Perfect Body Diet Planner" on page 100 if you'd like to calculate a daily intake total based on your customized calorie count.) The following fat-containing foods can be incorporated into your diet in various ways. You can eat them as quick snacks (nuts), add them to other dishes (such as avocado with tomatoes, or hummus on salads), or use them as the major component of meals (salmon for dinner, eggs for breakfast).

To obtain the correct balance of all the fatty acids in your diet, you should eat a wide variety of these fat-containing food equally throughout the week.

HIGHER-SATURATED-FAT FOODS	SERVING SIZE	CALORIES	TOTAL FAT (G)	SATURATED FAT (G)
Butter, real, nonhydrogenated	1 Tbsp	100	11.5	7
Coconut, shredded, unsweetened	1 Tbsp	30	3	2.5
Dairy, low-fat				
Cheese, cottage, 1% or 2%	½ c	80–100	1–2	1–1.5
Cheese, low-fat hard (Cheddar, mozzarella)	1 oz	50	1–2	1
Milk, 1% or 2%	1 c	100–120	2–4	1.5–3
Yogurt, plain	½ c	70	1–2	1
Dairy, higher-fat (try to limit these, but you don't have to completely avoid them)				
Cheese, cottage, full-fat	½ c	108	4.5	3
Cheese, feta, crumbled	⅓ c	131	10	7

HIGHER-SATURATED-FAT FOODS	SERVING SIZE	CALORIES	TOTAL FAT (G)	SATURATED FAT (G)
Cheese, full-fat hard and soft (Brie, Camembert)	1 oz	110	8–9	5
Cheese, ricotta cheese, part-skim	⅓ c	170	6	6
Milk, goat's	1 c	167	10	6.5
Milk, whole	1 c	150	8	5

HIGHER-MONOUNSATURATED-FAT FOODS	SERVING SIZE	CALORIES	TOTAL FAT (G)	MONOUNSAT FAT (G)
Avocado, Florida	⅓ each	110	9	5
Avocado, Hass	⅓ each	102	10	7
Egg, whole	1 medium	68	4.5	1.8
Hummus made with olive oil	¼ c	100	6	4
Lean meats and poultry, cooked (3 oz serving is equal in size to the palm of your hand)				
Beef, lean	3 oz	200	13–15	5–7
Chicken or turkey breasts, skinless	3 oz	135	2–3	1
Chicken or turkey, lean ground	3 oz	126	6–8	3–4
Lamb, lean	3 oz	180	10–14	4–6
Pork, lean	3 oz	175	7–10	3–5
Nuts and seeds, unsalted and raw				
Almonds	¼ c	210	15	11
Cashews	¼ c	187	16	9
Hazelnuts	¼ c	178	17	13
Macadamia nuts	¼ c	240	25	20
Peanuts	¼ c	210	18	9
Pecans	¼ c	186	20	11
Pistachios	¼ c	176	13	7
Nut butters, no sugar or other ingredients added				
Almond butter	2 Tbsp	202	18	12
Cashew butter	2 Tbsp	186	16	9
Peanut butter	2 Tbsp	186	16	8
Oils				
Canola oil	1 Tbsp	120	14	8
Extra-virgin olive oil	1 Tbsp	120	14	11
Peanut oil	1 Tbsp	120	14	6

(continued)

HIGHER-POLYUNSATURATED-FAT FOODS	SERVING SIZE	CALORIES	TOTAL FAT (G)	POLYUNSAT FAT (G)
Hummus made with canola oil (rich in omega-3 ALA and omega-6)	¼ c	100	6	3
Fish (rich in omega-3 EPA and DHA fat)				
Cod	4 oz cooked	120	1	0.3
Halibut	4 oz cooked	160	3	1
Herring	3.5 oz canned	210	8	3
Salmon	4 oz cooked	205	9	4
Sardines, canned in water	3.5 oz	175	9	3
Trout	4 oz cooked	160	4.5	1
Tuna, canned in water	6 oz can	150	1	0.5
Tuna, fresh	4 oz cooked	150	1.5	0.5
Nuts and seeds, raw and unsalted (rich in omega-3 ALA and omega-6)				
Brazil nuts	¼ c	230	23	9, mostly omega-6
Flaxseeds, ground	2 Tbsp	150	10	6, mostly omega-3 ALA
Hemp seeds	2 Tbsp	110	8	3, mostly omega-3 ALA
Pine nuts	¼ c	190	17	7, mostly omega-6
Pumpkin seeds	¼ c	186	15	7, mostly omega-6
Sesame seeds	2 Tbsp	110	10	4.5, mostly omega-6
Soy nuts	¼ c	140	7	4
Sunflower seeds	¼ c	186	16	10, mostly omega-6
Walnuts	¼ c	163	16	12, mostly omega-3 ALA
Tahini (sesame butter), no sugar or other ingredients added	2 Tbsp	177	16	7, rich in omega-6
Oils				
Enova oil	1 Tbsp	120	14	8, rich in omega-6
Flaxseed oil	1 Tbsp	120	14	9, rich in omega-3 ALA
Safflower oil	1 Tbsp	120	14	9, rich in omega-6
Sesame seed oil	1 Tbsp	120	14	6, rich in omega-6
Sunflower oil	1 Tbsp	120	14	10, rich in omega-6

FAT-BASED CONDIMENTS AND DRESSINGS

Of all the fat-based condiments you can choose, these are the better options.

》 Cheese sauces, made with low-fat cheese

》 Pesto (see recipe on page 204)

》 Peanut sauce, made with natural peanut butter (see recipe on page 195)

》 Mayonnaise made with olive oil or canola oil (see recipe on page 203)

>> Salad dressings, low-sugar, made with olive oil or canola oil

>> Hollandaise sauce, made low fat

Your Perfect Proteins

On the Greens and Berries Diet, 30 to 35 percent of your daily calories will come from protein, about 120 to 140 grams. (See "Your Perfect Body Diet Planner" on page 100 if you'd like to calculate a daily intake total based on your customized calorie count.) You're going to differentiate between foods that are *full* proteins and ones that are *partial* proteins. Full proteins are complete proteins, meaning that they contain all the essential amino acids in fairly equal quantities. Partial proteins are not complete, meaning that they are missing or limited in one or more of the essential amino acids.

Aim to eat at least three or more of your meals or snacks from the full-protein list and two to three of your snacks and some meals from the partial-protein list. You need to have one or the other form of protein every time you eat, and if you have both in one meal, that's perfect too.

PERFECT *FULL*-PROTEIN CHOICES

These protein choices are complete and contain a high quantity of dietary protein per serving. Try to incorporate these into your three main meals every day.

FOOD	SERVING SIZE	CALORIES	PROTEIN (G)
Beef and bison (buffalo)	**3–4 oz cooked**		
Lean ground		140	18–22
Steaks, round		180	22–27
Tenderloin, lean		180	24–26
Cheese, low-fat	**2 oz unless otherwise noted**		
American		140	14
Cheddar		100	13
Cottage, 1%	½ c	80	14
Feta		100	10
Goat		80	4
Mozzarella		140	16
Ricotta	½ c	170	14
Swiss		108	13
Eggs			
Egg, whole	1 medium	68	5.5
Egg whites, liquid	½ c	105	15

(continued)

FOOD	SERVING SIZE	CALORIES	PROTEIN (G)
Fish	4 oz cooked unless otherwise noted		
Catfish		190	22
Cod		120	26
Eel		260	27
Halibut		160	25
Pike		128	28
Salmon, canned and fresh		205	28
Snapper		145	29
Tilapia		145	29
Trout		160	28
Tuna, canned in water	6 oz can	150	32
Tuna, fresh		150	32
Lamb	3 oz cooked	170–190	22–27
Milk			
Cow's milk, 1% or 2%	1 c	100–120	8
Goat's milk	1 c	167	8
Pork	3 oz cooked		
Canadian-style bacon		157	21
Chops, lean		175	24
Ham, lean		125	17
Lean ground		190	21
Tenderloin, lean		140	24
Poultry and fowl	3 oz cooked		
Chicken and turkey: breasts, ground, tenderloins, thighs, wings		140–200	21–27
Duck		170	20
Ostrich, lean ground		120	23
Protein powders			
Hemp protein powder, such as Manitoba Harvest	1 oz, 2 scoops	134	15
Rice protein powder, such as Nutribiotic Rice Protein	1 heaping Tbsp	57	12
Soy protein powder	1 oz, 1 scoop	120–150	14–20
Whey protein powder	1 oz, 1 scoop	90–120	17–25

FOOD	SERVING SIZE	CALORIES	PROTEIN (G)
Shellfish	**3 oz cooked**		
Clams		100	22
Crab, not imitation		82	16
Lobster		100	17
Mussels		146	20
Oysters		60	7
Scallops		120	22
Shrimp		85	17
Soy			
Edamame (soybeans)	½ c	126	12
Soy nuts	¼ c	140	12
Tempeh	3 oz	165–185	15–18
Tofu, firm	½ c	100	10–14
Yogurt			
Greek, 2%	5 oz container	80	12–13
Plain, low-fat	½ c	120–150	8–12

PERFECT PARTIAL-PROTEIN CHOICES

These *partial* proteins are not complete, meaning that they are limited or devoid of one or more of the essential amino acids. You can choose these for your two or three daily snacks between your main meals, if you don't feel like eating a full protein. If you are vegetarian, choose from these options more often.

FOOD	SERVING SIZE	CALORIES	PROTEIN (G)
Falafel	2 oz	220	9–11
Hummus (see recipe on page 182)	2 Tbsp	100	5
Beans and legumes	**½ c cooked**		
Adzuki		147	8
Black		113	7
Black-eyed peas		100	7
Chickpeas		134	7
Fava		93	6
Great Northern		104	7
Kidney		110	8

(continued)

FOOD	SERVING SIZE	CALORIES	PROTEIN (G)
Lentils		114	9
Lima		95	6
Navy		129	8
Pink		125	8
Pinto		117	7
Refried, canned, no added fats		100	6
Split peas		115	8
White beans		127	8

Nuts and seeds, unsalted raw

FOOD	SERVING SIZE	CALORIES	PROTEIN (G)
Almonds	¼ c	210	8
Brazil nuts	¼ c	230	5
Cashews	¼ c	187	5
Flaxseeds	2 Tbsp	150	6
Hazelnuts	¼ c	178	4
Hemp seeds	2 Tbsp	110	6
Macadamia nuts	¼ c	240	3
Pecans	¼ c	186	2.5
Pine nuts	¼ c	190	8
Pistachios	¼ c	176	6
Pumpkin seeds	¼ c	186	8
Sesame seeds	2 Tbsp	110	5
Sunflower seeds	¼ c	186	6
Walnuts	¼ c	163	3

Nut butters, no sugar or other ingredients added

FOOD	SERVING SIZE	CALORIES	PROTEIN (G)
Almond butter	2 Tbsp	202	5
Cashew butter	2 Tbsp	186	5
Peanut butter	2 Tbsp	186	8

Your Perfect Body Meal Plans

Here are 14 days' worth of meal plans based on a 1,600-calorie daily diet. You can follow these plans exactly and you should reach your weight-less goal. But you can optimize your results by customizing these plans to fit your specific calorie needs as determined on page 100. Make changes by referring to "Your 100-Calorie Cheat Sheet" on page 79 or to the lists of perfect foods in this chapter. Chapter 10 provides the recipes for the dishes included here.

DAY 1

MEAL	DISH	PROTEIN (G)	CARBS (G)	FIBER (G)	TOTAL FAT (G)	SAT FAT (G)	CALORIES
Breakfast	Balanced-Body Smoothie (page 185)	24	22	12	22	2.5	382
	2 fish oil capsules	0	0	0	2	0	18
Snack	Creamy Garlic Hummus (page 182)	4	7	4	7	1	107
	1 medium red bell pepper, sliced	1	7	2	0	0	32
Lunch	Stuffed Peppers with Tuna Salad (page 169)	35	21	7	3	0	251
Snack	½ c fresh raspberries	0	7	4	0	0	28
	3 Tbsp raw whole almonds	5	4	3	11	0	135
Dinner	Salmon with Cucumber Dill Sauce (page 171)	47	10	8	19	3	399
	⅔ c steamed green beans	1	6	2	0	0	28
Snack	Chocolate Protein Pudding (page 208)	21	10	6	4	1	160
	Totals	138	94	48	68	7.5	1,540
	Percentages	36	24	12	40	4	100

THE GREENS AND BERRIES DIET

DAY 2

MEAL	DISH	PROTEIN (G)	CARBS (G)	FIBER (G)	TOTAL FAT (G)	SAT FAT (G)	CALORIES
Breakfast	High-Fiber Cottage Cheese and Yogurt (page 202)	35	17	6	10	3	320
	2 fish oil capsules	0	0	0	2	0	18
Snack	Bodacious Spinach and Bean Dip (page 182), 1 serving	10	22	3	10	1	218
	8 celery sticks	1	5	2	0	0	24
Lunch	Chicken Taco Salad (page 197)	43	12	6	7	3	283
Snack	1 scoop whey protein powder	23	3	0	1	0	113
	mixed with ½ c water	0	0	0	0	0	0
	and 2 tsp flaxseed oil	0	0	0	9	0	81
	and 2 g glucomannan	0	0	2	0	0	0
Dinner	Turkey and Cauliflower Casserole (page 198)	28	22	9	28	8	452
	1 fish oil capsule	0	0	0	1	0	9
Snack	Gluco-Berry Protein Sorbet (page 191)	11	8	5	0	0	76
	Totals	151	89	33	70.5	15	1,595
	Percentages	38	22	8	40	8	100

DAY 3

MEAL	DISH	PROTEIN (G)	CARBS (G)	FIBER (G)	TOTAL FAT (G)	SAT FAT (G)	CALORIES
Breakfast	**Super Fiber Breakfast Bowl (page 201)**	12	25	16	16	3	296
	1 fish oil capsule	0	0	0	1	0	9
Snack	½ c edamame (soybeans)	14	8	5	7	1	151
Lunch	**Dijon Chicken Salad (page 164), 1 serving**	29	8	4	10	2	238
	2 c baby spinach leaves	1	2	1	0	0	12
Snack	**Pumpkin Pie Smoothie (page 187)**	22	12	6	15	3	271
Dinner	**Slow-Cooker Split-Pea Soup (page 175), 1 serving**	19	53	14	3	1	315
	3 oz baked skinless chicken breast	26	0	0	2	0.5	122
	2 fish oil capsules	0	0	0	2	0	18
Snack	**2 Glucoroons (page 208)**	2	6	3	9	8	113
	Totals	**125**	**114**	**49**	**65.5**	**17.5**	**1,545**
	Percentages	32	30	13	38	10	100

THE GREENS AND BERRIES DIET

DAY 4

MEAL	DISH	PROTEIN (G)	CARBS (G)	FIBER (G)	TOTAL FAT (G)	SAT FAT (G)	CALORIES
Breakfast	Scrambled Egg Whites with Spinach (page 162)	17	13	6	8	1	192
	2 fish oil capsules	0	0	0	2	0	18
	1 slice sprouted grain bread	4	14	3	0	0	72
Snack	Easy Vanilla Protein Pudding (page 207)	37	6	2	2	1	190
Lunch	Slow-Cooker Split-Pea Soup (page 175), 1 serving	19	53	14	3	1	315
Snack	Creamy Ranch Dip (page 203), 1 serving	1	1	1	9	1	89
	½ cucumber, sliced	0	2	1	0	0	8
Dinner	Chicken with Pistachio Pesto (page 196), 1 serving	27	7	4	38	5	478
	1 c steamed broccoli	4	8	4	0	0	48
	1 fish oil capsule	0	0	0	1	0	9
Snack	1 scoop whey protein powder	23	3	0	1	0	113
	mixed with ½ c water	0	0	0	0	0	0
	and 2 g glucomannan	0	0	2	0	0	0
	Totals	132	107	37	64	9	1,532
	Percentages	34	28	10	38	5	100

DAY 5

MEAL	DISH	PROTEIN (G)	CARBS (G)	FIBER (G)	TOTAL FAT (G)	SAT FAT (G)	CALORIES
Breakfast	**Walnut Yogurt Smoothie (page 205)**	15	19	11	18.5	3	302
	2 fish oil capsules	0	0	0	2	0	18
Snack	1 Tbsp natural peanut butter	4	3	1	8	1	100
	8 celery sticks	1	5	2	0	0	24
	1 medium apple	0	20	3	0	0	80
Lunch	**Rainbow Broccoli Slaw (page 177), 1 serving**	2	10	5	7	1	111
	5 oz (16–20 large) boiled shrimp, peeled, deveined	31	0	0	1	0	133
Snack	**Spicy Gluco Guacamole (page 183), 1 serving**	1	4	3	7	1	83
	8 celery sticks	1	5	2	0	0	24
	1 cheese-string snack, 2% milk fat	8	1	0	4	2.5	72
Dinner	**Tilapia with Cucumber Salsa (page 172), 2 servings**	48	6	6	8	2	288
	Milk-Free Creamed Cauliflower (page 179), 1 serving	3	9	6	0	0	48
	1 fish oil capsule	0	0	0	1	0	9
Snack	**Chocolate Protein Pudding (page 208)**	21	10	6	4	1	160
	1 Tbsp almond butter	2	3	1	9	1	101
	Totals	**137**	**95**	**46**	**69.5**	**12.5**	**1,553.5**
	Percentages	**35**	**24**	**12**	**40**	**7**	**100**

THE GREENS AND BERRIES DIET

DAY 6

MEAL	DISH	PROTEIN (G)	CARBS (G)	FIBER (G)	TOTAL FAT (G)	SAT FAT (G)	CALORIES
Breakfast	No-Crust Vegetable Quiche (page 192), 1 serving	27	8	5	7	2	203
	1 c fresh cherries	0.5	19	3	0	0	80
	2 fish oil capsules	0	0	0	2	0	18
Snack	Easy Vanilla Protein Pudding (page 207)	37	6	2	2	1	190
Lunch	3 Turkey and Bean Burgers (page 167)	30	12	6	15	3	303
	1 medium pear	0	25	4	0	0	100
Snack	Crab-Stuffed Mushroom Caps (page 173), 1 serving	8	3	3	10	1	134
	1 Pumpkin Protein Fiber Muffin (page 191)	7	12	4	13	1	193
Dinner	Chicken Satay with Peanut Dipping Sauce (page 195)	28	7	4	14	3	266
	1 fish oil capsule	0	0	0	1	0	9
Snack	Sweet Egg White Splendor (page 209)	4	13	3	5	5	113
	Totals	141.5	105	30	69	16	1,609
	Percentages	35	26	7	39	9	100

DAY 7: LOWER-CALORIE DAY

MEAL	DISH	PROTEIN (G)	CARBS (G)	FIBER (G)	TOTAL FAT (G)	SAT FAT (G)	CALORIES
Breakfast	**1 Pumpkin Protein Fiber Muffin (page 191)**	7	12	4	13	1	193
	1 tsp butter	0	0	0	4	2	36
	2 fish oil capsules	0	0	0	2	0	18
Snack	**2 Turkey and Bean Burgers (page 167)**	20	8	4	10	2	202
Lunch	**Creamy Broccoli Soup (page 200), 1 serving**	2	8	4	3	0.5	67
	3 oz baked skinless chicken breast	26	0	0	2	0.5	122
Snack	**Sun-Dried Tomato Pesto (page 204), 1 serving**	3	5	4	12	2	140
	1 c steamed broccoli	4	8	4	0	0	48
Dinner	**Curried Chickpea Stew (page 174), 1 serving**	6	28	7	10	4	226
	4 oz lean, trimmed baked or grilled pork chop	35	0	0	7	2	203
	1 fish oil capsule	0	0	0	1	0	9
Snack	**2 Glucoroons (page 208)**	2	6	3	9	8	113
	1 medium apple	0	20	3	0	0	80
	Totals	105	95	33	73	22	1,457
	Percentages	29	26	9	45	14	100

THE GREENS AND BERRIES DIET

DAY 8

MEAL	DISH	PROTEIN (G)	CARBS (G)	FIBER (G)	TOTAL FAT (G)	SAT FAT (G)	CALORIES
Breakfast	Coconut Macaroon Smoothie (page 186)	26	12	7	13	8	269
	2 fish oil capsules	0	0	0	2	0	18
Snack	1 Pumpkin Protein Fiber Muffin (page 191)	7	12	4	13	1	193
Lunch	Tuna Salad (page 199)	33	0	2	12	1	240
	1 slice sprouted grain bread	4	14	3	0	0	72
	½ c fresh raspberries	0	7	4	0	0	28
Snack	Creamy Garlic Hummus (page 182)	4	7	4	7	1	107
	1 medium red bell pepper, sliced	1	7	2	0	0	32
Dinner	Slow-Cooker Chicken Cacciatore (page 165)	33	16	5	8	1	268
	1 c cooked spinach	2	3	3	0	0	20
	1 fish oil capsule	0	0	0	1	0	9
Snack	Almond Joy Smoothie (page 205)	26	8	7	15	5	271
	10 medium fresh strawberries	0	9	3	0	0	36
	Totals	136	95	44	71	17	1,563
	Percentages	35	24	11	41	10	100

DAY 9

MEAL	DISH	PROTEIN (G)	CARBS (G)	FIBER (G)	TOTAL FAT (G)	SAT FAT (G)	CALORIES
Breakfast	**Gluco-Granola (page 181), 1 serving**	9	19	5	15	3	247
	½ c plain low-fat yogurt	6	8	0	1.5	1	70
	mixed with 2 g glucomannan	0	0	2	0	0	0
	2 fish oil capsules	0	0	0	2	0	18
Snack	**Crab-Stuffed Mushroom Caps (page 173), 1 serving**	8	3	3	10	1	134
Lunch	**Slow-Cooker Chicken Cacciatore (page 165)**	33	16	5	8	1	268
Snack	6–8 (⅛ c) walnut halves	2	1	1	7	1	75
	1½ scoops whey protein powder	34	4	0	2	0	170
	mixed with ½ c water	0	0	0	0	0	0
	and 2 g glucomannan	0	0	2	0	0	0
Dinner	**Curried Chickpea Stew (page 174), 1 serving**	6	28	7	10	4	226
	Asparagus with Dill Mustard Sauce (page 176), 1 serving	7	12	5	1	0	85
	1 fish oil capsule	0	0	0	1	0	9
Snack	**Carrot Cake Smoothie (page 206)**	28	13	4	11	4	263
	Totals	**133**	**104**	**34**	**68.5**	**15**	**1,565**
	Percentages	**34**	**27**	**9**	**39**	**9**	**100**

THE GREENS AND BERRIES DIET

DAY 10

MEAL	DISH	PROTEIN (G)	CARBS (G)	FIBER (G)	TOTAL FAT (G)	SAT FAT (G)	CALORIES
Breakfast	**Ricotta Mango Breakfast (page 202)**	28	24	3	19	12	379
	2 fish oil capsules	0	0	0	2	0	18
Snack	**Sun-Dried Tomato Pesto (page 204), 1 serving**	3	5	4	12	2	140
	1 c steamed zucchini	2	5	2	0	0	28
	3 oz (8–12 large) boiled shrimp, peeled, deveined	23	0	0	1	0	101
Lunch	**Mixed Greens with Strawberries, Feta, and Walnuts (page 178)**	19	32	8	12.5	5	317
	¾ c plain low-fat yogurt	10	12	0	2.5	2	110.5
	mixed with 2 g glucomannan	0	0	2	0	0	0
Snack	½ c edamame (soybeans)	14	8	5	7	1	151
Dinner	**Thick and Hearty Beef Chili (page 168)**	29	29	10	10	2	322
	1 fish oil capsule	0	0	0	1	0	9
Snack	1 Tbsp natural peanut butter	4	3	1	8	1	100
	8 celery sticks	1	5	2	0	0	24
Totals		**123**	**111**	**35**	**72**	**23**	**1,589.5**
Percentages		**31**	**28**	**9**	**41**	**13**	**100**

DAY 11

MEAL	DISH	PROTEIN (G)	CARBS (G)	FIBER (G)	TOTAL FAT (G)	SAT FAT (G)	CALORIES
Breakfast	**Goat Cheese and Herb Gluco-Omelette (page 193)**	24	2	2	10	5	194
	⅓ c no-sugar-added salsa	1	5	1	0	0	24
	mixed with 2 g glucomannan	0	0	2	0	0	0
	1 slice sprouted grain bread	4	14	3	0	0	72
	2 fish oil capsules	0	0	0	2	0	18
Snack	**Gluco-Granola (page 181), 1 serving**	9	19	5	15	3	247
Lunch	**Egg Salad Wraps (page 194), 1 serving**	15	2	2	23	4	275
	1 medium apple	0	20	3	0	0	80
Snack	1 scoop whey protein powder	23	3	0	1	0	113
	mixed with ½ c water	0	0	0	0	0	0
	and 2 g glucomannan	0	0	2	0	0	0
Dinner	**Tilapia with Cucumber Salsa (page 172), 1 serving**	24	3	3	4	1	144
	Milk-Free Creamed Cauliflower (page 179)	3	9	6	0	0	48
	1 fish oil capsule	0	0	0	1	0	9
Snack	**Walnut Yogurt Smoothie (page 205)**	15	19	11	18.5	3	302
	Totals	**118**	**96**	**40**	**74.5**	**16**	**1,526**
	Percentages	**31**	**25**	**10**	**44**	**9**	**100**

THE GREENS AND BERRIES DIET

DAY 12

MEAL	DISH	PROTEIN (G)	CARBS (G)	FIBER (G)	TOTAL FAT (G)	SAT FAT (G)	CALORIES
Breakfast	Super Fiber Breakfast Bowl (page 201)	12	25	16	16	3	296
	2 fish oil capsules	0	0	0	2	0	18
Snack	Garden Asparagus Leek Soup (page 176), 1 serving	4	12	6	9	1	145
Lunch	Chicken Satay with Peanut Dipping Sauce (page 195)	28	7	4	14	3	266
	1 fish oil capsule	0	0	0	1	0	9
Snack	Perfect Fruit and Vegetable Smoothie (page 184)	21	39	14	12	2	348
Dinner	Salmon with Sage Sauce and Steamed Spinach (page 170), 1 serving	52	11	7	18	3	450
	1 fish oil capsule	0	0	0	1	0	9
Snack	¼ c edamame (soybeans)	7	4	3	3	1	71
	Totals	124	98	50	76.5	12	1,611
	Percentages	31	24	12	43	7	100

DAY 13

MEAL	DISH	PROTEIN (G)	CARBS (G)	FIBER (G)	TOTAL FAT (G)	SAT FAT (G)	CALORIES
Breakfast	**2 Whole Wheat Buttermilk Gluco-Pancakes (page 180)**	14	30	6	6	1	230
	2 tsp butter	0	0	0	8	5	72
	2 Tbsp unsweetened applesauce	0	3	0.5	0	0	12
	mixed with 2 g glucomannan	0	0	2	0	0	0
	2 fish oil capsules	0	0	0	2	0	18
Snack	**Spicy Gluco Guacamole (page 183), 1 serving**	1	4	3	7	1	83
	1 medium red bell pepper, sliced	1	7	2	0	0	32
	½ medium pear	0	13	2	0	0	52
Lunch	**Tuna Salad (page 199)**	33	0	2	12	1	240
	3 c mixed greens	2	5	4	0	0	28
	Balsamic vinegar	0	0	0	0	0	
Snack	**2 Turkey and Bean Burgers (page 167)**	20	8	4	10	2	202
Dinner	**Bangers and Cauliflower Mash (page 200)**	35	16	6	16	5	348
	1 fish oil capsule	0	0	0	1	0	9
Snack	**Carrot Cake Smoothie (page 206)**	28	13	4	11	4	263
	Totals	**134**	**102**	**35.5**	**73**	**19**	**1,601**
	Percentages	**33**	**25**	**9**	**41**	**11**	**100**

DAY 14: LOWER-CALORIE DAY

MEAL	DISH	PROTEIN (G)	CARBS (G)	FIBER (G)	TOTAL FAT (G)	SAT FAT (G)	CALORIES
Breakfast	No-Crust Vegetable Quiche (page 192), 1 serving	27	8	5	7	2	203
	½ c fresh raspberries	0	7	4	0	0	28
	2 fish oil capsules	0	0	0	2	0	18
Snack	Garden Asparagus Leek Soup (page 176), 1 serving	4	12	6	9	1	145
Lunch	Rainbow Broccoli Slaw (page 177), 1 serving	2	10	5	7	1	111
	5 oz (16–20 large) boiled shrimp, peeled, deveined	31	0	0	1	0	133
Snack	Gluco-Berry Protein Sorbet (page 191)	11	8	5	0	0	76
	3 Tbsp raw whole almonds	5	4	3	11	0	135
Dinner	Coconut Curry Shrimp (page 199)	25	4	3	16	11	260
	1 c steamed Brussels sprouts	4	13	4	0	0	68
Snack	Chocolate Cake Smoothie (page 206)	39	10	8	6	0	250
	Totals	148	76	43	59	15	1,427
	Percentages	41	21	12	37	9	100

Shopping List

This list includes most of the food items you will need to have on hand to prepare the dishes specified in the meal plans. A few words about freshness: Since it's best to buy fruits, vegetables, and fresh herbs immediately before use, we have not included every type here. Keep in mind that nuts and seeds stay freshest in the refrigerator or freezer; grains and flours are best stored in airtight containers and used within a couple of months.

- [ ] 1% milk
- [ ] Fat-free buttermilk
- [ ] Plain low-fat or fat-free yogurt
- [ ] Fat-free sour cream
- [ ] Low-fat soft cheeses (fat-free cream cheese, reduced-fat feta, part-skim ricotta, 1% or fat-free cottage cheese)
- [ ] Soft goat cheese
- [ ] Low-fat Cheddar cheese
- [ ] Grated Parmesan cheese
- [ ] Cheese string snacks, individually wrapped
- [ ] Medium or omega-3 eggs
- [ ] Pasteurized liquid egg substitute
- [ ] Pasteurized egg whites, such as Eggology
- [ ] Lean ground turkey and lean ground beef
- [ ] Lean pork chops
- [ ] Boneless, skinless chicken breasts
- [ ] Fresh or frozen raw shrimp, peeled and deveined
- [ ] Fresh fish fillets (salmon, tilapia)
- [ ] Canned chunk light tuna, packed in water
- [ ] Canned crabmeat
- [ ] Fresh berries and fruit in season (keep apples, lemons, and limes on hand)
- [ ] Fresh vegetables (keep garlic, onions, and 10-oz packages of spinach on hand)

- [ ] Edamame (green soybeans in the pod; found fresh at sushi counters and Asian markets or frozen in the natural foods section)
- [ ] Unsweetened carrot juice, such as Odwalla
- [ ] Fresh herbs
- [ ] Frozen berries
- [ ] Frozen peas and corn
- [ ] Canned diced low-salt tomatoes, whole peeled tomatoes, and tomato paste
- [ ] Canned mandarin oranges in juice, canned pumpkin puree, and jarred unsweetened applesauce
- [ ] Jarred capers and canned or jarred pimiento-stuffed green olives
- [ ] Sun-dried tomatoes
- [ ] No-sugar-added salsa
- [ ] Canned and dried beans (pinto, white, red kidney, chickpeas; dried split green peas)
- [ ] Chocolate, vanilla, and strawberry whey protein powders
- [ ] Sugar-free strawberry jam
- [ ] Natural creamy peanut butter and almond butter
- [ ] Sesame tahini
- [ ] Variety of nuts and seeds (unsalted raw whole almonds; unsalted walnuts, pecans, pine nuts, sunflower seeds; salted pistachios)
- [ ] Ground flaxseeds
- [ ] Graham crackers
- [ ] Almond and vanilla extracts
- [ ] Nonalkalinized cocoa powder
- [ ] Unsweetened shredded coconut
- [ ] Raisins

- [ ] High-fiber cereal, such as Fiber One
- [ ] Sprouted grain bread
- [ ] SteviaPlus or Splenda sweetener
- [ ] Granulated sugar (a small box)
- [ ] Baking soda
- [ ] Steel-cut oats
- [ ] Oat bran
- [ ] Whole wheat pastry flour
- [ ] Rye flour
- [ ] Unsweetened wheat germ (Wheat germ is the "heart" of the wheat kernel—a concentrated source of several essential nutrients including vitamin E, folate, phosphorus, thiamin, zinc, and magnesium. For the most health-promoting benefits, such as decreased cardiovascular disease risk, look for one with no added sugars.)
- [ ] Flaxseed oil
- [ ] Extra virgin olive oil
- [ ] Canola oil
- [ ] Nonstick cooking spray
- [ ] Canola oil–based mayonnaise, such as Cains All Natural Mayonnaise with Omega-3
- [ ] Vinegars (white and red wine, unsweetened rice, and balsamic)
- [ ] Light raspberry vinaigrette
- [ ] Hot-pepper sauce
- [ ] Worcestershire sauce
- [ ] Dijon and yellow mustard
- [ ] Liquid Smoke seasoning

- [ ] Dried herbs and spices (ground cardamom, cinnamon, coriander, and cumin; pumpkin pie spice; chili powder and curry powder; paprika; black peppercorns for grinding; ground white pepper; crushed red pepper flakes; fajita seasoning; bay leaves, oregano, and thyme)
- [ ] Sea salt
- [ ] Chicken stock (regular) and fat-free, reduced-sodium vegetable broth
- [ ] Canned sugar-free coconut milk, red curry paste, and Thai fish sauce (sold in the Asian food aisle)
- [ ] Sherry and red wine for cooking

CHAPTER 9

The Grains and Fruits Diet

Get ready: Here's the part where we tell you what to eat if the test in Chapter 5 indicated that you should follow the Grains and Fruits version of the *Women's Health Perfect Body Diet*. First we'll give you lists of your prescribed foods in each of the macronutrient groups. Starting on page 143, we'll give you 14 days' worth of sample meal plans. You can follow these as presented, making adjustments only as needed to hit your customized calorie count. Or you can use the prescribed foods lists (which include serving sizes, calorie counts, and grams of carbs, protein, and fat, as relevant) to build your own meals. Because after all, that's the beauty of the *Perfect Body Diet*: It helps you eat in the way that works best for *you*.

Your Perfect Carbs

The Grains and Fruits Diet contains 35 to 45 percent of calories from carbs. You'll choose from a list of carbohydrate foods that are digested a little faster but still make you feel full. You can have 150 to 185 daily grams of carbohydrates. (See "Your Perfect Body Diet Planner" on page 130 if you'd like to calculate a daily total intake based on your customized calorie count.) Your intake of carbohydrates should be higher in your main meals and lower in snacks. Remember, you'll be eating five or six times a day.

>>Your Perfect Body Diet Planner

You can use the following calculations to personalize your daily balance of the three macronutrients based on the calorie count you determined in "Customize Your Calorie Count in Three Simple Steps" on page 77.

FOR CARBOHYDRATES

Your ideal daily carb intake is 35 to 45 percent of calories. Multiply your customized calorie count by 0.35. Then divide the result by 4, since a gram of carbohydrate provides 4 calories. For example:

$$1{,}500 \text{ daily calories} \times 0.35 = 525$$

$$525 \div 4 = 131.25$$

On a 1,500-calorie diet, the minimum daily carb intake is about 131 grams.

To find the upper limit of your range, multiply your customized calorie count by 0.45. Then divide the result by 4. For example:

$$1{,}500 \text{ daily calories} \times 0.45 = 675$$

$$675 \div 4 = 168.75$$

So the maximum daily carb intake is about 169 grams.

FOR FATS

Your ideal daily fat intake is 25 to 35 percent of calories. Multiply your customized calorie count by 0.25. Then divide the result by 9, since a gram of fat provides 9 calories. For example:

VEGETABLES

You can eat the vegetables in the following list at any time of day. They have few calories, contain a lot of fiber, and provide a lot of water, so you can eat lots of them and not gain weight or add body fat. Eat them with most of your meals so that you fill up your stomach without filling out your thighs. Indulge in these foods as much as you want, as long as you stay within your daily calorie count and carb limit.

$$1{,}500 \text{ daily calories} \times 0.25 = 375$$
$$375 \div 9 = 41.66$$

On a 1,500-calorie diet, the minimum daily fat intake is about 42 grams.

To find the upper limit of your range, multiply your customized calorie count by 0.35. Then divide the result by 9. For example:

$$1{,}500 \text{ daily calories} \times 0.35 = 525$$
$$525 \div 9 = 58.33$$

So the maximum daily fat intake is about 58 grams.

FOR PROTEIN

Your ideal daily protein intake is 25 to 30 percent of calories. Multiply your customized calorie count by 0.25. Then divide the result by 4, since a gram of protein provides 4 calories. For example:

$$1{,}500 \text{ daily calories} \times 0.25 = 375$$
$$375 \div 4 = 93.75$$

On a 1,500-calorie diet, the minimum daily protein intake is about 94 grams.

To find the upper limit of your range, multiply your customized calorie count by 0.30. Then divide the result by 4. For example:

$$1{,}500 \text{ daily calories} \times 0.30 = 450$$
$$450 \div 4 = 112.5$$

So the maximum daily protein intake is about 113 grams.

VEGETABLE	SERVING SIZE	CALORIES	CARBS (G)	FIBER (G)
Artichoke	1 each, heart	60	9	4
Asparagus	12 spears	43	7	3
Bamboo shoots	½ c	12	2	1
Bean sprouts (adzuki, lentil, mung, etc.)	1 c raw	31	6	2
Bell peppers, (red, green, yellow)	1 medium, raw	32	7	2
Bok choy	1 c cooked	22	3	2

(continued)

VEGETABLE	SERVING SIZE	CALORIES	CARBS (G)	FIBER (G)
Broccoli	1 c cooked	44	8	4
Brussels sprouts	½ c cooked	32	13	4
Cabbage	1 c raw	22	4	2
Cauliflower	1 c cooked	28	5	3
Celery	3 medium stalks	30	7	3
Cherry tomatoes	10 each	35	7	2
Collards	1 c cooked	50	9	5
Cucumber	1 medium, peeled	24	5	1
Eggplant	1 c cooked	27	6	2
Endive	1 c raw	8	1	1
Garlic	1 clove	4	1	0
Green beans	1 c cooked	27	6	2
Kale	1 c cooked	36	7	3
Kohlrabi	1 c cooked	47	11	2
Leeks	1 c cooked	32	7	1
Lettuces (red, iceberg, romaine, radicchio, green leaf)	2 c raw	10	2	1
Mushrooms	10 raw	30	4	0
Okra	1 c cooked	51	11	4
Onions	½ c cooked	39	9	2
Radishes	1 c raw	15	3	1
Spaghetti squash	1 c cooked	41	10	2
Spinach	1 c cooked	41	6	4
Tomatoes	1 medium, raw	25	5	1
Zucchini and summer squash	1 c cooked	25	5	2

Although vegetables usually contain small amounts of carbohydrates, some contain more than others. The following vegetables are highest in carbohydrates and are acceptable at the specific serving sizes indicated.

VEGETABLE	SERVING SIZE	CALORIES	CARBS (G)	FIBER (G)
Baby carrots	15 each	57	12	2
Beets	1 c cooked	74	17	3
Corn, kernels (yellow or white)	½ c	72	17	2
Corn on the cob	1 cob	83	19	2
Jicama	½ small	69	16	9

VEGETABLE	SERVING SIZE	CALORIES	CARBS (G)	FIBER (G)
Parsnips	1 c cooked	126	30	6
Peas, green	⅔ c cooked	83	15	6
Potatoes (red, white or gold)	1 medium baked	132	30	3
Pumpkin	1 c canned	83	19	7
Sweet potatoes	1 medium baked	117	27	3
Turnips	2 c cooked	96	23	9
Winter squash (acorn, butternut)	1 c cooked	98–114	25–29	6–9

FRUITS

Fruits, the other namesake of the Grains and Fruits Diet, are a basis of the plan because they are loaded with healthy antioxidants. They also satisfy your sweet tooth without totally blowing your diet. For all fruits, always choose fresh, not dried, varieties. And stick with whole fruit, not fruit juice, whenever possible. Don't add sugar or artificial sweetener to your fruits either, because they're sweet enough in their natural state. One exception is grapefruit, which can use a little extra sweetness from Splenda or stevia.

FRUIT	SERVING SIZE	CALORIES	CARBS (G)	FIBER (G)
Apples	1 medium	80	22	5
Applesauce, unsweetened	½ c	52	14	1.5
Apricots	1 medium	16	4	1
Bananas	1 medium	100	27	3
Blackberries	½ c	37	9	4
Blueberries	½ c	40	10	2
Cantaloupe and other melons	¼ medium	50	12	1
Cherries	1 c, with pits	84	19	3
Cranberries, unsweetened	¼ c	23	11	2
Figs	2 each	100	24	4.5
Grapefruit	½ medium	45	11	2
Grapes	1 c	112	28	1.5
Guava	1 each	45	11	4.5
Kiwifruit	1 each	50	12	2
Mangos	1 each	130	35	3.5
Nectarine	1 each	70	16	2
Oranges	1 each	64	16	3
Papayas	½ each	118	15	2.5

(continued)

FRUIT	SERVING SIZE	CALORIES	CARBS (G)	FIBER (G)
Peaches	1 medium	42	10	2
Pears	1 medium	97	25	4
Pineapple	1 c	75	19	1.5
Plums	1 medium	36	9	1
Raspberries	½ c	30	7	4
Strawberries	½ c	22	5	2
Tangerines	1 each	36	10	1.5
Watermelon	1 slice, ⅛ melon	90	20	1

BEANS AND LEGUMES

Beans and legumes have extremely high fiber content and are perfect carbs for the Grains and Fruits Diet. Beans are very high in fiber and lower in usable calories than other carbohydrate foods, so they're great slow-digesting carbohydrates. The following nutritional information is for a ½-cup serving of cooked beans (either canned and rinsed, or fresh).

BEAN/LEGUME	CALORIES	CARBS (G)	FIBER (G)
Adzuki	147	28	8
Black	113	20	7
Black-eyed peas	100	17	6
Chickpeas	134	22	6
Fava/broadbeans	93	16	5
Great Northern	104	19	8
Kidney	110	19	9
Lentils	114	19	8
Lima	94	18	7
Navy	129	24	6
Pink	125	23	4
Pinto	117	21	7
Refried, canned, no added fats	100	18	6
Soy (edamame)	126	10	4
Split peas	115	20	8
White	127	23	9

> # What Are Sprouted Grain Breads?

We recommend breads made with sprouted grains instead of with typical refined flour. Compared with regular whole wheat bread, sprouted grain breads have greater nutritional value, including more essential protein, fiber and B vitamins, and fewer carbohydrates. Each slice explodes with flavor: We find that it tastes best when it's toasted and used for sandwiches. This type of bread must be kept cold because it has no preservatives and will spoil more easily than regular breads, so look for it in the freezer section of your local health food store or supermarket.

WHOLE GRAINS, CEREALS, BREADS, AND BAKED GOODS

Besides the foods in this chart, you can also choose whole grain breads, bagels, and English muffins made from 100 percent wheat, rye, spelt, etc. Check Nutrition Facts labels for carb and fiber content.

FOOD	SERVING SIZE	CALORIES	CARBS (G)	FIBER (G)
Barley, pearled	½ c cooked	96	22	3
Brown rice	½ c cooked	109	23	2
Bulgur (cracked wheat)	⅔ c cooked	100	22	5
Corn grits, yellow, enriched	¼ c dry	144	31	1
Couscous, whole wheat	⅔ c cooked	87	18	1
Cream of Rice	¼ c dry	160	35	1
Cream of Wheat	¼ c dry	160	33	1
Kamut	½ c cooked	173	35	9
Manna bread	¾" slice	151	29	5
Millet	½ c cooked	142	28	2
Oat bran	⅓ c dry	77	21	5
Oats, steel-cut or slow-cooking	⅓ c dry	148	27	2
Orzo, whole wheat	¼ c dry	148	30	1
Quinoa	¼ c dry	158	29	3
Sprouted grain breads, bagels, and English muffins	2 slices	160	28	6
Tortilla, corn	6", 2 each	140	28	2
Tortilla, 100% whole wheat	1 large	73	19	3
Vermicelli noodles (aka mung bean noodles)	⅔ c cooked	131	26	2
Wheat bran	2 Tbsp	15	4	3

(continued)

FOOD	SERVING SIZE	CALORIES	CARBS (G)	FIBER (G)
Wheat germ	2 Tbsp	53	5	2
Whole grain pastas	⅔ c cooked	115	24	2
Wild rice	⅔ c cooked	110	23	2

WHOLE GRAIN BREAKFAST CEREALS

Although the supermarket cereal aisle is loaded with food that could make your teeth fall out upon just reading the label, there are still a bunch of options that are great for attaining your perfect body. The following are the boxed cereals highest in fiber and lowest in sugar and other processed ingredients. When deciding how much of a cereal to eat, use the suggested serving sizes on the Nutrition Facts label as a guide. Modify as needed if the serving has more or less than 20 to 35 grams of carbohydrates or less than 10 to 12 grams of sugar.

Other great high-fiber breakfasts include hot cereals such as oatmeal and other breakfast grains. They are also high in fiber and low on the glycemic index. But if you don't have the time it takes to zap a hot cereal in the microwave, there are plenty of good cold alternatives below.

FOOD	SERVING SIZE	CALORIES	CARBS (G)	FIBER (G)
All-Bran Bran Buds	⅓ c	75	24	13
Bran flakes (add your own raisins to make a healthier, less sweet raisin bran)	¾ c	92	22	5
Cheerios	1 c	110	22	3
Corn grits, yellow, enriched	¼ c dry	144	31	1
Cream of Rice	¼ c dry	160	35	1
Cream of Wheat	¼ c dry	160	33	1
Fiber One	½ c	61	25	14
Grape-Nuts	¼ c	100	24	3
Kashi Go Lean	1 c	140	30	10
Oats, steel-cut or slow-cooking	⅓ c dry	148	27	2
Puffed rice	1 c	56	13	1
Puffed wheat	1 c	50	10	1
Shredded wheat	½ c	80	20	3

SNACKS

Although many processed carbohydrate snacks are undesirable for most women because they usually include bad fat pitfalls or too many simple sugars, the following list includes carbohydrate snacks that are acceptable for followers of the Grains and Fruits Diet. Remember to combine your carbohydrate snacks with fats, fibers, or full or partial proteins to make them a balanced and more slowly digesting treat.

FOOD	SERVING SIZE	CALORIES	CARBS (G)	FIBER (G)
Popcorn, air-popped	3 c popped	91	18	3
Triscuit crackers	8 crackers	120	21	3
Wasa Rye crackers	4 crackers	120	27	6
100% Whole Grain Wheat Thins crackers	16 crackers	140	21	2

Your Perfect Fats

The Grains and Fruits Diet gets 25 to 35 percent of its daily calories from fat. This comes out to 50 to 55 grams a day. (See "Your Perfect Body Diet Planner" on page 130 if you'd like to calculate a daily total based on your customized calorie count.) To obtain the correct balance of all the fatty acids in your diet, you should eat a wide variety of these fat-containing foods equally throughout the week. The foods can be incorporated into your diet in various ways: You can eat them as quick snacks (nuts), add them to other dishes (avocado with tomatoes, or hummus on salads), and use them as the major component of meals (salmon for dinner, eggs for breakfast).

HIGHER-SATURATED-FAT FOODS	SERVING SIZE	CALORIES	TOTAL FAT (G)	SATURATED FAT (G)
Butter, real, nonhydrogenated	1 Tbsp	100	11.5	7
Coconut, shredded, unsweetened	1 Tbsp	30	3	2.5
Dairy, low-fat				
Cheese, cottage, 1% or 2%	½ c	80–100	1–2	1–1.5
Cheese, low-fat hard (Cheddar, mozzarella)	1 oz	50	1–2	1
Milk, 1% or 2%	1 c	100–120	2–4	1.5–3
Yogurt, plain	½ c	70	1–2	1
Dairy, higher-fat (try to limit these, but you don't have to completely avoid them)				
Cheese, cottage, full-fat	½ c	108	4.5	3
Cheese, feta, crumbled	⅓ c	131	10	7
Cheese, full-fat hard and soft (Brie, Camembert)	1 oz	110	8–9	5
Cheese, ricotta, part-skim	⅓ c	170	6	6
Milk, goat's	1 c	167	10	6.5
Milk, whole	1 c	150	8	5

HIGHER-MONOUNSATURATED-FAT FOODS	SERVING SIZE	CALORIES	TOTAL FAT (G)	MONOUNSAT FAT (G)
Avocado, Florida	⅓ each	110	9	5
Avocado, Hass	⅓ each	102	10	7
Egg, whole	1 medium	68	4.5	1.8
Hummus made with olive oil	¼ c	100	6	4
Lean meats and poultry, cooked (3 oz serving is equal in size to the palm of your hand)				
Beef, lean	3 oz	200	13–15	5–7
Chicken or turkey breasts, skinless	3 oz	135	2–3	1
Chicken or turkey, lean ground	3 oz	126	6–8	3–4
Lamb, lean	3 oz	180	10–14	4–6
Pork, lean	3 oz	175	7–10	3–5
Nuts and seeds, unsalted and raw				
Almonds	¼ c	210	15	11
Cashews	¼ c	187	16	9
Hazelnuts	¼ c	178	17	13
Macadamia nuts	¼ c	240	25	20
Peanuts	¼ c	210	18	9
Pecans	¼ c	186	20	11
Pistachios	¼ c	176	13	7
Nut butters, no sugar or other ingredients added				
Almond butter	2 Tbsp	202	18	12
Cashew butter	2 Tbsp	186	16	9
Peanut butter	2 Tbsp	186	16	8
Oils				
Canola oil	1 Tbsp	120	14	8
Extra-virgin olive oil	1 Tbsp	120	14	11
Peanut oil	1 Tbsp	120	14	6

HIGHER-POLYUNSATURATED-FAT FOODS	SERVING SIZE	CALORIES	TOTAL FAT (G)	POLYUNSAT FAT (G)
Hummus made with canola oil (rich in omega-3 ALA and omega-6)	¼ c	100	6	3
Fish (rich in omega-3 EPA and DHA fat)				
Cod	4 oz cooked	120	1	0.3
Halibut	4 oz cooked	160	3	1
Herring	3.5 oz canned	210	8	3
Salmon	4 oz cooked	205	9	4
Sardines, canned in water	3.5 oz	175	9	3
Trout	4 oz cooked	160	4.5	1

HIGHER-POLYUNSATURATED-FAT FOODS	SERVING SIZE	CALORIES	TOTAL FAT (G)	POLYUNSAT FAT (G)
Tuna, canned in water	6 oz can	150	1	0.5
Tuna, fresh	4 oz cooked	150	1.5	0.5
Nuts and seeds, raw and unsalted (rich in omega-3 ALA and omega-6)				
Brazil nuts	¼ c	230	23	9, mostly omega-6
Flaxseeds, ground	2 Tbsp	150	10	6, mostly omega-3 ALA
Hemp seeds	2 Tbsp	110	8	3, mostly omega-3 ALA
Pine nuts	¼ c	190	17	7, mostly omega-6
Pumpkin seeds	¼ c	186	15	7, mostly omega-6
Sesame seeds	2 Tbsp	110	10	4.5, mostly omega-6
Soy nuts	¼ c	140	7	4
Sunflower seeds	¼ c	186	16	10, mostly omega-6
Walnuts	¼ c	163	16	12, mostly omega-3 ALA
Tahini (sesame butter), no sugar or other ingredients added	2 Tbsp	177	16	7, rich in omega-6
Oils				
Enova oil	1 Tbsp	120	14	8, rich in omega-6
Flaxseed oil	1 Tbsp	120	14	9, rich in omega-3 ALA
Safflower oil	1 Tbsp	120	14	9, rich in omega-6
Sesame seed oil	1 Tbsp	120	14	6, rich in omega-6
Sunflower oil	1 Tbsp	120	14	10, rich in omega-6

FAT-BASED CONDIMENTS AND DRESSINGS

Of all the fat-based condiments you can choose, these are the better options.

>> Cheese sauces, made with low-fat cheese

>> Pesto (see recipe on page 204)

>> Peanut sauce, made with natural peanut butter (see recipe on page 195)

>> Mayonnaise made with olive oil or canola oil (see recipe on page 203)

>> Salad dressings, low-sugar, made with olive oil or canola oil

>> Hollandaise sauce, made low fat

Your Perfect Proteins

On the Grains and Fruits Diet, 25 to 30 percent of your total daily calories will be protein, 100 to 120 grams per day. (See "Your Perfect Body Diet Planner" on page 130 if you'd like to calculate a daily total based on your customized calorie count.) You're going to differentiate between foods that are *full* proteins and ones that are *partial* proteins. Not every complete animal or plant product is a full-protein food; milk, for instance, contains only a small amount of protein, so it's considered a partial protein source in the *Women's Health Perfect Body Diet,* even though it's a complete source of protein.

Aim to eat at least three or more of your meals from the full-protein list and three of your meals from the partial-protein list. You need to have one or the other form of protein every time you eat, and if you have both in one meal, that's perfect too.

PERFECT *FULL*-PROTEIN CHOICES

These protein choices are complete and contain a high quantity of dietary protein per serving. Try to incorporate these into your three main meals every day.

FOOD	SERVING SIZE	CALORIES	PROTEIN (G)
Beef and bison (buffalo)	**3–4 oz cooked**		
Lean ground		140	18–22
Steaks, round		180	22–27
Tenderloin, lean		180	24–26
Cheese, low-fat	**2 oz unless otherwise noted**		
American		140	14
Cheddar		100	13
Cottage, 1%	½ c	80	14
Feta		100	10
Goat		80	4
Mozzarella		140	16
Ricotta	½ c	170	14
Swiss		108	13
Eggs			
Egg, whole	1 medium	68	5.5
Egg whites, liquid	½ c	105	15
Fish	**4 oz cooked unless otherwise noted**		
Catfish		190	22
Cod		120	26
Eel		260	27
Halibut		160	25
Pike		128	28
Salmon, canned and fresh		205	28
Snapper		145	29
Tilapia		145	29
Trout		160	28

FOOD	SERVING SIZE	CALORIES	PROTEIN (G)
Tuna, canned in water	6 oz can	150	32
Tuna, fresh		150	32
Protein powders			
Hemp protein powder, such as Manitoba Harvest	1 oz, 2 scoops	134	15
Rice protein powder, such as Nutribiotic Rice Protein	1 heaping Tbsp	57	12
Soy protein powder	1 oz, 1 scoop	120–150	14–20
Whey protein powder	1 oz, 1 scoop	90–120	17–25
Lamb	3 oz cooked	170–190	22–27
Milk			
Cow's milk, 1% or 2%	1 c	100–120	8
Goat's milk	1 c	167	8
Pork	**3 oz cooked**		
Canadian-style bacon		157	21
Chops, lean		175	24
Ham, lean		125	17
Lean ground		190	21
Tenderloin, lean		140	24
Poultry and fowl	**3 oz cooked**		
Chicken and turkey: breasts, ground, tenderloins, thighs, wings		140–200	21–27
Duck		170	20
Ostrich, lean ground		120	23
Shellfish	**3 oz cooked**		
Clams		100	22
Crab, not imitation		82	16
Lobster		100	17
Mussels		146	20
Oysters		60	7
Scallops		120	22
Shrimp		85	17
Soy			
Edamame (soybeans)	½ c	126	12
Soy nuts	¼ c	140	12
Tempeh	3 oz	165–185	15–18
Tofu, firm	½ c	100	10–14
Yogurt			
Greek, 2%	5 oz container	80	12–13
Plain, low-fat	½ c	120–150	8–12

PERFECT *PARTIAL*-PROTEIN CHOICES

These *partial* proteins are not complete, meaning that they are limited in or devoid of one or more of the essential amino acids. You can choose these for your two or three daily snacks between your main meals, if you don't feel like eating a full protein. If you are vegetarian, choose from these options more often.

FOOD	SERVING SIZE	CALORIES	PROTEIN (G)
Falafel	2 oz	220	9–11
Hummus (see recipe on page 182)	2 Tbsp	100	5
Beans and legumes	**½ c cooked**		
Adzuki		147	8
Black		113	7
Black-eyed peas		100	7
Chickpeas		134	7
Fava		93	6
Great Northern		104	7
Kidney		110	8
Lentils		114	9
Lima		95	6
Navy		129	8
Pink		125	8
Pinto		117	7
Refried, canned, no added fats		100	6
Split peas		115	8
White beans		127	8
Nuts and seeds, unsalted raw			
Almonds	¼ c	210	8
Brazil nuts	¼ c	230	5
Cashews	¼ c	187	5
Flaxseeds	2 Tbsp	150	6
Hemp seeds	2 Tbsp	110	6
Hazelnuts	¼ c	178	4
Macadamia nuts	¼ c	240	3
Pecans	¼ c	186	2.5
Pine nuts	¼ c	190	8
Pistachios	¼ c	176	6
Pumpkin seeds	¼ c	186	8
Sesame seeds	2 Tbsp	110	5
Sunflower seeds	¼ c	186	6
Walnuts	¼ c	163	3
Nut butters, no sugar or other ingredients added			
Almond butter	2 Tbsp	202	5
Cashew butter	2 Tbsp	186	5
Peanut butter	2 Tbsp	186	8

Your Perfect Body Meal Plans

Here are 14 days' worth of meal plans based on a 1,600-calorie daily diet. You can follow these plans exactly and you should reach your weight-less goal. But you can optimize your results by customizing these plans to fit your specific calorie needs as determined on page 130. Make changes by referring to "Your 100-Calorie Cheat Sheet" on page 79 or to the lists of perfect foods in this chapter. Chapter 10 provides the recipes for the dishes included here.

DAY 1

MEAL	DISH	PROTEIN (G)	CARBS (G)	FIBER (G)	TOTAL FAT (G)	SAT FAT (G)	CALORIES
Breakfast	Balanced-Body Smoothie (page 185)	19	24	13	14	1	378
	2 fish oil capsules	0	0	0	2	0	18
Snack	Creamy Garlic Hummus (page 182)	4	7	4	7	1	107
	12 baby carrots	1	10	2	0	0	44
Lunch	Caribbean Sweet Potato Salad (page 216), 1 serving	2	18	4	9	1	161
	3 oz baked, skinless chicken breast	26	0	0	2	0.5	122
	½ c seedless grapes	0	14	1	0	0	56
Snack	¼ c (1 oz) seedless raisins	0	22	2	0	0	88
	⅛ c whole unsalted almonds	2	2	1	7	0	79
Dinner	New Orleans Chicken with Red Beans and Rice (page 211)	33	40	9	7	1	355
	½ c cooked green peas	4	11	4	0	0	60
	1 fish oil capsule	0	0	0	1	0	9
Snack	½ c fresh raspberries	0	7	4	0	0	28
	1 c 1% milk	8	10	0	2	1	90
	Totals	99	185	44	51	5.5	1,595
	Percentages	25	46	11	29	3	100

THE GRAINS AND FRUITS DIET

DAY 2

MEAL	DISH	PROTEIN (G)	CARBS (G)	FIBER (G)	TOTAL FAT (G)	SAT FAT (G)	CALORIES
Breakfast	Gluco-Granola (page 181), 1 serving	9	19	5	15	3	247
	½ c low-fat plain yogurt	6	8	0	1.5	1	70
	mixed with 2 g glucomannan	0	0	2	0	0	0
	1 fish oil capsule	0	0	0	1	0	9
Snack	Bodacious Spinach and Bean Dip (page 182), 1 serving	10	22	3	10	1	218
	6 reduced-fat Triscuit crackers	3	18	3	3	0	111
Lunch	Chicken Taco Salad (page 212)	36	22	6	9	3	313
	1 medium apple	0	20	3	0	0	80
Snack	1 scoop whey protein powder	23	3	0	1	0	113
	mixed with ½ c water	0	0	0	0	0	0
	and 2 g glucomannan	0	0	2	0	0	0
Dinner	Turkey Shepherd's Pie (page 213), 1 serving	19	31	6	12	4	308
	Savory Poultry Gravy (page 225), 1 serving	0.5	0	1	0	0	2
	1 fish oil capsule	0	0	0	1	0	9
Snack	Gluco-Berry Protein Sorbet (page 191)	11	8	5	0	0	76
	1 fish oil capsule	0	0	0	1	0	9
	Totals	117.5	151	36	54.5	12	1,565
	Percentages	30	39	9	31	7	100

DAY 3

MEAL	DISH	PROTEIN (G)	CARBS (G)	FIBER (G)	TOTAL FAT (G)	SAT FAT (G)	CALORIES
Breakfast	**Super Fiber Breakfast Bowl (page 220)**	12	45	18	3	2	255
	1 fish oil capsule	0	0	0	1	0	9
Snack	**Creamy Garlic Hummus (page 182)**	4	7	4	7	1	107
	12 baby carrots	1	10	2	0	0	44
Lunch	**Dijon Chicken Salad (page 164), 1 serving**	29	8	4	10	2	238
	⅛ c whole unsalted almonds	2	2	1	7	0	79
Snack	**Blueberry Beet Almond Smoothie (page 224)**	7	32	10	16	1	300
Dinner	**Slow-Cooker Split-Pea Soup (page 175), 1 serving**	19	53	14	3	1	315
	1 slice sprouted grain bread	4	14	3	0	0	72
	2 fish oil capsules	0	0	0	2	0	18
Snack	**Chocolate Protein Pudding (page 228)**	21	15	6	4	1	180
	Totals	99	186	62	53	8	1,617
	Percentages	24	46	15	29	4	100

THE GRAINS AND FRUITS DIET

DAY 4

MEAL	DISH	PROTEIN (G)	CARBS (G)	FIBER (G)	TOTAL FAT (G)	SAT FAT (G)	CALORIES
Breakfast	**Scrambled Egg Whites with Spinach (page 162)**	17	13	6	8	1	192
	1 large banana	1	30	3	0	0	124
	1 fish oil capsule	0	0	0	1	0	9
Snack	**Gluco-Granola (page 181), 1 serving**	9	19	5	15	3	247
	¼ c low-fat plain yogurt	3	4	0	1	0	37
	mixed with 2 g glucomannan	0	0	2	0	0	0
	1 fish oil capsule	0	0	0	1	0	9
Lunch	**Quick Turkey, Bean, and Pea Chili (page 166)**	37	28	12	6	3	314
Snack	**Super Fiber Applesauce (page 225)**	2	15	5	7	1	131
Dinner	**Coconut Curry Shrimp with Rice (page 215)**	27	27	5	16	11	360
	1 fish oil capsule	0	0	0	1	0	9
Snack	**Ginger-Apricot Scone (page 227), 1 serving**	17	25	6	2	0.5	186
	Totals	**113**	**161**	**44**	**58**	**19.5**	**1,618**
	Percentages	**28**	**40**	**11**	**32**	**11**	**100**

DAY 5

MEAL	DISH	PROTEIN (G)	CARBS (G)	FIBER (G)	TOTAL FAT (G)	SAT FAT (G)	CALORIES
Breakfast	**Banana-Walnut Smoothie (page 223)**	15	35	12	14	3	330
	1 fish oil capsule	0	0	0	1	0	9
Snack	5 dried unsweetened prunes	0	26	3	0	0	104
	⅛ c whole unsalted almonds	2	2	1	7	0	79
Lunch	**Rainbow Broccoli Slaw (page 177), 1 serving**	2	10	5	7	1	111
	3 oz baked skinless chicken breast	26	0	0	2	0.5	122
Snack	**Spicy Gluco Guacamole (page 183), 1 serving**	1	4	3	7	1	83
	4 reduced-fat Triscuit crackers	1	12	1.5	2	0	70
Dinner	**Tasty Orzo Pilaf (page 221)**	5	29	3	2	0	154
	4 oz broiled top round steak	40	0	0	5	2	205
	⅔ c cooked green peas	5	15	5	0	0	80
	2 fish oil capsules	0	0	0	2	0	18
Snack	1 medium pear	0	25	4	0	0	100
	1 c 1% milk	8	10	0	2	1	90
	Totals	**105**	**168**	**37.5**	**51.5**	**8.5**	**1,555**
	Percentages	**27**	**43**	**10**	**30**	**5**	**100**

THE GRAINS AND FRUITS DIET

DAY 6

MEAL	DISH	PROTEIN (G)	CARBS (G)	FIBER (G)	TOTAL FAT (G)	SAT FAT (G)	CALORIES
Breakfast	**Egg and Corn Tortillas (page 210)**	19	36	7	11	3	319
	1 fish oil capsule	0	0	0	1	0	9
Snack	**1 Bran Date Muffin (page 228)**	4	19	7	7	0.5	155
Lunch	**3 Turkey and Bean Burgers (page 167)**	30	12	6	15	3	303
	½ c yellow corn kernels	2	17	2	0	0	76
	1 medium kiwifruit	0	12	2	0	0	48
Snack	½ scoop whey protein powder	11	1	0	0	0	48
	mixed with ½ c water	0	0	0	0	0	0
	and 2 g glucomannan	0	0	2	0	0	0
Dinner	**Vegetable-Stuffed Peppers (page 218), 1 serving**	23	53	15	3	1	331
	2 fish oil capsules	0	0	0	2	0	18
Snack	**Strawberry Cheesecake (page 189), 1 serving**	25	32	6	6	1	282
	Totals	**114**	**182**	**47**	**45**	**8.5**	**1,589**
	Percentages	**29**	**46**	**12**	**25**	**5**	**100**

DAY 7: LOWER-CALORIE DAY

MEAL	DISH	PROTEIN (G)	CARBS (G)	FIBER (G)	TOTAL FAT (G)	SAT FAT (G)	CALORIES
Breakfast	**1 Bran Date Muffin (page 228)**	4	19	7	7	0.5	155
	1 cheese-string snack, 2% milk fat	8	1	0	4	2.5	72
	1 fish oil capsule	0	0	0	1	0	9
Snack	**2 Turkey and Bean Burgers (page 167)**	20	8	4	10	2	202
	1½ c low-sodium V8 vegetable juice	1	18	3	0	0	76
Lunch	**Pumpkin Pie Smoothie (page 187)**	22	24	7	10	2	274
Snack	**Creamy Mushroom Soup (page 217), 1 serving**	6	18	3	7	4	159
	1 medium pear	0	25	4	0	0	100
Dinner	**Curried Chickpea Stew (page 174), 1 serving**	6	28	7	10	4	226
	3 oz cooked skinless chicken breast	26	0	0	2	0.5	122
	10 medium fresh strawberries	0	9	3	0	0	36
	2 fish oil capsules	0	0	0	2	0	18
	Totals	93	150	38	53	15.5	1,449
	Percentages	26	41	10	33	10	100

DAY 8

MEAL	DISH	PROTEIN (G)	CARBS (G)	FIBER (G)	TOTAL FAT (G)	SAT FAT (G)	CALORIES
Breakfast	**Coconut Macaroon Smoothie (page 186)**	28	26	9	11	8	315
	1 fish oil capsule	0	0	0	1	0	9
Snack	**Gluco-Granola (page 181), 1 serving**	9	19	5	15	3	247
Lunch	**Tuna Salad (page 214)**	33	0	2	6	1	186
	2 slices sprouted grain bread	8	28	6	0	0	144
Snack	**Zucchini Bread (page 226), 1 slice**	21	23	8	6	1	230
Dinner	**Brown Rice and Salmon Salad (page 214)**	25	41	5	7	1	327
	2 fish oil capsules	0	0	0	2	0	18
Snack	**Creamy Grapefruit Protein Smoothie (page 188)**	13	18	4	1	0	133
	Totals	137	155	39	49	14	1,609
	Percentages	34	39	10	27	8	100

THE GRAINS AND FRUITS DIET

DAY 9

MEAL	DISH	PROTEIN (G)	CARBS (G)	FIBER (G)	TOTAL FAT (G)	SAT FAT (G)	CALORIES
Breakfast	**Simple Oats with Whey (page 220)**	29	21	5.5	10	1	290
	1 fish oil capsule	0	0	0	1	0	9
Snack	**1 Turkey and Bean Burger (page 167)**	10	4	2	5	1	101
	½ pink grapefruit	0	11	2	0	0	44
	Splenda or stevia sweetener	0	0	0	0	0	0
Lunch	**Creamy Mushroom Soup (page 217), 1 serving**	6	18	3	7	4	159
	3 oz boiled shrimp, peeled and deveined	23	0	0	1	0	101
	with ⅓ c no-sugar-added salsa	1	6	1	0	0	28
	and 2 g glucomannan	0	0	2	0	0	0
Snack	½ c 1% cottage cheese	14	3	0	1	1	77
	¼ c (1 oz) seedless raisins	0	22	2	0	0	88
	2 g glucomannan	0	0	2	0	0	0
Dinner	**New Orleans Chicken with Red Beans and Rice (page 211)**	33	40	9	7	1	355
	1 c cooked spinach	2	3	3	0	0	20
	2 fish oil capsules	0	0	0	2	0	18
Snack	**Apple and Blackberry Fiber Crumble (page 190)**	4	34	10	14	4	278
	Totals	122	162	41.5	48	12	1,568
	Percentages	31	41	11	28	7	100

THE GRAINS AND FRUITS DIET

DAY 10

MEAL	DISH	PROTEIN (G)	CARBS (G)	FIBER (G)	TOTAL FAT (G)	SAT FAT (G)	CALORIES
Breakfast	**Ricotta Mango Breakfast (page 222)**	19	20	3	12	8	264
	1 fish oil capsule	0	0	0	1	0	9
Snack	**Spicy Gluco Guacamole (page 183), 1 serving**	1	4	3	7	1	83
	4 reduced-fat Triscuit crackers	1	12	1.5	2	0	70
Lunch	**Mixed Greens with Strawberries, Feta, and Walnuts (page 178)**	19	32	8	12.5	5	317
	2 c air-popped salted popcorn	2	13	3	0	0	60
Snack	½ scoop whey protein powder	11	1	0	0	0	48
	mixed with ½ c water	0	0	0	0	0	0
	and 2 g glucomannan	0	0	2	0	0	0
	2 fish oil capsules	0	0	0	2	0	18
Dinner	**Thick and Hearty Beef Chili (page 168)**	29	29	10	10	2	322
	2 c cooked broccoli, carrots, and cauliflower combo (fresh or frozen)	4	14	6	0	0	72
Snack	**Zucchini Bread (page 226), 1 slice**	21	23	8	6	1	230
	1 c 1% milk	8	10	0	2	1	90
	Totals	**115**	**158**	**44.5**	**54.5**	**18**	**1,583**
	Percentages	**29**	**40**	**11**	**31**	**10**	**100**

DAY 11

MEAL	DISH	PROTEIN (G)	CARBS (G)	FIBER (G)	TOTAL FAT (G)	SAT FAT (G)	CALORIES
Breakfast	**Pumpkin-Spiced Oatmeal (page 221)**	22	33	14.5	12	0	328
	1 fish oil capsule	0	0	0	1	0	9
Snack	**Zucchini Bread (page 226), 1 slice**	21	23	8	6	1	230
Lunch	**Slow-Cooker Split-Pea Soup (page 175), 1 serving**	19	53	14	3	1	315
	2 Wasa rye crackers	1	14	3	0	0	60
Snack	1 cheese-string snack, 2% milk fat	8	1	0	4	2.5	72
	1 medium kiwifruit	0	12	2	0	0	48
Dinner	**Chicken Orzo Salad (page 212)**	33	23	4	16	4	368
	2 fish oil capsules	0	0	0	2	0	18
Snack	**Chocolate Protein Pudding (page 228)**	21	15	6	4	1	180
	Totals	**125**	**174**	**51.5**	**48**	**9.5**	**1,628**
	Percentages	**31**	**43**	**13**	**27**	**5**	**100**

THE GRAINS AND FRUITS DIET

DAY 12

MEAL	DISH	PROTEIN (G)	CARBS (G)	FIBER (G)	TOTAL FAT (G)	SAT FAT (G)	CALORIES
Breakfast	**Super Fiber Breakfast Bowl (page 220)**	12	45	18	3	2	255
	1 fish oil capsule	0	0	0	1	0	9
Snack	**Pumpkin Soup (page 219), 1 serving**	4	22	10	1	0	113
	3 oz baked skinless chicken breast	26	0	0	2	0.5	122
Lunch	**Perfect Fruit and Vegetable Smoothie (page 184)**	21	39	14	12	2	348
Snack	¼ c (1 oz) seedless raisins	0	22	2	0	0	88
	2 Tbsp unsalted sunflower seeds	3	3	2	8	1	96
Dinner	**Salmon with Sage Sauce and Steamed Spinach (page 170), 1 serving**	52	11	7	18	3	450
	2 fish oil capsules	0	0	0	2	0	18
Snack	**Suspiciously Delicious Rice Pudding (page 226), 1 serving**	9	31	5	1	0	169
	Totals	127	173	58	48	8.5	1,667
	Percentages	30	42	14	26	5	100

DAY 13

MEAL	DISH	PROTEIN (G)	CARBS (G)	FIBER (G)	TOTAL FAT (G)	SAT FAT (G)	CALORIES
Breakfast	**2 Whole Wheat Buttermilk Gluco-Pancakes (page 180)**	14	30	6	6	1	230
	Super Fiber Applesauce (page 225)	2	15	5	7	1	131
	1 fish oil capsule	0	0	0	1	0	9
Snack	**1 Pumpkin Protein Fiber Muffin (page 191)**	7	12	4	13	1	193
Lunch	**Stuffed Peppers with Tuna Salad (page 169)**	35	21	7	3	0	251
	1 c pineapple chunks in water	1	21	2	0	0	88
Snack	**Crab-Stuffed Mushroom Caps (page 173), 1 serving**	8	3	3	10	1	134
	1½ c low-sodium V8 vegetable juice	1	18	3	0	0	76
Dinner	4 oz broiled top round steak	40	0	0	5	2	205
	Asparagus with Dill Mustard Sauce (page 176), 1 serving	7	12	5	1	0	85
	½ c cooked brown rice	2	23	1	0	0	100
Snack	**Gluco-Berry Protein Sorbet (page 191)**	11	8	5	0	0	76
	2 fish oil capsules	0	0	0	2	0	18
	Totals	**128**	**163**	**41**	**47**	**6**	**1,587**
	Percentages	**32**	**41**	**10**	**27**	**3**	**100**

THE GRAINS AND FRUITS DIET

DAY 14: LOWER-CALORIE DAY

MEAL	DISH	PROTEIN (G)	CARBS (G)	FIBER (G)	TOTAL FAT (G)	SAT FAT (G)	CALORIES
Breakfast	**Eggs with Gluco-Salsa (page 163)**	15	6	3	9	2	165
	1 slice sprouted grain bread	4	14	3	0	0	72
	½ c fresh blueberries	0	10	1	0	0	40
	2 fish oil capsules	0	0	0	2	0	18
Snack	**Apple Pie Smoothie (page 223)**	24	28	7	9	1	289
Lunch	**Garden Asparagus Leek Soup (page 176), 1 serving**	4	12	6	9	1	145
	4 oz broiled tilapia or snapper	29	0	0	1	0	125
Snack	2 c air-popped salted popcorn	2	13	3	0	0	60
	1 cheese-string snack, 2% milk fat	8	1	0	4	2.5	72
Dinner	**Slow-Cooker Chicken Cacciatore (page 165)**	33	16	5	8	1	268
	⅔ c cooked bulgur	3	22	2	0	0	100
	1 fish oil capsule	0	0	0	1	0	9
	Totals	**122**	**122**	**30**	**43**	**7.5**	**1,363**
	Percentages	**36**	**36**	**9**	**28**	**5**	**100**

Shopping List

This list includes most of the food items you will need to have on hand to prepare the dishes specified in the meal plans. A few words about freshness: Since it's best to buy fruits, vegetables, and fresh herbs immediately before use, we have not included every type here. Keep in mind that nuts and seeds stay freshest in the refrigerator or freezer; grains and flours are best stored in airtight containers and used within a couple of months.

☐ 1% milk

☐ Low-fat buttermilk

☐ Half-and-half

☐ Butter, salted and unsalted

☐ Fat-free or low-fat plain yogurt

☐ Fat-free sour cream

☐ Low-fat soft cheeses (fat-free cream cheese, reduced-fat feta, part-skim ricotta, 1% cottage cheese)

☐ Soft goat cheese

☐ Low-fat Cheddar cheese

☐ Grated Parmesan cheese

☐ Cheese string snacks, individually wrapped

☐ 4½"-diameter corn tortillas

☐ Medium or omega-3 eggs

☐ Pasteurized liquid egg substitute

☐ Pasteurized liquid egg whites, such as Eggology

☐ Top round steak

☐ Lean ground turkey and lean ground beef

☐ Boneless, skinless chicken breasts

☐ Fresh fish fillets (salmon, tilapia)

☐ Canned chunk light tuna, packed in water

☐ Pouches of salmon, packed in water

- [ ] Canned crabmeat
- [ ] Fresh berries and fruit in season (keep apples, bananas, lemons, and limes on hand)
- [ ] Fresh vegetables (keep garlic, onions, and 10-bags of spinach on hand)
- [ ] Fresh tubers and root vegetables (keep Yukon gold potatoes, sweet potatoes, and parsnips on hand)
- [ ] Fresh herbs
- [ ] Unsweetened carrot juice, such as Odwalla
- [ ] Frozen berries
- [ ] Frozen peas, corn, and spinach
- [ ] Canned tomato paste, no-salt-added tomato sauce, whole peeled tomatoes, and diced, low-salt, no-sugar-added tomatoes
- [ ] Canned mandarin oranges in juice, pineapple in water, and pumpkin puree
- [ ] Jarred unsweetened applesauce
- [ ] Jarred capers and canned or jarred pimiento-stuffed green olives
- [ ] Canola oil–based mayonnaise, such as Cains All Natural Mayonnaise with Omega-3
- [ ] Light mayonnaise
- [ ] Dijon and yellow mustards
- [ ] Liquid Smoke seasoning
- [ ] Hot-pepper sauce
- [ ] Worcestershire sauce
- [ ] Vinegars (white and red wine, and unsweetened rice)
- [ ] Light raspberry vinaigrette
- [ ] Low-sodium V8 100% vegetable juice
- [ ] Canned unsweetened pineapple juice

- ☐ Canned diced tomatoes, no sugar-added
- ☐ Canned and dried beans (black, pinto, white, red kidney, chickpeas; dried split green peas)
- ☐ Chocolate, vanilla, and strawberry whey protein powders
- ☐ Sugar-free strawberry jam
- ☐ Natural creamy peanut butter
- ☐ Variety of nuts and seeds (unsalted raw whole almonds; unsalted walnuts, pecans, pine nuts, and sunflower seeds)
- ☐ Ground flaxseeds
- ☐ Unsweetened shredded coconut
- ☐ Unsweetened canned coconut milk
- ☐ Dried fruit (raisins, unsweetened prunes, unsweetened apricots, chopped dates)
- ☐ High-fiber cereal, such as Fiber One
- ☐ Sprouted grain bread
- ☐ Brown rice
- ☐ Bulgur
- ☐ Steel-cut oats
- ☐ Oat bran
- ☐ Whole wheat pastry flour and whole wheat all-purpose flour
- ☐ Stone ground rye flour
- ☐ Sweeteners (SteviaPlus or Splenda sweetener in sachets, Baking Splenda, Splenda brown sugar blend)
- ☐ Granulated sugar (a small box)
- ☐ Maple syrup
- ☐ Baking soda and baking powder
- ☐ Vanilla extract

- [ ] Dried herbs and spices (ground cinnamon, nutmeg, ginger, coriander, and cumin; pumpkin pie spice; chili powder and curry powder; paprika; black peppercorns for grinding; crushed red pepper flakes; celery salt; poultry seasoning; bay leaves, oregano, and thyme)
- [ ] Sea salt
- [ ] Fat-free, reduced-sodium chicken broth, regular chicken broth, and organic vegetable stock
- [ ] Unsweetened wheat germ
- [ ] Wheat bran
- [ ] Flaxseed oil
- [ ] Extra virgin olive oil
- [ ] Canola oil
- [ ] Nonstick cooking spray (olive oil and plain)
- [ ] Crackers (reduced-fat Triscuits, Wasa rye crackers, and graham crackers)
- [ ] Baked corn tortilla chips
- [ ] No-sugar-added salsa (mild and hot)
- [ ] Orzo
- [ ] Popcorn kernels or microwave popcorn, no flavorings added
- [ ] Sherry and red wine for cooking

CHAPTER 10

Your Perfect Recipes

We now present all the recipes included in the meal plans in Chapters 8 and 9. The first group of 33 recipes includes dishes that are appropriate for both the Greens and Berries Diet and the Grains and Fruits Diet. Recipes specially formulated for the Greens and Berries Diet are found on pages 192 to 208; there are 25 of these. Grains and Fruits girls will find 28 recipes designed just for them on pages 209 to 228.

Each recipe uses glucomannan as an ingredient. Since all of your food will get thicker and more satisfying with glucomannan, make sure to wash it down with plenty of water; drink at least 8 ounces of H_2O with every meal or snack. For the best taste and texture—clumps of glucomannan aren't exactly gourmet, and they could even get stuck in your throat—always mix the powder thoroughly into your grub and wait 2 to 3 minutes for it to soak up whatever sauce, broth, dressing, or other liquid is on your plate or in your bowl or glass. Sit back and watch your serving size expand without any extra calories.

Scrambled Egg Whites with Spinach

2⅔ cups 5 medium egg whites, separated from yolks

⅓ cup chopped spinach

2 tablespoons unsalted raw sunflower seeds

½ cup no-sugar-added salsa

2 grams glucomannan

1. Coat a small skillet with olive oil cooking spray. Heat to medium-high.

2. Add the egg whites, spinach, and sunflower seeds. Cook, stirring, to desired doneness.

3. In a small bowl, combine the salsa and glucomannan. Let stand for 1 minute to thicken.

4. Remove the eggs to a plate. Top with the gluco-salsa.

SERVES 1
PER SERVING:
192 calories, 17 g protein, 13 g carbs, 6 g fiber, 8 g total fat, 1 g saturated fat

Eggs with Gluco-Salsa

2 **medium or omega-3 eggs**

1 **egg white**

   Ground black pepper to taste (optional)

⅓ **cup no-sugar-added salsa**

2 **grams glucomannan**

1. Coat a small skillet with olive oil cooking spray and heat to medium-high.

2. Add the eggs and egg white. Cook, stirring, to desired doneness. Season with pepper, if desired.

3. In a small bowl, mix the salsa and glucomannan.

4. Remove the eggs to a plate. Top with the gluco-salsa.

SERVES 1
PER SERVING:
165 calories, 15 g protein, 6 g carbs, 3 g fiber, 9 g total fat, 2 g saturated fat

Dijon Chicken Salad

1½ tablespoons chicken broth, regular

1½ tablespoons Dijon mustard

1 tablespoon extra-virgin olive oil

4 grams glucomannan

2–3 ounces broiled boneless, skinless chicken breasts, chopped

½ cup chopped celery

⅓ cup peeled, chopped sweet apples (such as Golden Delicious)

1 tablespoon capers, drained (optional)

Salt and ground black pepper to taste

1. In a medium bowl, mix together the broth, mustard, oil, and glucomannan. Let stand for about 5 minutes to thicken.

2. Add the chicken, celery, apples, and capers (if using). Toss until well combined. Season with salt and pepper. Chill before serving.

SERVES 2
PER SERVING:
238 calories, 29 g protein, 8 g carbs, 4 g fiber, 10 g total fat, 2 g saturated fat

Slow-Cooker Chicken Cacciatore

- 3 pounds boneless,
  skinless chicken breasts
- ¼ cup + 2 tablespoons
  extra-virgin olive oil
- 1 medium yellow onion,
  coarsely chopped
- 1 large red bell pepper,
  coarsely chopped
- 1 cup white mushrooms, halved
- 1 can (28 ounces) whole peeled tomatoes, with juice
- 1 can (12 ounces) tomato paste
- ½ cup regular chicken stock
- ½ cup red cooking wine
- 3 cloves garlic, minced
- 1 bay leaf
- 2 tablespoons minced fresh oregano
- 2 tablespoons minced fresh parsley
- 1 tablespoon minced fresh basil
- 1 teaspoon salt
- ½ teaspoon ground black pepper
- 20 grams glucomannan

1. In a large nonstick saucepan over medium-high heat, brown the chicken in 2 tablespoons of the oil. Do not cook through.

2. In a large slow cooker, combine the remaining ingredients.

3. Add the chicken to the slow cooker.

4. Cook on high heat for 4 hours or on low heat for 8 hours.

5. Immediately before eating, add 2 grams of the glucomannan to each serving.

SERVES 10
PER SERVING:
268 calories, 33 g protein, 16 g carbs, 5 g fiber, 8 g total fat, 1 g saturated fat

Quick Turkey, Bean, and Pea Chili

¼ cup frozen green peas

3 ounces lean ground turkey

½ cup canned red kidney beans,
drained and rinsed

½ cup no-sugar-added tomato sauce

2 grams glucomannan

1. Cook the peas in the microwave oven according to the package directions.

2. Coat a nonstick skillet with olive oil cooking spray. Add the turkey and cook, breaking apart the meat, over medium-high heat for 10 minutes, until browned. Set aside to cool for at least 5 minutes.

3. In a medium microwaveable bowl, combine the peas, turkey, beans, tomato sauce, and glucomannan. Stir well. Heat in the microwave for 1 minute before serving.

SERVES 1
PER SERVING:
314 calories, 37 g protein, 28 g carbs, 12 g fiber, 6 g total fat, 3 g saturated fat

Turkey and Bean Burgers

1 tablespoon butter	2 pounds lean ground turkey
1 large yellow onion, chopped	2 large or omega-3 eggs
1 large carrot, grated	2 teaspoons chili powder
1½ cups canned dark red kidney beans, drained and rinsed	¼ teaspoon freshly ground black pepper
12 grams glucomannan	½ teaspoon sea salt
½ cup water	½ teaspoon dried oregano

1. Preheat the oven to 325°F. Coat a nonstick baking sheet with olive oil cooking spray.

2. In a large saucepan, over medium-high heat, melt the butter. Add the onion and carrot. Cook for 3 to 5 minutes, until the onion is lightly browned. Remove from the heat and set aside.

3. In a large bowl, mash the beans.

4. In a medium bowl, mix together the glucomannan and water to thicken. Add to the mashed beans.

5. Add the ground turkey, eggs, onion-and-carrot mixture, chili powder, pepper, salt, and oregano. Mix well.

6. Form the mixture into 18 patties, each about ½" thick and 3" in diameter, placing them on the prepared baking sheet. Bake for 45 minutes, or until a thermometer inserted in the center of a burger registers 165°F and the meat is no longer pink.

MAKES 18 SMALL BURGERS
PER BURGER:
101 calories, 10 g protein, 4 g carbs, 2 g fiber, 5 g total fat, 1 g saturated fat

Thick and Hearty Beef Chili

2 tablespoons extra-virgin olive oil

1½ pounds lean ground beef

Sea salt to taste

Freshly ground black pepper to taste

1 medium yellow onion, chopped

1 green or red bell pepper, seeded and chopped

3 cloves garlic, minced

2 cans (28 ounces each) no-sugar-added diced tomatoes

1 can (15 ounces) pinto beans, rinsed and drained

2 tablespoons chili powder

1 tablespoon fresh oregano or ½ teaspoon dried

2 teaspoons hot-pepper sauce

2 teaspoons ground cumin

2 teaspoons unsweetened cocoa powder

1 cup frozen corn kernels, thawed

2 tablespoons chopped fresh cilantro

1 tablespoon fresh lime juice

12 grams glucomannan

1. In a large pot over medium heat, heat 1 tablespoon of the olive oil. Add the beef. Season with the salt and black pepper. Cook, stirring, for 5 minutes, until lightly browned. Transfer to a medium bowl.

2. In the same pot, combine the onion, bell pepper, garlic, and the remaining 1 tablespoon oil. Cook for 5 minutes. Stir in the tomatoes (with juice), beans, chili powder, oregano, hot-pepper sauce, cumin, and cocoa powder. Reduce the heat to medium-low and cook, covered, for 30 minutes.

3. Add the beef, corn, cilantro, lime juice, and glucomannan. Cook, uncovered, for 15 minutes, until thick.

SERVES 6
PER SERVING:
322 calories, 29 g protein, 29 g carbs, 10 g fiber, 10 g total fat, 2 g saturated fat

Stuffed Peppers with Tuna Salad

- 1 can (6 ounces) chunk light tuna packed in water, drained slightly (keep some water so the glucomannan mixes easily)
- 4 small pimiento-stuffed green olives, chopped
- 2 grams glucomannan
- 1 small clove garlic, minced
- ½ cup mandarin oranges packed in juice, drained
- 1½ tablespoons red wine vinegar
- 2 teaspoons finely chopped red onion
- 1 medium red bell pepper, halved, seeded, and stem removed

1. In a medium bowl, mix together all of the ingredients except the pepper.

2. Spoon half of the tuna salad mixture into each pepper half. Serve immediately.

SERVES 1
PER SERVING:
251 calories, 35 g protein, 21 g carbs, 7 g fiber, 3 g total fat, 0 g saturated fat

Tip: Look for a red pepper with a flat bottom. Otherwise, the "bowl" will be hard to stuff and even trickier to eat.

Salmon with Sage Sauce and Steamed Spinach

1 pound salmon fillets

1 microwaveable bag (10 ounces) fresh spinach leaves

1 tablespoon extra-virgin olive oil

3 cloves garlic, minced

¼ large yellow onion, chopped

8 grams glucomannan

½ cup water

⅔ cup low-fat plain yogurt

⅓ cup sherry

10 fresh sage leaves, chopped

¼ cup fresh parsley, chopped

1 tablespoon fresh lemon juice

Fresh ground sea salt to taste

1 teaspoon white vinegar

1. In a large nonstick skillet over medium-high heat, cook the salmon for 7 minutes per side, until the middle is barely cooked through. Remove to a plate and set aside.

2. While salmon is cooking, add about ½" of water to a large cooking pot. Then, add the spinach. Cover the pot and bring the water to a boil over high heat. Once the water is boiling, open the lid and check to see if the spinach is reduced in volume and steamed down. If not, let boil a minute or two longer. Once the leaves are steamed down, remove from heat and let stand while covered, until the remaining steps of the recipe are complete.

3. Reduce the heat to medium. In the same skillet, combine the oil, garlic, and onion. Cook, stirring frequently, for 3 to 5 minutes, until lightly brown.

4. In a medium bowl, combine the glucomannan and water. Let stand to thicken, about 2 to 3 minutes.

5. Add the glucomannan, yogurt, sherry, sage, parsley, and lemon juice to the skillet. Stir well to mix. Season with the salt to taste.

6. Cook until the sauce becomes thick and creamy, about 7 minutes.

7. Add the salmon to the skillet and reheat until the meat is completely cooked though, about 4 to 5 minutes. Divide the salmon and sauce into two equal portions.

8. Season the spinach with the vinegar and add half to each serving plate.

SERVES 2
PER SERVING:
450 calories, 52 g protein, 11 g carbs, 7 g fiber, 18 g total fat, 3 g saturated fat

Salmon with Cucumber Dill Sauce

½ cup cucumber, peeled, seeded, and chopped

¼ cup fat-free sour cream

¼ cup fat-free plain yogurt

2 tablespoons finely chopped fresh dill

1 tablespoons canola oil–based mayonnaise

½ tablespoon white vinegar

½ teaspoon salt

8 grams glucomannan

1 pound salmon fillet with skin

1. In a medium bowl, mix together all of the ingredients except the salmon until well blended. Refrigerate for 1 to 2 hours to allow flavors to meld.

2. Preheat the broiler.

3. Place the salmon skin side up on a broiler pan. Broil 5" to 6" from the heat for 7 to 9 minutes per side, until the fish flakes easily with a fork.

4. Allow to cool slightly. Remove the skin if desired. Divide the salmon between two plates. Serve each plate with half of the dill sauce.

SERVES 2
PER SERVING:
399 calories, 47 g protein, 10 g carbs, 8 g fiber, 19 g total fat, 3 g saturated fat

Tilapia with Cucumber Salsa

TILAPIA

- 4 tilapia or red snapper fillets (about 4 ounces each)
- 2 tablespoons fresh lemon juice
- 1 tablespoon finely chopped fresh oregano
- ¼ teaspoon paprika
- ⅛ teaspoon salt

SALSA

- ¼ cup water
- 2 tablespoons fresh lemon juice
- 1 tablespoon extra-virgin olive oil
- 8 grams glucomannan
- ¾ cup peeled, finely chopped cucumber
- ¼ cup chopped fresh mint or snipped fresh parsley
- 2 tablespoons capers, rinsed and drained
- ⅛ teaspoon salt

TO MAKE THE TILAPIA

1. Preheat the oven to 400°F.

2. Lightly coat a 13" × 9" × 2" baking dish with olive oil cooking spray.

3. Rinse the fish and pat dry with paper towels. Arrange in a single layer in the dish. Spoon the lemon juice over the fish. Sprinkle with the oregano, paprika, and salt.

4. Bake for 10 minutes, or until the fish flakes easily.

TO MAKE THE SALSA

1. In a small bowl, stir together the water, lemon juice, oil, and glucomannan. Once thickened, add the cucumber, mint or parsley, capers, and salt.

2. Spoon ¼ cup of the salsa over each fillet.

SERVES 4
PER SERVING:
144 calories, 24 g protein, 3 g carbs, 3 g fiber, 4 g total fat, 1 g saturated fat

Crab-Stuffed Mushroom Caps

12 **large white mushrooms**

1 **tablespoon extra-virgin olive oil**

2 **tablespoons minced white onion**

4 **ounces canned crabmeat, drained**

2 **tablespoons canola oil–based mayonnaise**

2 **tablespoons grated Parmesan cheese**

1 **tablespoon chopped fresh parsley**

1 **teaspoon salt**

1 **teaspoon ground black pepper**

3 **drops hot-pepper sauce**

8 **grams glucomannan**

1. Preheat the oven to 400°F.

2. Wash the mushrooms and pat dry with a paper towel. Pull out the stems, leaving a hole where the filling will go. Chop the stems finely. Set aside.

3. In a nonstick skillet, heat the oil to medium. Add the reserved mushroom stems and the onion. Cook, stirring, for 3 to 4 minutes, until the vegetables are tender.

4. In a medium bowl, combine the mushroom mixture with the crabmeat, mayonnaise, cheese, parsley, salt, black pepper, hot-pepper sauce, and glucomannan. Let stand for a few minutes to thicken.

5. Using a teaspoon, stuff each mushroom with an equal amount of filling, mounding the filling on top.

6. Arrange the stuffed mushrooms in a single layer in a shallow baking pan. Bake for 15 minutes. Serve hot or at room temperature.

SERVES 4 (3 EACH)
PER SERVING:
134 calories, 8 g protein, 3 g carbs, 3 g fiber, 10 g total fat, 1 g saturated fat

Curried Chickpea Stew

2 tablespoons extra-virgin olive oil

1½ cups diced onion

1 teaspoon ground cumin

1 teaspoon curry powder

¾ teaspoon salt

3 cloves garlic, minced

12 grams glucomannan

1½ cups fat-free, reduced-sodium vegetable broth

1 can (28 ounces) no-salt-added diced tomatoes, drained

1 can (19 ounces) chickpeas, drained and rinsed

1 can (13.5 ounces) light coconut milk

1. In a large stockpot, heat the oil to medium-high.

2. Add the onion, cumin, curry powder, and salt. Cook, stirring, for 4 minutes. Add the garlic. Cook, stirring, for 1 minute.

3. In a medium bowl, mix together the glucomannan and broth. Add to the pot.

4. Add the tomatoes, chickpeas, and coconut milk. Stir well. Bring to a boil.

5. Reduce the heat to medium-low. Cook for 30 minutes, stirring occasionally.

6. Remove from the heat. Place 1 cup of the soup in a blender or food processor. Blend until smooth. Return the blended soup to the pot. Mix well.

SERVES 6
PER SERVING (ABOUT 1 CUP):
226 calories, 6 g protein, 28 g carbs, 7 g fiber, 10 g total fat, 4 g saturated fat

Slow-Cooker Split-Pea Soup

- 1 pound dried split green peas
- 3 stalks celery with leaves, chopped
- 2 cloves garlic, minced
- 1 large yellow onion, chopped
- 1 cup baby carrots, chopped
- ½ cup chopped fresh parsley
- 1 tablespoon dried thyme
- 2 bay leaves
- 2 teaspoons sea salt

  Freshly ground black pepper to taste
- 1 tablespoon extra-virgin olive oil
- 2 teaspoons liquid smoke seasoning
- 4 cups (32 ounces) vegetable stock
- 12 grams glucomannan
- 2 cups water

1. In a large bowl, soak the peas in enough water to cover them by 2" for 4 hours. Drain and rinse.

2. In a slow cooker, combine the peas, celery, garlic, onion, carrots, parsley, thyme, bay leaves, salt, pepper, oil, and liquid smoke. Add the stock.

3. In a medium bowl, combine the glucomannan and water. Stir to thicken. Add to the slow cooker. Mix.

4. Cook on low for 8 to 9 hours or on high for 4 to 5 hours, until the peas are completely cooked and softened.

SERVES 6
PER SERVING:
315 calories, 19 g protein, 53 g carbs, 14 g fiber, 3 g total fat, 1 g saturated fat

YOUR PERFECT RECIPES

Garden Asparagus Leek Soup

2 tablespoons extra-virgin olive oil

1 large leek, roughly chopped

1 bunch asparagus (about 1 pound), roughly chopped

2½ cups vegetable stock

2 cloves garlic, minced

1 teaspoon salt

1 teaspoon ground black pepper

8 grams glucomannan

1. In a skillet over low temperature, heat the oil. Add the leek and cook for 15 minutes, or until tender.

2. Transfer the leek to a large pot. Add the asparagus and stock. Cover and cook over medium heat for 15 minutes, until the asparagus is tender.

3. Transfer the soup to a food processor. Add the garlic, salt, pepper, and glucomannan. Blend until smooth.

SERVES 3
PER SERVING:
145 calories, 4 g protein, 12 g carbs, 6 g fiber, 9 g total fat, 1 g saturated fat

Asparagus with Dill Mustard Sauce

2 pounds asparagus stalks, ends trimmed off

½ cup low-fat plain yogurt

⅛ cup water

8 grams glucomannan

2 tablespoons finely chopped fresh dill

1 tablespoon Dijon mustard

¼ teaspoon salt

¼ teaspoon ground black pepper

1. Bring a large pot of water to boil over high heat. Add the asparagus. Boil for about 15 minutes, until tender.

2. In a small bowl, combine the remaining ingredients. Mix until smooth.

3. Evenly divide the asparagus among 4 plates. Top each with one-quarter of the mustard sauce.

SERVES 4
PER SERVING:
85 calories, 7 g protein, 12 g carbs, 5 g fiber, 1 g total fat, 0 g saturated fat

Note: The glucomannan will thicken the mustard sauce if left to sit too long; if this occurs, add a small amount of water to thin out the sauce to the desired consistency.

Rainbow Broccoli Slaw

1 bag (6 ounces) shredded broccoli coleslaw mixture

2 scallions, chopped

½ red bell pepper, cut into thin strips

½ yellow bell pepper, cut into thin strips

½ medium zucchini, cut into thin strips

⅓ small red onion, cut into thin strips

¼ pound snow peas, halved

4 tablespoons fresh cilantro, finely chopped

2 tablespoons extra-virgin olive oil

2 tablespoons unsweetened rice vinegar

2 tablespoons water

1 teaspoon granulated sugar

8 grams glucomannan

¼ teaspoon salt

¼ teaspoon ground black pepper

1. In a large bowl, combine the coleslaw mixture, scallions, red and yellow bell peppers, zucchini, onion, snow peas, and cilantro.

2. In a small bowl, whisk together the oil, vinegar, water, sugar, glucomannan, salt, and black pepper.

3. Add the vinaigrette to the vegetables. Cover and toss until well coated.

4. Refrigerator for 1 hour to allow the flavors to meld.

SERVES 4
PER SERVING:
111 calories, 2 g protein, 10 g carbs, 5 g fiber, 7 g total fat, 1 g saturated fat

Mixed Greens with Strawberries, Feta, and Walnuts

    3 cups mixed greens, washed and dried well

    4 medium fresh strawberries, sliced

    3 medium white mushrooms, sliced

    1 ounce (about ¼ cup) crumbled reduced-fat feta cheese

6–8 walnut halves

    2 tablespoons light raspberry vinaigrette

    ¾ cup low-fat plain yogurt

    2 grams glucomannan

1. In a large bowl, combine the greens, strawberries, mushrooms, feta, and walnuts. Toss.

2. Drizzle with the vinaigrette.

3. In a small bowl, mix together the yogurt and glucomannan. Let stand for 3 to 5 minutes to thicken. Serve the salad with the gluco-yogurt mixture on the side.

SERVES 1
PER SERVING:
317 calories, 19 g protein, 32 g carbs, 8 g fiber, 12.5 g total fat, 5 g saturated fat

Milk-Free Creamed Cauliflower

1 **large head cauliflower, separated into florets**

8 **grams glucomannan**

   Salt and ground black pepper to taste

1. Place a steamer basket in a large pot with 2" of water. Bring to a boil over high heat. Place the cauliflower in the basket and steam for 10 minutes, or until soft enough to easily pierce with a fork.

2. Transfer the cauliflower to a food processor or a blender. Process until smooth. Add the glucomannan, salt, and pepper. Pour from blender into a large bowl. Divide into 4 servings and enjoy.

SERVES 4
PER SERVING:
48 calories, 3 g protein, 9 g carbs, 6 g fiber, 0 g total and saturated fat

Whole Wheat Buttermilk Gluco-Pancakes

2 eggs, lightly beaten

1 cup low-fat buttermilk

2 tablespoons canola oil

¾ cup whole wheat pastry flour

¼ cup wheat germ

1 teaspoon baking soda

¼ teaspoon salt

8 grams glucomannan

1. In a medium bowl, combine the eggs, buttermilk, and oil. Stir in the flour, wheat germ, baking soda, salt, and glucomannan. Mix until blended.

2. Coat a skillet with olive oil cooking spray. Heat to medium-high.

3. Pour ¼ cup of the batter into the skillet. Cook until golden brown, 3 minutes per side, turning once. Repeat with the remaining batter to make a total of 6 pancakes.

SERVES 2 (3 PANCAKES EACH)
PER PANCAKE:
115 calories, 7 g protein, 15 g carbs, 3 g fiber, 3 g total fat, 0.5 g saturated fat

Gluco-Granola

1 cup steel-cut oats

½ cup unsalted, raw sunflower seeds

½ cup shredded unsweetened coconut

½ cup unsalted pecan halves

¼ cup toasted wheat germ

1 scoop vanilla whey protein powder

4 tablespoons water

1 tablespoon canola oil

8 grams glucomannan

1. Preheat the oven to 350°F.

2. In a large bowl, combine the oats, sunflower seeds, coconut, pecans, and wheat germ.

3. In a small bowl, mix together the whey protein powder, water, oil, and glucomannan. Stir until it becomes a viscous gel.

4. Add the glucomannan mixture to the oat mixture. Mix together until well coated.

5. Spread onto a baking sheet.

6. Bake for 20 minutes, until golden brown, stirring after 10 minutes.

SERVES 8
PER SERVING:
247 calories, 9 g protein, 19 g carbs, 5 g fiber, 15 g total fat, 3 g saturated fat

Variations: Try different types of nuts and seeds, such as almonds and pumpkin seeds. Chopped dried fruit can be added after baking.

Bodacious Spinach and Bean Dip

2 cups frozen spinach, cooked according to the package directions

1 can (15 ounces) white beans, drained and rinsed

2 tablespoons extra-virgin olive oil

2 teaspoons fresh lemon juice

1 tablespoon + ½ cup water

6 grams glucomannan

Salt and ground black pepper to taste

1. In a blender or food processor, combine the spinach, beans, oil, lemon juice, and 1 tablespoon of the water. Blend until creamy.

2. In a small bowl, combine the glucomannan and the remaining ½ cup water. Mix until blended evenly and smoothly. Add to the blender. Blend briefly. Season with salt and pepper.

SERVES 3
PER SERVING:
218 calories, 10 g protein, 22 g carbs, 3 g fiber, 10 g total fat, 1 g saturated fat

Creamy Garlic Hummus

1 can (15 ounces) chickpeas, drained and rinsed

¾ cup water

½ cup sesame tahini

¼ cup fresh lemon juice

2 cloves garlic

1 teaspoon sea salt

¼ teaspoon cumin

16 grams glucomannan

1 tablespoon chopped fresh parsley

¼ teaspoon paprika

1. In a blender or food processor, combine the chickpeas, water, tahini, lemon juice, garlic, sea salt, cumin, and glucomannan. Blend until smooth and creamy.

2. Add more water if needed to achieve desired consistency; the hummus will thicken slightly upon standing. Garnish with the parsley and paprika.

SERVES 10
PER SERVING:
107 calories, 4 g protein, 7 g carbs, 4 g fiber, 7 g total fat, 1 g saturated fat

Spicy Gluco Guacamole

2 ripe medium Hass avocados, chopped

Juice of 1 lime

½ jalapeño chile pepper, seeded and chopped

½ cup seeded and chopped tomato

¼ cup diced red onion

1 tablespoon chopped fresh cilantro

½ teaspoon salt

8 grams glucomannan

In a large bowl, combine all of the ingredients. Mash with a potato ricer or fork until you achieve the desired consistency.

SERVES 8
PER ⅓-CUP SERVING:
83 calories, 1 g protein, 4 g carbs, 3 g fiber, 7 g total fat, 1 g saturated fat

Perfect Fruit and Vegetable Smoothie

1 medium apple, peeled, cored and sliced

⅓ Hass avocado, ripe

½ cup frozen spinach

½ cup low-fat plain yogurt

½ cup pasteurized egg whites

¼ cup raspberries, frozen or fresh

¼ cup water

4 grams glucomannan

   Ice cubes

In a blender, combine all of the ingredients. Blend until smooth and creamy. Pour immediately into a large cup.

SERVES 1
PER SERVING:
348 calories, 21 g protein, 39 g carbs, 14 g fiber, 12 g total fat, 2 g saturated fat

Balanced-Body Smoothie

GREENS AND BERRIES DIET

- ½ cup fresh or frozen raspberries
- ⅓ cup 1% cottage cheese
- ⅓ cup low-fat plain yogurt
- 2 tablespoons natural creamy peanut butter
- 1 tablespoon ground flaxseeds
- 4 grams glucomannan

GRAINS AND FRUITS DIET

- ½ cup fresh or frozen raspberries
- 1 medium banana
- ⅓ cup 1% cottage cheese
- ¼ cup low-fat plain yogurt
- 1 tablespoon ground flaxseeds
- 1 tablespoon natural creamy peanut butter
- 4 grams glucomannan

In a blender, combine all of the ingredients. Blend until smooth and creamy. Pour immediately into a large cup.

SERVES 1

GREENS AND BERRIES DIET, PER SERVING:
382 calories, 24 g protein, 22 g carbs, 12 g fiber, 22 g total fat, 2.5 g saturated fat

GRAINS AND FRUITS DIET, PER SERVING:
378 calories, 19 g protein, 24 g carbs, 13 g fiber, 14 g total fat, 1 g saturated fat

Coconut Macaroon Smoothie

GREENS AND BERRIES DIET

- ½ cup pasteurized liquid egg whites
- ½ scoop vanilla whey protein powder
- ⅓ cup water
- 3 tablespoons dried unsweetened shredded coconut
- 1 tablespoon raisins
- 1 teaspoon flaxseed oil
- 4 grams glucomannan
  Ice cubes

GRAINS AND FRUITS DIET

- ½ cup pasteurized liquid egg substitute
- ⅓ cup water
- ¼ cup steel-cut oats
- 3 tablespoons dried unsweetened shredded coconut
- 1 tablespoon raisins
- ½ scoop vanilla whey protein powder
- 4 grams glucomannan
  Ice cubes

In a blender, combine all of the ingredients. Blend until smooth and creamy.
Pour immediately into a large cup.

SERVES 1
GREENS AND BERRIES DIET, PER SERVING:
269 calories, 26 g protein, 12 g carbs, 7 g fiber, 13 g total fat, 8 g saturated fat
GRAINS AND FRUITS DIET, PER SERVING:
315 calories, 28 g protein, 26 g carbs, 9 g fiber, 11 g total fat, 8 g saturated fat

Pumpkin Pie Smoothie

GREENS AND BERRIES DIET

- ⅔ cup water
- ⅓ cup pure pumpkin, canned
- 1 scoop vanilla whey protein powder
- 1 tablespoon extra-virgin olive oil
- 1 teaspoon ground cinnamon or pumpkin pie spice
- ½ teaspoon stevia or 1 tablespoon Splenda
- 4 grams glucomannan
  Ice cubes

GRAINS AND FRUITS DIET

- ½ cup canned pumpkin
- ⅔ cup water
- 2 teaspoons extra-virgin olive oil
- 1 teaspoon maple syrup
- 1 teaspoon ground cinnamon or pumpkin pie spice
- 1 scoop vanilla whey protein powder
- 4 grams glucomannan
  Ice cubes

In a blender, combine all of the ingredients. Blend until smooth and creamy. Pour immediately into a large cup.

SERVES 1

GREENS AND BERRIES DIET, PER SERVING:
271 calories, 22 g protein, 12 g carbs, 6 g fiber, 15 g total fat, 3 g saturated fat

GRAINS AND FRUITS DIET, PER SERVING:
274 calories, 22 g protein, 24 g carbs, 7 g fiber, 10 g total fat, 2 g saturated fat

Creamy Grapefruit Protein Smoothie

GREENS AND BERRIES DIET

- 11 unsalted raw whole almonds
- ½ pink grapefruit, peeled and segmented
- ⅓ cup low-fat plain yogurt
- ⅓ cup 1% cottage cheese
- ⅓ cup water
- 4 grams glucomannan

GRAINS AND FRUITS DIET

- ½ pink grapefruit, peeled and segmented
- ⅓ cup low-fat plain yogurt
- ⅓ cup 1% cottage cheese
- ⅓ cup water
- 4 grams glucomannan

In a blender, combine all of the ingredients. Blend until smooth and creamy. Pour immediately into a large cup.

SERVES 1
GREENS AND BERRIES DIET, PER SERVING:
273 calories, 18 g protein, 21 g carbs, 7 g fiber, 13 g total fat, 2 g saturated fat
GRAINS AND FRUITS DIET, PER SERVING:
133 calories, 13 g protein, 18 g carbs, 4 g fiber, 1 g total fat, 0 g saturated fat

Strawberry Cheesecake

CRUST

- 1 cup graham cracker crumbs
- ¼ cup ground flaxseeds
- ¼ cup oat bran
- ⅓ cup water
- 6 grams glucomannan

FILLING

- 2 cups 1% cottage cheese
- 6 grams glucomannan
- 3 ounces fat-free cream cheese
- 3 scoops strawberry or vanilla whey protein powder

TOPPING

- 1 cup sliced fresh strawberries
- 4 tablespoons sugar-free strawberry jam

TO MAKE THE CRUST

1. Coat a 9" pie pan with cooking spray.

2. In a large bowl, combine all of the crust ingredients. Stir this mixture until it's all the same consistency.

3. Press the crumb mixture into the pie pan, easing the crust up the sides of the pan.

TO MAKE THE FILLING

1. In a blender, combine all of the filling ingredients. Blend on high until smooth and creamy.

2. Pour the filling into the crust. Refrigerate for 1 hour.

TO MAKE THE TOPPING

1. In a small bowl, mix together the strawberries and jam.

2. Spread the topping over the chilled pie.

SERVES 6
PER SERVING:
282 calories, 25 g protein, 32 g carbs, 6 g fiber, 6 g total fat, 1 g saturated fat

Apple and Blackberry Fiber Crumble

FRUIT FILLING

- 3 medium tart apples,
  cored and cut into ¼" slices
- 1 pint blackberries, rinsed
- 1 tablespoon fresh lemon juice
- 8 grams glucomannan
- ½ cup water

CRUMBLE TOPPING

- ⅔ cup steel-cut oats
- ½ cup walnuts, crushed
- ¼ cup stone-ground rye flour
- 1 teaspoon ground cinnamon
- ½ teaspoon stevia
- 8 grams glucomannan
- 3 tablespoons salted butter, softened

TO MAKE THE FILLING

1. Preheat the oven to 375°F.

2. In an 8" × 8" baking dish, combine the apples, blackberries, and lemon juice.

3. In small bowl, combine the glucomannan and water. Stir to thicken.
Add to the apple mixture. Mix with your hands to thoroughly cover the fruit.

TO MAKE THE TOPPING

1. In a medium bowl, combine the oats, walnuts, flour, cinnamon,
stevia, and glucomannan. Add the butter. Mix to form crumbles.

2. Evenly cover the fruit mixture with crumble topping.

3. Bake for 45 minutes, until the apples are softened.

SERVES 6
PER SERVING:
278 calories, 4 g protein, 34 g carbs, 10 g fiber, 14 g total fat, 4 g saturated fat

Gluco-Berry Protein Sorbet

1 cup frozen unsweetened strawberries

1 scoop strawberry whey protein powder

6 grams glucomannan

½ cup water

1. In a blender or food processor, combine all of the ingredients. Blend until the mixture forms a smooth paste.

2. Evenly divide between two small glass bowls. Place in the freezer. Serve when hardened.

SERVES 2
PER SERVING:
76 calories, 11 g protein, 8 g carbs, 5 g fiber, 0 g total and saturated fat

Pumpkin Protein Fiber Muffins

¾ cup all-purpose rye flour

½ cup vanilla whey protein powder

2 tablespoons ground flaxseeds

2 teaspoons ground cinnamon

1 teaspoon salt

1 teaspoon ground nutmeg

1 teaspoon stevia

6 grams glucomannan

2 egg whites

1 medium egg

1 can (15 ounces) pumpkin puree

¾ cup unsweetened applesauce

½ cup canola oil

1 teaspoon pure vanilla extract

½ cup crushed walnuts and almonds

1. Preheat the oven to 350°F. Line a 12-cup muffin pan with paper muffin liners.

2. In a large bowl, mix together the flour, whey protein powder, flaxseeds, cinnamon, salt, nutmeg, stevia, and glucomannan.

3. Add the egg whites, egg, pumpkin, applesauce, oil, and vanilla extract. Mix well. Fold in the nuts.

4. Spoon the batter into the prepared muffin cups.

5. Bake for 20 minutes, until a toothpick inserted into center of a muffin comes out clean.

MAKES 12 MUFFINS
PER MUFFIN:
193 calories, 7 g protein, 12 g carbs, 4 g fiber, 13 g total fat, 1 g saturated fat

Recipes for the Greens and Berries Diet

The following recipes have been developed specifically for the Greens and Berries Diet. Many of them are featured in the meal plans in Chapter 8.

EGGS

No-Crust Vegetable Quiche

8 grams glucomannan

½ cup water

5 medium egg whites

3 medium or omega-3 eggs

¾ cup low-fat cottage cheese, drained through a colander

¼ teaspoon salt

¼ teaspoon ground black pepper

¼ cup chopped yellow onion

¼ cup chopped spinach

¼ cup chopped broccoli

¼ cup chopped white mushrooms

1. Preheat the oven to 400°F.

2. In a small bowl, combine the glucomannan and water. Let stand for a few minutes to thicken.

3. In a medium bowl, whisk together the egg whites, eggs, and cottage cheese. Season with the salt and pepper.

4. Add the onion and spinach to the egg mixture.

5. Add the glucomannan mixture to the egg mixture.

6. Coat an 8" × 8" baking dish with nonstick cooking spray. Arrange the broccoli and mushrooms in an even layer on the bottom of the dish.

7. Add the gluco-egg mixture to the dish. Bake for 30 minutes. Serve hot.

SERVES 2
PER SERVING:
203 calories, 27 g protein, 8 g carbs, 5 g fiber, 7 g total fat, 2 g saturated fat

Goat Cheese and Herb Gluco-Omelette

- **2 grams glucomannan**
- **2 tablespoons water**
- **4 egg whites**
- **1 medium or omega-3 egg**
- **1 tablespoon finely chopped chives**
- **1 tablespoon chopped fresh parsley**
- **1 teaspoon tarragon leaves**
- **1 ounce soft goat cheese, crumbled (about ¼ cup)**
- **Salt and freshly ground black pepper to taste**

1. In a medium bowl, mix together the glucomannan and water. Add the egg whites, egg, chives, parsley, and tarragon. Beat lightly with a fork until combined.

2. Coat a small nonstick skillet with olive oil cooking spray. Heat to medium-high. Add the egg mixture. Cook for about 5 minutes, or until set.

3. Sprinkle with the goat cheese. Carefully fold in half and cook through. Omelette should be very lightly browned. Season with salt and pepper.

SERVES 1
PER SERVING:
194 calories, 24 g protein, 2 g carbs, 2 g fiber, 10 g total fat, 5 g saturated fat

Tip: In a pinch, you can use dried herbs instead of fresh, but since dried herbs pack more flavor per tablespoon, decrease the amounts by one-third.

THE GREENS AND BERRIES DIET

Egg Salad Wraps

8 large eggs

4 tablespoons Glorious Gluco-Mayo (see page 189)
   or canola or olive oil–based mayonnaise

10 chives, finely chopped

3 celery stalks, finely chopped

Salt and freshly ground black pepper to taste

8 grams glucomannan

4 butter lettuce leaves

1. Place the eggs in a pan filled with enough cold water to cover them.

2. Bring the water to a boil over medium heat.

3. Reduce the heat to medium. Cook for 15 minutes.

4. Drain the eggs. Run under cold water until cool enough to peel.

5. Chop the peeled eggs and place in a large bowl. Add the gluco-mayo, chives, and celery. Season with the salt and pepper.

6. Add the glucomannan. Stir until well blended.

7. Evenly divide the egg salad among the lettuce leaves and serve.

SERVES 4
PER SERVING:
275 calories, 15 g protein, 2 g carbs, 2 g fiber, 23 g total fat, 4 g saturated fat

Chicken Satay with Peanut Dipping Sauce

CHICKEN SATAY

- ½ pound boneless, skinless chicken breast, cut lengthwise into 1" strips
- 1 tablespoon low-sodium soy sauce
- 1 tablespoon extra-virgin olive oil
- 1 teaspoon Thai fish sauce
- 1 teaspoon ground black pepper
- 1 teaspoon ground cumin
- 1 teaspoon ground coriander
- 1 teaspoon curry powder
- 2 cloves garlic, minced
- 1 teaspoon stevia

DIPPING SAUCE

- 1 tablespoon natural creamy peanut butter
- 1 tablespoon sugar-free canned coconut milk
- ½ tablespoon red curry paste
- ½ teaspoon fish sauce
- 4 grams glucomannan

TO MAKE THE CHICKEN SATAY

1. In a large bowl, combine all the chicken satay ingredients. Refrigerate for at least 1 hour and up to 24 hours.

2. Preheat the broiler.

3. Soak 10 bamboo skewers in water for 15 minutes to prevent them from burning.

4. Thread the marinated chicken strips onto the skewers and place on a baking sheet.

5. Broil for 3 minutes per side, until brown around the edges.

TO MAKE THE DIPPING SAUCE

Immediately before serving, combine all the ingredients for the dipping sauce in a small bowl. Mix until creamy.

SERVES 2

PER SERVING:
266 calories, 28 g protein, 7 g carbs, 4 g fiber, 14 g total fat, 3 g saturated fat

Note: The glucomannan will thicken the peanut sauce if it is left to sit; if this occurs, add a small amount of water to thin out the sauce to the desired texture.

THE GREENS AND BERRIES DIET

Chicken with Pistachio Pesto

⅔ cup shelled salted pistachios

2 cups (packed) fresh cilantro leaves

8 grams glucomannan

1 clove garlic, chopped

1 teaspoon ground cardamom

¾ teaspoon salt

3 tablespoons fresh lemon juice

½ cup extra-virgin olive oil

 Ground black pepper to taste

4 large (about 3½ ounces each) boneless, skinless chicken breasts

1. Preheat the oven to 400°F.

2. Spread the pistachios on a baking sheet and cook for about 7 minutes, until golden.

3. In a food processer, combine the pistachios, cilantro, glucomannan, garlic, cardamom, salt, and 2 tablespoons of the lemon juice. Process until a coarse paste forms.

4. With the processor running, gradually add ⅓ cup of the oil. Season with the pepper.

5. Brush 1 tablespoon of the pesto onto each chicken breast. Place the chicken in a baking dish. Bake for 25 to 30 minutes, or until a thermometer inserted in the thickest portion registers 160°F and the juices run clear.

6. Place the remaining pesto in a small bowl. Whisk in the remaining olive oil and 1 tablespoon lemon juice. Drizzle half of the pesto sauce over cooked chicken breasts and serve. Save the remaining pesto for snacks or other meals.

SERVES 4
PER SERVING:
478 calories, 27 g protein, 7 g carbs, 4 g fiber, 38 g total fat, 5 g saturated fat

Chicken Taco Salad

3 ounces sliced grilled chicken breast or tenderloins, seasoned with fajita seasoning

½ cup no-sugar-added salsa

2 grams glucomannan

2 cups baby spinach leaves

2 ounces shredded low-fat Cheddar cheese

1. In a medium bowl, mix together the chicken, salsa, and glucomannan. Let stand for 3 to 5 minutes to thicken.

2. Place the chicken mixture over the spinach leaves.

3. Sprinkle with the cheese.

SERVES 1
PER SERVING:
283 calories, 43 g protein, 12 g carbs, 6 g fiber, 7 g total fat, 3 g saturated fat

Turkey and Cauliflower Casserole

   4 links nitrite- and nitrate-free lean Italian turkey sausage

   2 cups regular chicken stock

   2 heads cauliflower, cubed, including stalks but trimmed of leaves

   1 tablespoon extra-virgin olive oil

   2 cloves garlic, minced

   1 small yellow onion, chopped

   1 cup white mushrooms, halved

 10 grams glucomannan

   ½ cup 1% milk

   1 tablespoon butter

   1 teaspoon ground black pepper

   ¼ cup grated Parmesan cheese

   ½ cup chopped walnuts

1. Preheat the oven to 400°F.

2. Remove the sausages from the casings. Crumble the meat into a skillet.
Cook over medium heat about 10 minutes until brown. Remove from skillet and set aside.

3. In a large pot, bring the stock to a boil over high heat. Add the cauliflower.
Boil for 10 minutes, until tender.

4. In the same skillet used to cook the sausage, heat the oil to medium-high.
Add the garlic, onion, and mushrooms. Cook for 3 minutes, until lightly browned.

5. Drain the cauliflower. In the pot, mash with a large spoon. Add the glucomannan, milk,
butter, and pepper. Mix until the glucomannan has fully dissolved. Add the reserved sausage
and the vegetable mixture. Mix well.

6. Coat a nonstick 8" × 8" baking dish with olive oil cooking spray. Spread the sausage-
vegetable mixture into the dish. Top with the cheese and walnuts.

7. Bake for 8 to 10 minutes, until the cheese has browned.

SERVES 4
PER SERVING:
452 calories, 28 g protein, 22 g carbs, 9 g fiber, 28 g total fat, 8 g saturated fat

Tuna Salad

1 can (6 ounces) chunk light tuna, packed in water

1 tablespoon canola oil–based mayonnaise

1 teaspoon yellow mustard

2 grams glucomannan

Drain the tuna and place into a bowl. Add the mayonnaise, mustard, and glucomannan, mixing to combine. Chill before serving, if desired.

SERVES 1
PER SERVING:
240 calories, 33 g protein, 0 g carbs, 2 g fiber, 12 g total fat, 1 g saturated fat

Coconut Curry Shrimp

1 tablespoon extra-virgin olive oil

½ cup chopped white onion

½ cup chopped red bell pepper

1 clove garlic, minced

1 teaspoon ground cumin

¾ teaspoon ground coriander

½ teaspoon curry powder

1 cup unsweetened coconut milk

¼ teaspoon crushed red-pepper flakes

1 pound raw shrimp, peeled and deveined

8 grams glucomannan

2 tablespoons water

2 tablespoons chopped fresh cilantro

1. In a large nonstick saucepan, heat the oil to medium. Add the onion, bell pepper, and garlic. Cook, stirring, for 3 minutes, until the vegetables begin to soften. Add the cumin, coriander, and curry powder. Cook for 1 minute. Add the coconut milk and red-pepper flakes. Bring to a boil. Reduce the heat to medium. Cook for 2 minutes.

2. Bring to a boil.

3. Add the shrimp. Raise the heat to medium-high. Cook, stirring, about 6 minutes, until the shrimp is opaque.

4. In a small bowl, combine the glucomannan and water. Once thickened, add to the saucepan. Cook for 1 minute, until the sauce is bubbly and thickened.

5. Stir in the cilantro just before serving.

SERVES 4
PER SERVING:
260 calories, 25 g protein, 4 g carbs, 3 g fiber, 16 g total fat, 11 g saturated fat

Creamy Broccoli Soup

1 tablespoon extra-virgin olive oil

1 large yellow onion, quartered

3½ cups water

3 cups broccoli stems and tops, cut into large chunks

1 teaspoon salt

1 teaspoon ground black pepper

10 grams glucomannan

2 cloves garlic, minced

1. In a large pot, heat the oil to medium. Add the onion and cook for 15 minutes, until soft.

2. Add the water, broccoli, salt, and pepper. Cook for 20 minutes, until the broccoli is tender.

3. Transfer the warm soup to a food processor. Add the glucomannan and garlic. Blend until the soup is creamy. Let sit for a few minutes to cool down before consuming. Divide into 4 servings.

SERVES 4
PER SERVING:
67 calories, 2 g protein, 8 g carbs, 4 g fiber, 3 g total fat, 0.5 g saturated fat

Bangers and Cauliflower Mash

1 large head cauliflower, separated into florets

½ cup 1% milk

2 cloves garlic, minced

8 grams glucomannan

Salt and ground black pepper to taste

4 links natural (nitrite- and nitrate-free) lean Italian turkey sausage, cooked according to the package directions

1. Preheat the oven to 300°F.

2. Place a steamer basket in a large pot with 2" of water. Bring to a boil over high heat. Place the cauliflower in the basket and steam for 10 minutes, until soft enough to easily pierce with a fork. Remove from the heat and drain.

3. Transfer the cauliflower to a food processor or a blender. Process until smooth. Add the milk, garlic, glucomannan, salt, and pepper.

4. Pour into a 1½-quart Pyrex baking dish. Bake for about 10 minutes, until the top is lightly browned.

5. Serve one-quarter of the mixture on a plate alongside 2 sausages. Save the remaining mash for a later meal or snack.

SERVES 4
PER SERVING, WITH SAUSAGE:
348 calories, 35 g protein, 16 g carbs, 6 g fiber, 16 g total fat, 5 g saturated fat

Super Fiber Breakfast Bowl

½ cup Fiber One cereal

¾ cup plain low-fat yogurt

1 tablespoon flaxseed oil

2 grams glucomannan

1. Pour the cereal into a medium bowl.

2. In a small bowl, combine the yogurt, flaxseed oil, and glucomannan. Immediately pour over the cereal. Stir and eat.

SERVES 1

PER SERVING:

296 calories, 12 g protein, 25 g carbs, 16 g fiber, 16 g total fat, 3 g saturated fat

Her Perfect Body

WHO: MISCHA A.

WHAT: THE GREENS AND BERRIES DIET HELPED CONTROL THIS DIABETIC'S BLOOD SUGAR

In her first 2 weeks on the diet, Mischa A. commented that all she was missing was "a pizza now and then." After dropping 12 pounds in 6 weeks, she can't even finish a whole slice. "Fatty foods have become kind of a turn-off," Mischa says.

A few months before starting the diet, Mischa was diagnosed with diabetes, and her blood sugar was on a virtual roller coaster. "I skipped breakfast all the time during the work week, and on weekends I would eat a big breakfast and then not eat again until dinner," Mischa says. Following the Greens and Berries Diet has changed her routine. "Eating every few hours allows me to eat less, because I'm never hungry. I'm also making a conscious effort to eat slower. All this has also helped a lot with keeping my blood sugar levels even."

Mischa appreciated that knowing the proper ratios of macronutrients allowed her to create her own meals for the day. "The diet was easy," she says. "I have a better sense of what I can eat and what I need to stay away from."

Mischa has also become more body aware. She's following the workout program and seeing results. Her clothes are fitting better, and she's noticed that her bras aren't uncomfortable anymore. Others are noticing Mischa's success as well. "A coworker told me that she could tell immediately that I've lost weight. Compliments always make me feel good. So I'm more motivated than ever to stick with the diet."

High-Fiber Cottage Cheese and Yogurt

½ cup 1% cottage cheese

½ cup low-fat plain yogurt

1 tablespoon almond butter

1 tablespoon wheat germ

½ scoop vanilla whey protein powder

2 grams glucomannan

1. In a medium bowl, mix together all the ingredients.

2. Let stand for 3 to 5 minutes to thicken, then eat.

SERVES 1

PER SERVING:
320 calories, 35 g protein, 17 g carbs, 6 g fiber, 10 g total fat, 3 g saturated fat

Ricotta Mango Breakfast

1 cup part-skim ricotta cheese

⅓ cup diced fresh mango

2 grams glucomannan

1. In a medium bowl, mix together all the ingredients.

2. Let stand for 3 to 5 minutes to thicken, then eat.

SERVES 1

PER SERVING:
379 calories, 28 g protein, 24 g carbs, 3 g fiber, 19 g total fat, 12 g saturated fat

Glorious Gluco-Mayo

2 large eggs

Juice of ½ lemon

1 teaspoon red wine vinegar

½ teaspoon salt

¼ teaspoon ground white pepper

Dash of Worcestershire sauce

1 cup extra-virgin olive oil or canola oil

10 grams glucomannan

1. In a large bowl, combine the eggs, lemon juice, vinegar, salt, pepper, and Worcestershire sauce. With a handheld blender, process until smooth.

2. Add the oil very gradually in a thin stream, blending constantly.

3. Blend in the glucomannan. Adjust the seasonings to taste and refrigerate until ready to serve. Keeps approximately 1 week.

SERVES APPROXIMATELY 20
PER 1-TABLESPOON SERVING:
100 calories, 0.5 g protein, 0 g carbs, 0.5 g fiber, 11 g total fat, 1.5 g saturated fat

Creamy Ranch Dip

½ cup low-fat plain yogurt

½ cup canola oil–based mayonnaise

¼ cup fat-free buttermilk

1 tablespoon chopped fresh parsley

1 clove garlic, minced

1 tablespoon chopped chives

½ teaspoon celery salt

⅛ teaspoon ground black pepper

10 grams glucomannan

In a medium bowl, combine all the ingredients. Mix until creamy. Refrigerate for at least 30 minutes to let the flavors meld.

MAKES 10 SERVINGS FOR SALAD OR DIPPING
PER SERVING:
89 calories, 1 g protein, 1 g carbs, 1 g fiber, 9 g total fat, 1 g saturated fat

Note: Glucomannan will thicken the dressing when left to sit in the refrigerator. Add water as desired to thin out the dressing to the desired texture.

Sun-Dried Tomato Pesto

½ cup water

½ cup sun-dried tomatoes

2 tablespoons pine nuts

2 cloves garlic

2 cups fresh basil

1 cup fresh parsley

¼ cup grated Parmesan cheese

3 tablespoons extra-virgin olive oil

8 grams glucomannan

1. In a medium saucepan, bring ¼ cup of the water to a boil over high heat.

2. Remove the pan from the heat. Add the sun-dried tomatoes. Let stand for 20 minutes, until the tomatoes have rehydrated.

3. Drain the tomatoes. Place in a food processor. Blend until pastelike.

4. Add the pine nuts and garlic. Blend thoroughly. Add the basil, parsley, and cheese. Blend thoroughly. Drizzle in the oil, the glucomannan, and the remaining ¼ cup water. Blend until smooth. Add more water if you prefer a thinner consistency.

SERVES 4
PER SERVING:
140 calories, 3 g protein, 5 g carbs, 4 g fiber, 12 g total fat, 2 g saturated fat

Almond Joy Smoothie

- 11 unsalted raw whole almonds
- 1 scoop chocolate whey protein powder
- ⅔ cup water
- 1 tablespoon dried unsweetened shredded coconut
- ½ teaspoon almond extract
- 4 grams glucomannan
- Ice cubes

In a blender, combine all of the ingredients. Blend until smooth and creamy.
Pour immediately into a large cup.

SERVES 1
PER SERVING:
271 calories, 26 g protein, 8 g carbs, 7 g fiber, 15 g total fat, 5 g saturated fat

Walnut Yogurt Smoothie

- ½ cup low-fat plain yogurt
- ½ cup 1% milk
- 6–8 unsalted raw walnut halves
- 1 tablespoon ground flaxseeds
- 2 teaspoons flaxseed oil
- ¼ teaspoon ground cinnamon
- 6 ice cubes
- 4 grams glucomannan

In a blender, combine all of the ingredients. Blend until smooth and creamy.
Pour immediately into a large cup.

SERVES 1
PER SERVING:
302 calories, 15 g protein, 19 g carbs, 11 g fiber, 18.5 g total fat, 3 g saturated fat

Carrot Cake Smoothie

½ cup unsweetened carrot juice

1 scoop vanilla whey protein powder

2 tablespoons toasted wheat germ

1 tablespoon soft cream cheese, regular fat

1 teaspoon flaxseed oil

¼ teaspoon ground cinnamon

2 grams glucomannan

Ice cubes

In a blender, combine all of the ingredients. Blend until smooth and creamy. Pour immediately into a large cup.

SERVES 1
PER SERVING:
263 calories, 28 g protein, 13 g carbs, 4 g fiber, 11 g total fat, 4 g saturated fat

Chocolate Cake Smoothie

½ cup 1% cottage cheese

⅓ cup water

1 scoop chocolate whey protein powder

1 tablespoon ground flaxseeds

4 grams glucomannan

Ice cubes

In a blender, combine all of the ingredients. Blend until smooth and creamy. Pour immediately into a large cup.

SERVES 1
PER SERVING:
250 calories, 39 g protein, 10 g carbs, 8 g fiber, 6 g total fat, 0 g saturated fat

Chocolate Raspberry Smoothie

½ cup unsweetened raspberries, fresh or frozen

⅔ cup low-fat plain yogurt

1 tablespoon nonalkalinized cocoa powder

⅙ cup whole unsalted raw almonds

¼ cup water

4 grams glucomannan

Ice cubes

In a blender, combine all of the ingredients. Blend until smooth and creamy.
Pour immediately into a large cup.

SERVES 1
PER SERVING:
294 calories, 14 g protein, 28 g carbs, 12 g fiber, 14 g total fat, 2 g saturated fat

Easy Vanilla Protein Pudding

½ cup 1% cottage cheese

1 scoop vanilla whey protein powder

2 grams glucomannan

In a small bowl, combine all of the ingredients. Mix well.

SERVES 1
PER SERVING:
190 calories, 37 g protein, 6 g carbs, 2 g fiber, 2 g total fat, 1 g saturated fat

THE GREENS AND BERRIES DIET

Chocolate Protein Pudding

1⅓ cups 1% cottage cheese

1 cup water

6 grams glucomannan

1 tablespoon ground flaxseeds

2 teaspoons unsweetened cocoa powder

½ teaspoon stevia sweetener or Splenda

In a blender or food processor, combine the cottage cheese, water, and glucomannan. Blend. Add the flaxseeds, cocoa, and stevia or Splenda.

SERVES 2
PER SERVING:
160 calories, 21 g protein, 10 g carbs, 6 g fiber, 4 g total fat, 1 g saturated fat

Glucoroons

4 egg whites, at room temperature

⅔ cup Splenda Sugar Blend for Baking

½ teaspoon pure vanilla extract

¼ teaspoon salt

10 grams glucomannan

2 cups shredded unsweetened coconut

1. Preheat the oven to 325°F. Lightly coat a baking sheet with cooking spray.

2. In a large bowl, beat the egg whites with an electric mixer until peaks begin to form.

3. Add the Splenda, vanilla extract, salt, and glucomannan. Beat until stiff peaks form.

4. Fold in the coconut.

5. Drop 20 tablespoon-size mounds about 1" apart on the prepared baking sheet. Bake for 17 minutes, or until the tops are golden brown. Let cool before eating.

MAKES APPROXIMATELY 20 MACAROONS
PER MACAROON:
56 calories, 1 g protein, 3 g carbs, 1.5 g fiber, 4.5 g total fat, 4 g saturated fat

Recipes for the Grains and Fruits Diet

The following recipes were developed specifically for the Grains and Fruits Diet. Many of them are featured in the meal plans in Chapter 9.

Sweet Egg White Splendor

- 1 cup (about 8 medium) egg whites, at room temperature
- ⅔ cup Splenda
- ½ teaspoon pure vanilla extract
- 6 grams glucomannan
- ¼ teaspoon salt
- ½ apple, finely chopped
- ⅔ cup grated shredded unsweetened coconut
- ¼ cup raisins
  Ground cinnamon

1. Preheat the oven to 325°F. Coat a 6-cup muffin pan with cooking spray.

2. In a large bowl, beat the egg whites with an electric mixer on medium speed, until medium peaks form. Gradually beat in the Splenda, vanilla extract, glucomannan, and salt. Turn the mixer to high speed and beat until stiff (but not dry) peaks form.

3. Gently fold in the apple, coconut, and raisins.

4. Fill each muffin cup halfway with batter mixture. Lightly sprinkle cinnamon over each cup.

5. Bake for 15 minutes. Remove from the oven. Let cool for 1 minute. Transfer to a wire rack to cool completely. The meringues will have expanded and risen as they baked, but once out of the oven, they will settle.

SERVES 6
PER SERVING:
113 calories, 4 g protein, 13 g carbs, 3 g fiber, 5 g total fat, 5 g saturated fat

Egg and Corn Tortillas

1 medium or omega-3 egg

1 egg white

2 grams glucomannan

2 tablespoons chopped yellow onion

2 tablespoons chopped red bell pepper

1 tablespoon chopped fresh parsley

3 corn tortillas (4½" diameter)

¼ cup canned black beans, drained and rinsed

¼ cup mild no-sugar-added salsa, such as Tostitos All Natural

1. In a small bowl, mix together the egg, egg white, and glucomannan. Add the onion, pepper, and parsley.

2. Coat a nonstick medium skillet with olive oil cooking spray. Heat to medium-high. Add the egg-and-vegetable mixture. Cook, stirring, for about 4 minutes, until the eggs are firm.

3. In a small skillet or in the microwave oven, warm the tortillas with a sprinkle of water until soft.

4. Place the tortillas on a plate, and top each one with an equal amount of the scrambled eggs, beans, and salsa. Fold the tortillas in half to eat.

SERVES 1
PER SERVING:
319 calories, 19 g protein, 36 g carbs, 7 g fiber, 11 g total fat, 3 g saturated fat

New Orleans Chicken with Red Beans and Rice

⅔ cup brown rice

4 large boneless, skinless chicken breasts, approximately 3½ ounces each

10 grams glucomannan

1 cup water

1 tablespoon extra-virgin olive oil

½ large yellow onion, chopped

1 clove garlic, minced

¼ teaspoon chili powder

⅛ teaspoon fresh ground black pepper

1 tablespoon hot sauce

1 tablespoon coarsely chopped fresh parsley

1 can (15 ounces) red kidney beans, drained and rinsed

1. Preheat the broiler.

2. Cook the rice according to the package directions.

3. In a broiler pan, broil the chicken for 4 minutes on each side, or until a thermometer inserted in the thickest portion registers 160°F and the juices run clear. Set aside.

4. In a medium bowl, combine the glucomannan and water. Let stand for 3 to 5 minutes to thicken.

5. Heat the oil in a large saucepan over medium-high heat. Add the onion. Cook, stirring frequently, for 3 to 5 minutes, until lightly browned.

6. Add the glucomannan mixture to the saucepan. Add the garlic. Cook for 2 minutes.

7. Add the rice. Mix. Add the chili powder, pepper, hot sauce, and parsley. Evenly divide the rice and beans and the reserved chicken breasts among four plates.

SERVES 4
PER SERVING:
355 calories, 33 g protein, 40 g carbs, 9 g fiber, 7 g total fat, 1 g saturated fat

Chicken Orzo Salad

¼ cup orzo

2 grams glucomannan

⅔ cup diced cooked chicken breast

2 teaspoons extra-virgin olive oil

1 teaspoon red wine vinegar

¼ teaspoon dried oregano

Salt and ground
black pepper to taste

1 scallion, thinly sliced,
green parts only

1 tablespoon crumbled
soft goat cheese

1½ cups baby spinach leaves

1. Bring a medium saucepan of salted water to a boil over high heat. Add the orzo. Return to a boil. Cook for 6 minutes, or until the orzo is al dente. Drain most of the water, leaving the orzo slightly wet. Add the glucomannan. Stir until absorbed by the orzo.

2. Immediately add the chicken, oil, vinegar, oregano, salt, and pepper. Toss. Add the scallion and cheese. Mix. Serve on a bed of the spinach leaves.

SERVES 1
PER SERVING:
368 calories, 33 g protein, 23 g carbs, 4 g fiber, 16 g total fat, 4 g saturated fat

Chicken Taco Salad

3 ounces sliced grilled chicken breast,
seasoned with fajita seasoning

½ cup no-sugar-added salsa

2 grams glucomannan

2 cups baby spinach leaves

½ ounce (approximately 8)
baked corn tortilla chips, broken

1 ounce shredded low-fat
Cheddar cheese

1. In a medium bowl, mix together the chicken, salsa, and glucomannan. Let stand for 3 to 5 minutes to thicken.

2. Place the chicken mixture over the spinach leaves and chips.

3. Sprinkle with the cheese.

SERVES 1
PER SERVING:
313 calories, 36 g protein, 22 g carbs, 6 g fiber, 9 g total fat, 3 g saturated fat

Turkey Shepherd's Pie

1 tablespoon extra-virgin olive oil

1 small yellow onion, chopped

1 clove garlic, minced

1 pound lean ground turkey

3 tablespoons Worcestershire sauce

1 tablespoon water

10 grams glucomannan

1 teaspoon ground cumin

2 large sweet potatoes, peeled and cubed

1 medium parsnip, peeled and cubed

⅓ cup 1% milk

2 tablespoons butter

½ cup frozen peas

½ cup frozen corn

4 tablespoons chopped fresh parsley

1. Preheat the oven to 350°F.

2. Heat the oil in a large nonstick saucepan over medium-high heat. Add the onion and garlic. Cook, stirring frequently, for 3 to 5 minutes, until lightly browned.

3. Add the turkey. Cook, breaking apart the meat, for 10 minutes, until browned.

4. In a small bowl, mix together the Worcestershire sauce, water, and 6 grams of the glucomannan. Add to the turkey mixture. Add the cumin. Allow to thicken for 2 to 3 minutes. Remove from the heat.

5. Bring a large pot of water to a boil over high heat. Add the sweet potatoes and parsnip. Boil for 8 to 9 minutes, until tender. Drain. Add the milk, butter, and the remaining 4 grams glucomannan. Mash.

6. In an 8" × 8" nonstick baking dish, the layer ground turkey mixture, peas, corn, and the mashed sweet potato and parsnips.

7. Bake for 20 minutes. Then broil for 5 minutes, until top is browned to your liking. Garnish with the parsley.

SERVES 5
PER SERVING:
308 calories, 19 g protein, 31 g carbs, 6 g fiber, 12 g total fat, 4 g saturated fat
Serving suggestion: Serve with Savory Poultry Gravy (page 225).

Tuna Salad

1 can (6 ounces) chunk light tuna, packed in water

1 tablespoon light mayonnaise

1 teaspoon yellow mustard

2 grams glucomannan

Drain the tuna and place into a bowl. Add the mayonnaise, mustard, and glucomannan, mixing to combine. Chill before serving if desired.

SERVES 1
PER SERVING:
186 calories, 33 g protein, 0 g carbs, 2 g fiber, 6 g total fat, 1 g saturated fat

Brown Rice and Salmon Salad

2 grams glucomannan

⅓ cup unsweetened pineapple juice

¼ cup water

½ cup cooked brown rice

1 teaspoon white vinegar

1 tablespoon fresh lemon juice

3 drops hot-pepper sauce

Salt and ground black pepper to taste

1½ cups finely chopped raw spinach leaves

1 tablespoon minced fresh dill

1 pouch (3 ounces) pink salmon packed in water

1. In a small bowl, mix together the glucomannan, pineapple juice, and water about 3 minutes until thickened.

2. In a medium bowl, mix together the rice, vinegar, lemon juice, hot-pepper sauce, salt and pepper, spinach, and dill. Add the glucomannan mixture. Stir well. Top with the crumbled salmon.

SERVES 1
PER SERVING:
327 calories, 25 g protein, 41 g carbs, 5 g fiber, 7 g total fat, 1 g saturated fat

Coconut Curry Shrimp with Rice

- 1 tablespoon extra-virgin olive oil
- ½ cup chopped white onion
- ½ cup chopped red bell pepper
- 1 clove garlic, minced
- 1 teaspoon ground cumin
- ¾ teaspoon ground coriander
- ½ teaspoon curry powder
- 1 cup unsweetened coconut milk
- ¼ teaspoon crushed red-pepper flakes
- 1 pound raw shrimp, peeled and deveined
- 8 grams glucomannan
- 2 tablespoons water
- 2 tablespoons chopped fresh cilantro
- 2 cups cooked brown rice

1. In a large nonstick saucepan over medium-high heat, heat the oil. Add the onion, bell pepper, and garlic. Cook, stirring, for 3 minutes, or until the vegetables begin to soften. Add the cumin, coriander, and curry powder. Cook for 1 minute. Add the coconut milk and red-pepper flakes. Bring to a boil. Reduce the heat to medium. Cook for 2 minutes.

2. Add the shrimp. Raise the heat to medium-high. Cook, stirring, about 6 minutes, until the shrimp is cooked through.

3. In a small bowl, combine the glucomannan and water. Once thickened, add to the saucepan. Cook for 1 minute, until the sauce is bubbly and thickened.

4. Stir in the cilantro just before serving. Serve one-quarter of the curry over ½ cup of the rice.

SERVES 4
PER SERVING:
360 calories, 27 g protein, 27 g carbs, 5 g fiber, 16 g total fat, 11 g saturated fat

THE GRAINS AND FRUITS DIET

Caribbean Sweet Potato Salad

1 large sweet potato, peeled and chopped into 1" cubes

½ medium cucumber, sliced thin

¼ red onion, chopped

½ cup frozen yellow corn, cooked according to the package directions

1 clove garlic, minced

3 tablespoons finely chopped fresh cilantro

2 tablespoons extra-virgin olive oil

1 tablespoon fresh lime juice

1 teaspoon Dijon mustard

½ teaspoon hot-pepper sauce

¼ teaspoon salt

⅛ teaspoon ground black pepper

6 grams glucomannan

1. Bring a large pot of water to a boil over high heat. Add the sweet potato. Boil for 10 minutes, until tender.

2. Drain the sweet potato. In a large bowl, combine the sweet potato, cucumber, onion, and corn.

3. In a small bowl, combine the garlic, cilantro, oil, lime juice, mustard, hot-pepper sauce, salt, pepper, and glucomannan. Add to the potato mixture. Cover and toss until evenly coated with the lime-mustard sauce.

SERVES 3
PER SERVING:
161 calories, 2 g protein, 18 g carbs, 4 g fiber, 9 g total fat, 1 g saturated fat

Creamy Mushroom Soup

1 cup half-and-half

1 cup water

12 grams glucomannan

½ teaspoon salt

1 large Yukon gold potato, peeled and thinly sliced

1 tablespoon butter

½ cup diced onion

2 cloves garlic, minced

1½ pounds assorted mushrooms, chopped

3 cups fat-free, reduced-sodium chicken broth

1. In a large saucepan, combine the half-and-half, water, glucomannan, salt, and potato. Bring to a boil over high heat.

2. Reduce the heat to medium. Cook for 18 minutes, until the potato slices are tender.

3. In a stockpot, melt the butter over medium-high heat. Add the onion and garlic. Cook, stirring frequently, about 3 to 5 minutes, until lightly browned. Add the mushrooms. Cook, stirring, for another 5 minutes. Add the broth. Bring to a boil.

4. Reduce the heat to medium. Cook for 6 minutes.

5. Add the potato mixture to the mushroom mixture. In a food processor or blender, puree the soup in batches.

SERVES 6
PER 1¼-CUP SERVING
159 calories, 6 g protein, 18 g carbs, 3 g fiber, 7 g total fat, 4 g saturated fat
Serving suggestion: Garnish with chopped fresh thyme.

Vegetable-Stuffed Peppers

½ cup bulgur

1 cup water

2 large red bell peppers, halved lengthwise, with seeds removed

2 large green bell peppers, halved lengthwise, with seeds removed

½ pound lean ground beef

⅓ cup finely chopped white onion

1 can (15 ounces) kidney beans, drained and rinsed

1 cup frozen whole kernel yellow corn, thawed and drained

¾ cup no-sugar-added hot salsa

1 clove garlic, minced

2 tablespoons chopped fresh parsley

1 teaspoon chili powder

1 teaspoon ground cumin

Salt and ground black pepper to taste

12 grams glucomannan

1. Preheat the oven to 350°F.

2. Cook the bulgur according to the package directions. Remove from the heat and set aside, covered.

3. In a small saucepan bring the water to boil over high heat. Add the red and green bell peppers. Boil for 3 minutes, until slightly soft. Drain and set aside.

4. In a large nonstick skillet over medium-high heat, combine the ground beef and onion. Cook about 10 minutes, until the beef is no longer pink. Add the reserved bulgur, beans, corn, salsa, garlic, parsley, chili powder, and cumin, salt and black pepper. Cook until bubbling. Add the glucomannan. Mix well until thickened.

5. Place the bell peppers cut side up on a baking sheet. Spoon an equal amount of the beef mixture into each pepper. Cover with aluminum foil. Bake for 35 to 40 minutes. Remove and serve. One whole pepper (two halves) plus stuffing serves 1 person.

SERVES 4
PER SERVING:
331 calories, 23 g protein, 53 g carbs, 15 g fiber, 3 g total fat, 1 g saturated fat
Serving suggestion: Serve with a tossed green salad with balsamic vinegar dressing.

Pumpkin Soup

½ cup bulgur

1 can (15 ounces) pumpkin

12 baby carrots, sliced, or 2 whole carrots, peeled and sliced

½ cup chopped yellow onion

4 cups vegetable stock, regular

1 teaspoon curry powder

½ teaspoon ground cinnamon

½ teaspoon ground nutmeg

½ teaspoon paprika

½ teaspoon ground ginger

8 grams glucomannan

Hot-pepper sauce to taste

Salt to taste

1. Cook the bulgur according to the package directions.

2. Add the pumpkin, carrots, onion, stock, curry powder, cinnamon, nutmeg, paprika, and ginger. Mix well. Bring to a boil over high heat. Cook for 5 minutes.

3. Reduce the heat to medium-low. Add the glucomannan. Stir. Cook for 30 minutes. Season with the hot-pepper sauce and salt. Cool before serving.

SERVES 4
PER SERVING:
113 calories, 4 g protein, 22 g carbs, 10 g fiber, 1 g total fat, 0 g saturated fat

Super Fiber Breakfast Bowl

½ cup Fiber One cereal

1 medium apple, cored, peeled, and cut into cubes

¾ cup low-fat plain yogurt

2 grams glucomannan

1. Pour the cereal into a medium bowl. Add the apple.

2. In a small bowl, combine the yogurt and glucomannan and immediately pour over the cereal. Stir everything together and eat.

SERVES 1
PER SERVING:
255 calories, 12 g protein, 45 g carbs, 18 g fiber, 3 g total fat, 2 g saturated fat

Simple Oats with Whey

1 cup water

Pinch of salt

⅓ cup steel-cut oats

2 grams glucomannan

1 scoop whey protein powder

6–8 unsalted walnut halves

1. In a small pot, bring the water to a boil over high heat. Add the salt and oats. Cook, stirring, for 15 minutes, until the oatmeal is soft. Remove from the heat.

2. Stir in the glucomannan and let thicken for about 2 minutes. Stir in the whey protein powder and walnuts.

SERVES 1
PER SERVING:
290 calories, 29 g protein, 21 g carbs, 5.5 g fiber, 10 g total fat, 1 g saturated fat

Pumpkin-Spiced Oatmeal

1 cup water	½ scoop vanilla whey protein powder
Pinch of salt	2 tablespoons ground flaxseeds
⅓ cup steel-cut oats	2 grams glucomannan
¼ cup canned pure pumpkin	Dash of ground cinnamon

1. In a small pot, bring the water to a boil over high heat. Add the salt and oats. Cook, stirring, for 15 minutes, until the oatmeal is soft.

2. In a medium bowl, combine the pumpkin, whey protein powder, flaxseeds, glucomannan, and cinnamon. Mix well.

3. Add the pumpkin mixture to the oatmeal. Reduce the heat to low. Cook for 3 minutes, stirring frequently.

SERVES 1
PER SERVING:
328 calories, 22 g protein, 33 g carbs, 14.5 g fiber, 12 g total fat, 0 g saturated fat

Tasty Orzo Pilaf

1 teaspoon extra-virgin olive oil	6 grams glucomannan
½ cup orzo (see note)	1 cup vegetable stock, regular
2 cloves minced garlic	Salt and ground black pepper to taste
1 scallion, thinly sliced, white and light green parts only	

1. In a large skillet, heat the oil on medium-high. Add the orzo, garlic, and scallions. Cook, stirring occasionally, for 4 minutes, until the orzo is golden brown.

2. In a small bowl, mix together the glucomannan and stock to thicken.

3. Add the vegetable stock mixture, salt, and pepper to the skillet. Cover. Reduce the heat to medium-low. Cook for 15 minutes, until the stock has been absorbed and the orzo is tender.

SERVES 3
PER SERVING:
154 calories, 5 g protein, 29 g carbs, 3 g fiber, 2 g total fat, 0 g saturated fat

Note: "Orzo" is the Italian word for barley; however, the orzo sold in North America is a barley-shaped pasta.

Ricotta Mango Breakfast

⅔ cup part-skim ricotta cheese

⅓ cup diced fresh mango

2 grams glucomannan

1. In a medium bowl, mix together all of the ingredients.

2. Let stand for 3 to 5 minutes to thicken, then eat.

SERVES 1
PER SERVING:
264 calories, 19 g protein, 20 g carbs, 3 g fiber, 12 g total fat, 8 g saturated fat

Apple Pie Smoothie

- 1 medium apple, peeled, cored, and sliced
- 6–8 unsalted raw walnut halves
- 1 scoop vanilla whey protein powder
- 1 tablespoon steel-cut oats
- 1 teaspoon ground cinnamon
- ⅔ cup water
- 4 grams glucomannan
- Ice cubes

In a blender, combine all of the ingredients. Blend until smooth and creamy.
Pour immediately into a large cup.

SERVES 1
PER SERVING:
289 calories, 24 g protein, 28 g carbs, 7 g fiber, 9 g total fat, 1 g saturated fat

Banana-Walnut Smoothie

- ½ large banana
- ½ cup low-fat plain yogurt
- ½ cup 1% milk
- 6–8 unsalted raw walnut halves
- 1 tablespoon ground flaxseeds
- ¼ teaspoon ground cinnamon
- 6 ice cubes
- 4 grams glucomannan

In a blender, combine all of the ingredients. Blend until smooth and creamy.
Pour immediately into a large cup.

SERVES 1
PER SERVING:
330 calories, 15 g protein, 35 g carbs, 12 g fiber, 14 g total fat, 3 g saturated fat

Blueberry Beet Almond Smoothie

½ cup unsweetened carrot juice

¼ cup frozen or fresh blueberries

¼ cup peeled and grated raw beet

¼ cup unsweetened applesauce

¼ cup unsalted raw whole almonds

⅓ cup ice cubes

½ teaspoon fresh lime juice

2 grams glucomannan

   Dash of ground ginger

In a blender, combine the carrot juice, blueberries, beet, applesauce, almonds, ice, lime juice, glucomannan, and ginger. Blend until smooth and creamy. Pour immediately into a large cup.

SERVES 1
PER SERVING:
300 calories, 7 g protein, 32 g carbs, 10 g fiber, 16 g fat, 1 g saturated fat

Savory Poultry Gravy

- 1¼ cups chicken stock, regular
- 6 grams glucomannan
- ½ cup water
- ½ teaspoon poultry seasoning
- ½ teaspoon salt
- ¼ teaspoon ground black pepper
- ⅛ teaspoon celery salt

1. In a medium saucepan, bring the stock to a boil over high heat.

2. In a small bowl, combine the glucomannan and water. Gradually whisk into the stock.

3. Add the poultry seasoning, salt, pepper, and celery salt.

4. Bring to a boil. Reduce the heat to medium. Cook for 8 to 10 minutes, to the desired consistency.

SERVES 5
PER SERVING:
2 calories, 0.5 g protein, 0 g carbs, 1 g fiber, 0 g total and saturated fat

Super Fiber Applesauce

- ½ cup unsweetened applesauce
- 6–8 unsalted walnut halves
- 2 grams glucomannan
- Pinch of ground cinnamon

In a small bowl, combine the applesauce, walnuts, glucomannan, and cinnamon. Let stand for 3 to 5 minutes to thicken.

SERVES 1
PER SERVING:
131 calories, 2 g protein, 15 g carbs, 5 g fiber, 7 g total fat, 1 g saturated fat

Suspiciously Delicious Rice Pudding

½ cup brown rice

1 ripe banana

2 tablespoons raisins

1 tablespoon Splenda
   Brown Sugar Blend

1 scoop vanilla whey protein powder

½ teaspoon ground cinnamon

⅛ teaspoon ground nutmeg

⅛ teaspoon ground ginger

6 grams glucomannan

1. Cook the rice according to the package directions.

2. In a medium bowl, mash the banana. Add the mashed banana and the raisins, Splenda, protein powder, cinnamon, nutmeg, ginger, and glucomannan to the rice. Mix together until smooth and creamy. Divide into 3 portions and serve.

SERVES 3
PER SERVING:
169 calories, 9 g protein, 31 g carbs, 5 g fiber, 1 g total fat, 0 g saturated fat

Zucchini Bread

1 medium zucchini, shredded

5 large egg whites

1 tablespoon flaxseed oil

12 grams glucomannan

⅔ cup water

1 large apple, shredded

4 scoops vanilla whey protein powder

½ cup ground flaxseeds

½ cup whole wheat all-purpose flour

½ cup Splenda Sugar Blend for Baking

1½ teaspoons ground cinnamon

½ teaspoon baking powder

½ teaspoon baking soda

1. Preheat the oven to 325°F. Lightly coat an 8" × 4" loaf pan with olive oil cooking spray.

2. Place the zucchini in a large bowl. Fold in the egg whites and oil.

3. In a medium bowl, combine the glucomannan and water. Add to the zucchini mixture.

4. In another medium bowl, mix together the apple, whey protein powder, flaxseeds, flour, Splenda, cinnamon, baking powder, and baking soda. Add to the zucchini mixture. Mix well.

5. Pour the batter into the prepared loaf pan. Bake for 45 to 50 minutes, until a toothpick inserted in the middle comes out clean. Cut into 6 slices.

SERVES 6
PER SERVING:
230 calories, 21 g protein, 23 g carbs, 8 g fiber, 6 g total fat, 1 g saturated fat

Ginger-Apricot Scones

 1 cup steel-cut oats

12 grams glucomannan

 6 scoops vanilla whey protein powder

1¼ teaspoons baking powder

 1 teaspoon SteviaPlus or 2 tablespoons Splenda Sugar Blend for Baking

 ¾ cup chopped dried, unsweetened apricots

 2" cube fresh gingerroot, peeled and chopped

 ¼ teaspoon salt

1½ cups whole wheat all-purpose flour

 ½ cup unsweetened applesauce

 ½ cup water

1. Preheat the oven to 350°F. Coat a baking sheet with olive oil cooking spray.

2. In a blender, process the oats on high, until ground into a fine powder.

3. In a large bowl, combine the glucomannan, whey protein powder, baking powder, stevia or Splenda, apricots, ginger, salt, and 1 cup of the flour. Mix well.

4. Add the applesauce and water. Mix until it forms a soft dough.

5. Spoon out one-third of the dough and place on a surface floured with some of the remaining ½ cup flour.

6. Sprinkle flour over the top of the dough and flatten into a ¾"-thick, circular patty.

7. Cut the circle crosswise into four quarters and place each wedge on the prepared baking sheet.

8. Repeat for the remaining thirds of dough. Bake for 10 to 12 minutes, until a toothpick inserted into the center of each scone comes out clean.

MAKES 12 SCONES
PER SCONE:
186 calories, 17 g protein, 25 g carbs, 6 g fiber, 2 g total fat, 0.5 g saturated fat

Chocolate Protein Pudding

1⅓ cups 1% cottage cheese

1 cup water

6 grams glucomannan

1 tablespoon ground flaxseeds

1 tablespoon granulated sugar

2 teaspoons unsweetened cocoa powder

1. In a blender or food processor, combine the cottage cheese, water, and glucomannan. Blend.

2. Add the flaxseeds, sugar, and cocoa. Blend until smooth and creamy. Pour immediately into 2 medium bowls.

SERVES 2
PER SERVING:
180 calories, 21 g protein, 15 g carbs, 6 g fiber, 4 g total fat, 1 g saturated fat

Bran Date Muffins

1½ cups wheat bran

1 cup low-fat buttermilk

1 large egg

⅓ cup canola oil

½ teaspoon pure vanilla extract

1 cup whole wheat flour

½ cup chopped dates

5 tablespoons + 1 teaspoon Splenda Brown Sugar Blend

1 teaspoon baking soda

1 teaspoon baking powder

½ teaspoon salt

24 grams glucomannan

1. Preheat the oven to 375°F. Line a 12-cup muffin pan with paper liners.

2. In a large bowl, combine the wheat bran and buttermilk. Let stand for 10 minutes, until the bran is softened.

3. In a small bowl, gently whisk together the egg, oil, and vanilla extract. Add to the bran mixture.

4. In a medium bowl, combine the remaining ingredients. Slowly add to the bran mixture, mixing well until the batter appears smooth.

5. Evenly divide the batter among the muffin cups. Bake for 15 minutes, until a toothpick inserted into the center of a muffin comes out clean.

MAKES 12 MUFFINS
PER SERVING:
155 calories, 4 g protein, 19 g carbs, 7 g fiber, 7 g total fat, 0.5 g saturated fat

CHAPTER 11

Keeping Track
of Your Perfect Body

So . . . how's it going?

Keeping a detailed record of your progress is the best way to determine how close you are to your perfect body. After the first week, you'll probably notice your clothes are a little roomier, but that's not exactly a scientific way to measure your progress. Although every woman's specific results will depend on many factors, such as her starting weight, her age, and how closely she follows the diet, you should notice that the scale dips down by at least a pound or two after the first week. You'll continue on this path until the 8 weeks are up. The record-keeping tools in this chapter will allow you to track what you eat and how much you weigh. Later on, you'll track your workouts as well as your body measurements. Together, all these figures will be motivation on the road to your goal: getting your perfect body.

Studies have shown that keeping a food diary greatly improves your chances of weight-loss success. A diary helps you control how much you eat and minimizes cheating—mostly because it forces you to take note of what's going into your mouth. Often, we don't realize how much we eat over the course of a day, especially if we think that we have good eating habits. But this "ghost eating" is where unwanted calories add up. When you write it down, you're forced to face up to eating two handfuls of jelly beans when you pass a co-worker's candy dish.

Teddie, a woman we worked with for 3 months, unconsciously snacked on nachos and salsa while she cooked, then ate a full meal with her family when her casserole was finished. She mindlessly put candies in her mouth, tasted her daughter's sundae, or ate a chocolate bar while she was grocery shopping. She never realized she was doing all of this until she started writing down everything she ate. Now she understands why her weight never changed, no matter how hard she worked out.

Within your food diary, you'll be recording when, what, and how much you eat. Include the beverages you drink, the supplements you take, and the number of meals in which you include glucomannan. You should also write down how you feel each morning and at the end of each day. By recording what you consume and how you feel, you can identify which areas are lacking and which are working great as the weeks progress. Photocopy the worksheet on page 232 to easily keep track of all this vital info.

In the weigh-in section, you'll chart your progress daily. Record your weight at the same

*Her*PerfectBody

WHO: MEREDITH S.

WHAT: HER PERFECT BODY FOOD DIARY SPARKED A 10-POUND WEIGHT LOSS

Meredith S. has lots to be happy about. This 28-year-old New York City speech pathologist just got married. Interestingly, she didn't start the *Women's Health Perfect Body Diet* until *after* the wedding and the honeymoon. "I thought I looked great at my wedding, but I was fed up with how I looked in pictures. I didn't want to be the dumpy wife. I wanted to look good for myself and my husband. The program has been great for both of us. We agree that we like this new way of eating much better than what we were eating before."

The first weeks of any marriage are challenging. Add to that the tension of starting a new diet. But Meredith says that after the first week things went relatively smoothly, and she progressed to losing close to 2 pounds a week, for a total of 10 pounds and more than two clothing sizes. "I was really opposed to the food diary because I never wanted to know exactly what I was eating. But once I got the hang of it, I realized that it was the key to the whole program. I am so much more aware of what I eat, because it's written down right in front of me. It really kept me honest. Before I used to time each day. Weigh yourself right after you've woken up and used the bathroom so that the number on the scale won't be affected by your clothing, a full bladder, or breakfast.

Food Diary

Each morning, write down how you feel about your progress. Then document every food item you eat and drink over the course of the day. Also document the calorie total for each meal and the grams of protein, carbs, and fats. You can use the caloric and macronutrient information in the tables and menu plans in Chapters 8 and 9 to determine these values. You can also use package labels from the food you're eating, or look at various Web sites that provide accurate nutrient information, such as the USDA nutrient database at www.nal.usda.gov/fnic/foodcomp/search, www.calorieking.com, www.fitday.com, or www.nutritiondata.com.

eat too much; my portions were too high. I look back through the diary and compare all the good things that I'm eating to the way I was eating before. I can't believe what I had been eating. It was a real wake-up call."

Meredith admits that she has been dieting for most of her life. She was even thinking about liposuction because she had never gotten the weight-loss results she was after. But this diet was different. "This one was fitting the best into my lifestyle," Meredith raves. "I just increased my protein, cut down the carbs, and cut out desserts. I loved that I could eat real food—not the processed stuff you have to eat on some other programs. I loved that I was encouraged to snack! I think it taught me better eating habits and how to choose food wisely without being too stringent. As soon as I learned that I could incorporate the glucomannan into foods that I buy, it was no problem at all."

Now married life is all good. Meredith beamed when she told us, "I fit into a pair of my college pants today. My husband asked if they were new, but they were 8 years old! A lot of people are noticing the weight change, especially my husband. All these positive comments really make me feel great: I'm finally happy with the way I look."

Date: _____

This morning I feel _____

Meal	Food	Carbs (g)	Protein (g)	Fat (g)	Calories
1: Breakfast					
TIME:					
2: Snack					
TIME:					
3: Lunch					
TIME:					
4: Snack					
TIME:					
5: Dinner					
TIME:					
6: Snack/Dessert					
TIME:					

Supplements: _____

Total number of meals with glucomannan: _____

Finally, determine your overall grade for each day. Grade yourself on the following scale:

A+ = Ate all the right foods and didn't cheat or overeat

B = Kept to eating goals for five of the six meals

C = Overate at more than one meal

D = Cheated and overate at least twice during the day

F = Completely off track

Enter your overall grade for the day: _____

Today I felt: _____

_____

Weekly Weigh-In

The first step is to record your weight daily and then determine your weekly loss. Keep track of your progress and, at the end of the 8 weeks, compare your total weight loss with your weight-loss goal to see how you made out.

TOTAL WEIGHT LOSS GOAL (IN POUNDS):

	WEEK 1	WEEK 2	WEEK 3	WEEK 4	WEEK 5	WEEK 6	WEEK 7	WEEK 8
Sunday								
Monday								
Tuesday								
Wednesday								
Thursday								
Friday								
Saturday								
TOTAL WEIGHT lost this week:								
TOTAL WEIGHT lost to date:								

POUNDS LEFT TO LOSE to Reach Your Perfect Body:

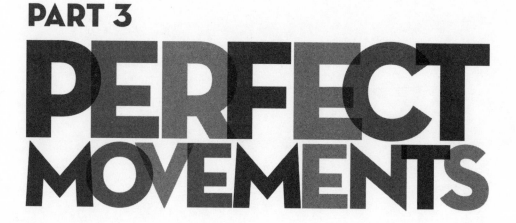

PART 3
PERFECT MOVEMENTS

CHAPTER 12

The Perfect Body Exercise Program

Let's get ready to sweat.

In this chapter we're going to go over the exercise portion of the *Women's Health Perfect Body Diet*. We'll cover not only what workouts we want you to do but also— just as important—*why* we want you to do them.

Let's tackle the "why" first. Lots of diets work pretty well in the short term. You reduce the number of calories you eat and pretty quickly start to notice that your tummy is a little tighter than it was and your hips aren't quite as broad. But often-times, something strange soon starts to happen: Even though you're still sticking to your new lower-calorie diet, your weight loss slows to a crawl—and then stops completely. Instead of being motivated to keep moving all the way to your perfect weight, you feel hungry, cranky, and frustrated (which, trust us, is *not* the formula for successful weight loss).

Turns out there's a reason this happens. Your body is pretty smart: When you eat fewer calories than it needs to maintain its weight, your body thinks it's starv-ing and responds by lowering its metabolic rate, reducing the number of calories you burn. So now you have to eat even less just to avoid putting the pounds back on—and forget about *losing* more weight.

We know what you're thinking: Damned if you diet, damned if you don't.

This is why exercise is so important for weight loss and, more important, for fat loss. Regular exercise keeps your metabolism running at a high level, which allows those pounds and fat stores to keep dropping off. But exercise and what you might consider to be physical activity are really two different things. Physical activity is any movement that expends energy. It's usually related to everyday tasks, such as cleaning the house or mowing the lawn. While you might work up a sweat doing these, we don't consider them to be exercise, which is a structured physical activity that is performed with intensity for a specified duration of time. Examples of exercise include a basketball game, mountain biking, or a weight-lifting workout. Exercise is performed specifically to increase physical fitness, which is what we're here to do.

You need to move every day if you really want to change your body. This means at least 30 minutes of exercise and physical activity 7 days a week. On the Perfect Body exercise program, you'll do strength-training workouts 3 days a week and cardio workouts another 3 days a week; on the remaining day, you'll engage in some kind of vigorous physical activity—a night out dancing or an outdoor hike would count—for at least 30 minutes to keep your metabolic rate high and help you lose the fat you want. And in case you can't make it to the gym, we provide two options for working out at home.

Perfect Body Workout Plans

Like the eating plans in this book, the workouts are customized for your life. Our exercise plans feature both resistance training and cardio, and they can be done either in the gym or at home, whichever works better for you.

Weight lifting is an important component of this plan because it's essential for building and sculpting your Perfect Body. The weight-training workouts are distinct for each body type. While each workout provides full-body training, you'll put extra emphasis on particular areas depending on whether you're an Apple, Pear, or Avocado. The goal is to whittle away the fat from the places you don't want it, while building muscle everywhere else. For example, if you're a Pear with a slender top and a well-defined waist that's topping off a larger butt, you're going to subtly reshape your body so that your lower half is not quite as prominent. You'll focus on upper-body resistance exercise to build and sculpt your shoulders, arms, and chest. And you'll do less heavy weight lifting for your lower body to concentrate on toning that area without making it any bigger.

All of the weight-training programs use a well-researched training method known as *periodization*. This refers to a change in exercises, sets, reps, and load (the amount of weight

The Perfect Body Workout for Bananas

If you're already a lean, slender Banana, you don't have as much fat to lose as the other body types. Follow the Avocado and Banana plan in Chapter 15 to build muscle in your entire body, but limit your cardiovascular work to just 2 days a week instead of 3. If you do too much cardio, you'll never give your muscles time to grow. Keep track of how much weight you use for each exercise. Follow the strength-training workout with 10 to 15 minutes of light cardiovascular exercise (such as walking on a flat treadmill).

lifted) over time. You'll do a full 8 weeks of different exercises instead of just 1 week's worth repeated eight times. Periodized programs are proven to promote more muscle growth and more fat loss than any other type of weight-training program.

You'll also include aerobic exercise in your training in a form known as *interval training*. Instead of maintaining a steady pace throughout every session (like jogging or biking at the same speed for an extended length of time), devote some workouts to intervals, mixing up lower-intensity periods with higher-intensity ones. In exercise physiology circles, this is termed *high-intensity-interval training* (HIIT). In HIIT, you alternate a slow, low-intensity aerobic activity with a very fast, high-intensity aerobic activity, such as walking at 4 miles per hour on a treadmill and then cranking it up to a sprint at 8 miles per hour. You alternate back and forth between low-intensity and high-intensity activity, usually in a 2:1 or 1:1 ratio (2 minutes of walking and 1 minute of sprinting, say, or 1 minute of each) until your session is complete. The purpose of HIIT training is to both shorten your workout time and increase the number of calories you burn during and after the exercise.

For the Perfect Body workout program, we've created seven different HIIT routines to keep you from getting bored with the same old, same old. You'll do these on your non-weight-training days to help you burn the most body fat and improve your cardiovascular fitness. You can do these cardio workouts on machines at the gym, at home, or outside biking or running. We've even designed two of them as home cardio/weight-lifting workouts so you don't have to rely on gym machines for your weight-lifting workout.

This exercise plan also includes a separate abdominal routine specifically created for each body type. You'll do this workout on your non-weight-training days, either before or after your aerobic exercise of choice. This ensures that your abs get the attention they need to be beach ready.

Before beginning any intense cardio or strength-training workout, you need to loosen your muscles and prepare them for intense movements. A static stretch (the traditional reach-and-hold stretch) is not the best means to accomplish this. Because it forces the target muscle to relax, it temporarily makes it weaker. And that may make you more susceptible to muscle strains, pulls, and tears in the short term. Static stretching also reduces blood-flow to your muscles and decreases the activity of your central nervous system—meaning that it inhibits your brain's ability to communicate with your muscles, which limits your capacity to generate force. The bottom line: Never perform static stretching before you work out or play sports.

Instead, we recommend an *active dynamic warmup* (ADW). In an active dynamic stretch, you quickly move a muscle in and out of a stretched position (rather than holding a stretch). Here's why the difference matters: Weight training requires your muscles to stretch at fast speeds in various body positions, so your warmup must consist of stretches that prepare them to do that. Dynamic stretching improves this "active" flexibility. It also excites your central nervous system and increases bloodflow, strength, and power. So it's the ideal warmup for the Perfect Body exercise plan.

Workout Calendar

Week 1 of the weight program begins with straight-set training performed on just 2 days, to help your body adjust to weight lifting. In the straight-set format, you perform 2 or 3 sets of the first individual exercise with 30 seconds to 1 minute of rest between sets. You then rest for 2 minutes before moving on to the next exercise, also for 2 or 3 sets. Your goal is to use a weight that challenges you to complete the prescribed number of repetitions for that exercise in each set. Some exercises (such as pushups) don't require you to use any additional weight, but you should try to complete all the prescribed reps.

If you've been working out on a regular basis and doing the same program for a while, Week 1 will provide a change-up that will spark new challenges and new gains and that will prepare your body for the upcoming changes. On 3 or 4 days this week, instead of weight training, you'll do one of the cardio options, pairing it with one of the Perfect Body Ab routines for your body type.

For Weeks 2 and 3, you'll weight train 3 days a week, and on 3 other days you'll do one of the cardio options combined with one of the Perfect Body Ab routines. Try to choose one of the more intense cardio options (#2, 3, or 4) for at least 2 of those days and a less intense option (#1 or 5) on the remaining day. This will ensure that you don't overwork yourself with too many intense workouts per week. Instead of weight training 3 days in a row, you should alternate weight workouts with cardio, so your muscles have enough time to recover.

Week 4 is a back-off week—you will lift only 2 days but still do cardio on 3 or 4 days. Use the extra day away from weight training to recuperate. In week 5, you'll return to 3 days of weight training with a rep range of 10 to 12 or 12 to 15, depending on your body type.

During Weeks 6 through 8, start focusing more on physical strength. Instead of increasing your muscles' endurance with higher reps during every weight-lifting session, we want you to really challenge your body to perform either 4 to 6 or 6 to 8 reps using heavier weights, depending on the exercise. Lifting heavier weights will make your muscles stronger and more powerful. So this program will not only make you firmer and more toned in the places where you want to be, it will also give you extra strength and energy for your favorite activities—whether that means dancing all night, walking all over the shopping district with armloads of bags, or wrestling with your guy (and winning!).

Your Body Knows Best

To determine how intensely you should train on any given workout day, listen to your body. If you push yourself too hard when you're stressed or tired, you risk increasing your body's levels of cortisol, a hormone that will prompt you to store more fat in favor of burning a higher percentage of carbohydrates for fuel–the opposite of your goal. On days when you're dragging, choose the lower-intensity cardio options or complete two sets of resistance exercises instead of three. You may even want to replace your workout with a brisk walk around the neighborhood or a yoga class.

Here's an example of what your workout week will look like, based on the guidelines.

Monday: ADW + Weight-Training Day 1

Tuesday: Cardio Option #2, 3, or 4 + Perfect Body Ab Workout

Wednesday: ADW + Weight-Training Day 2

Thursday: Cardio Option #1 or 5 (less intense) + Perfect Body Ab Workout

Friday: ADW + Weight-Training Day 3

Saturday: Cardio Option #2, 3, or 4 + Perfect Body Ab Workout

Sunday: Take the day off from the gym, but make sure you do some sort of activity—whether it's yard work, walking, hiking, or vigorous cleaning—for at least 30 minutes. Sometimes, the weekends can be the hardest days to stay on track with your nutrition, so adding a bit of structured activity can help prevent those spontaneous trips to the kitchen.

*Her*Perfect Body

WHO: MICHELLE B., CSCS

WHAT: THE WOMEN'S HEALTH PERFECT BODY EXERCISE PROGRAM GAVE HER MORE CONFIDENCE

There have been many times when I have asked myself why I get up so early to work out, or why I don't just have a piece of cake, or why I don't just skip a workout. I know that if I follow my plan, it will make me feel great about myself and increase my self-confidence.

There are many psychological games you might have to play with yourself to keep going, but don't ever lose sight of your perfect body goals. Trust me, once you have your perfect body, it's much better than that piece of chocolate cake—and it can last a lifetime.

Why ADW Is the Best Warmup

1. It increases body temperature, allowing your muscles to work more efficiently.

2. It gets your heart and lungs ready for vigorous activity.

3. It stretches your muscles, preparing them for the weight-lifting session.

4. It ingrains proper movement patterns and the coordination needed to lift weights.

5. It wakes up your nervous system and gets your brain communicating with your muscles.

The Active Dynamic Warmup

Prior to every weight-lifting workout, as we described above, you will complete an Active Dynamic Warmup (ADW) to raise your body temperature, increase your dynamic flexibility, and decrease your chance of injury. By increasing bloodflow and warming up the specific muscle groups that are going to be worked, you will actually engage more motor units (groups of muscle fibers, each with its own motor neuron), which in turn will enhance the quality of your lifting and prevent injuries or strains.

The ADW exercises replace any other warmup you would normally do. For each exercise, complete the specified number of reps in a row for 1 set. If you find that a couple of the exercises are quite difficult, do an extra set of those exercises until they become fairly effortless.

Perform the following exercises one after the other, using your body weight or very light weights.

Prisoner Squat: 10 reps

Y Squat: 10 reps

Lateral Lunge: 8 reps per leg

Hip-Pop on Floor: 10 reps

Single-Leg Hip-Pop on Floor: 10 reps per leg

Bird Dog or Single-Arm, Single-Leg Superman: 10 reps per side

Y's: 10 reps

T's: 10 reps

I's: 10 reps

Wall Arm Slide: 15 reps

Walking Quad Stretch: 10 reps per leg

Knee Grab: 10 reps per leg

Walking Straight-Leg Kick: 8 reps per leg

Forward Lunge with Outside Twist: 8 reps per leg

Scapular Pushup: 10 to 15 reps

Windmill: 12 per side

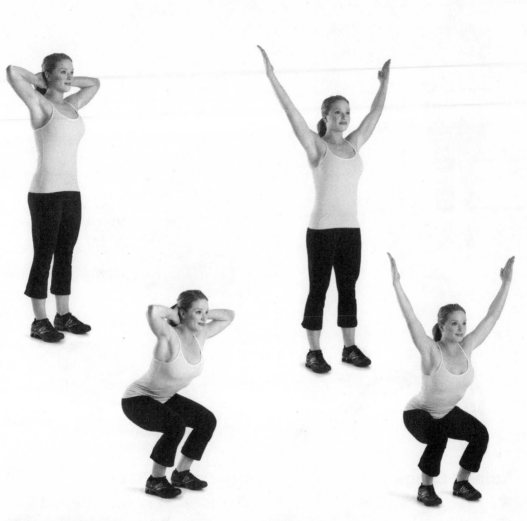

Prisoner Squat

1 Stand with your feet shoulder-width apart and your hands behind your head, fingers interlocked and chest out.

2 Bend your knees and lower your body as if you were sitting back into a chair. Stop when your thighs are parallel to the floor. Return to the starting position. Do 10 reps.

Y Squat

1 Stand with your feet shoulder-width apart and your arms extended above your head at 45-degree angles, as if forming the "Y" in "YMCA."

2 Bend your knees and lower your body as if you were sitting back into a chair. Stop when your thighs are parallel to the floor. Return to the starting position. Do 10 reps.

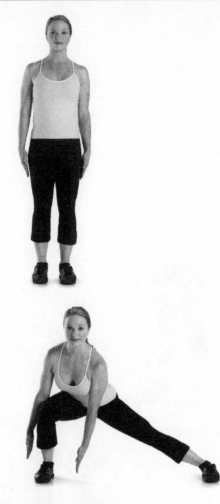

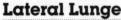

Lateral Lunge

1 Stand with your feet together.

2 Step out to the side, keeping the toes of both feet facing forward and your stationary leg straight with its foot flat on the floor. Be sure that your weight falls to the heel of your outside leg and that your foot is flat on the floor once you step out. Return to the starting position. Repeat to the other side. Do 8 reps with each leg, continuing to alternate legs.

Hip-Pop on Floor

1 Lie faceup on the floor with your knees bent and your heels close to your butt. Raise your toes off the floor so only your heels are pressed against the ground. Cross your arms over your chest and keep your head and shoulders on the floor.

2 Raise your hips toward the ceiling, creating a straight line from your shoulders to your knees and back down again. Return to the starting position. Do 10 reps.

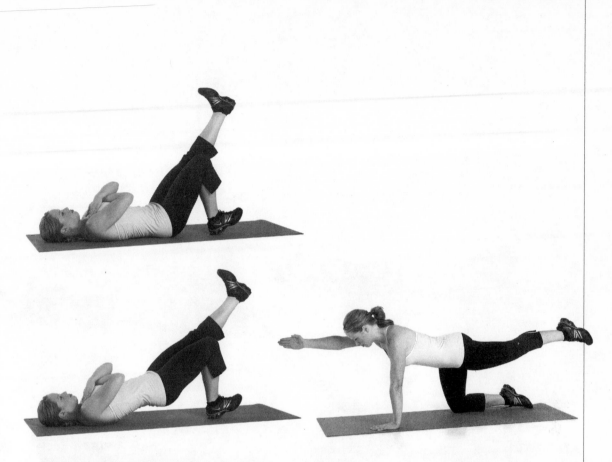

Single-Leg Hip-Pop on Floor

1 Lie faceup on the floor with one knee bent and the heel close to your butt and the other leg extended up in the air, heel toward the ceiling and knee relatively straight. Raise the toes of your planted foot off the floor so only your heel is pressed against the ground. Cross your arms over your chest and keep your head and shoulders on the floor.

2 Raise your hips toward the ceiling, creating a straight line from your shoulders to your knees and back down again. Return to the starting position. Do 10 reps, then switch legs and repeat.

Bird Dog

From an all-fours position, extend one leg and the opposite arm so that they are parallel to the floor. Hold this position for 3 to 4 seconds, and then repeat with the opposite arm and leg. Perform 10 reps on each side, ensuring that your back does not sag at any time.

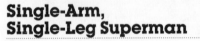

Single-Arm, Single-Leg Superman

1 Lie facedown on the floor with your arms extended in front of you, palms facing in and thumbs toward the ceiling. Flex your ankles so your toes are on the floor.

2 Keeping your eyes looking straight at the floor in front of you, simultaneously raise your left arm and right leg, keeping your knees straight and your hips square to the floor. Return to the starting position. Do 10 reps on one side before switching to the other.

Y's

1 Lie facedown on the floor with your ankles flexed and your toes on the ground. Extend your arms in front of you in a Y position with your thumbs facing up.

2 Pressing your shoulder blades down and back, lift your arms, keeping a 45-degree angle to form a Y. Return to the starting position. Do 10 reps.

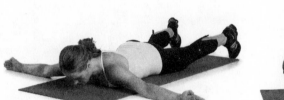

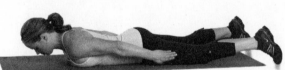

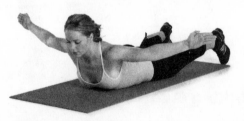

T's

1 Lie facedown on the floor with your ankles flexed and your toes on the ground. Extend your arms out to your sides in a T position with your thumbs facing up.

2 Pressing your shoulder blades down and back, lift your arms. Return to the starting position. Do 10 reps.

I's

1 Lie facedown on the floor with your ankles flexed and your toes on the ground. Extend your arms down next to your sides, forming an I shape with your body. Rotate your hands so your pinky fingers are facing up.

2 Pressing your shoulder blades down and back, lift your arms. Return to the starting position. Do 10 reps.

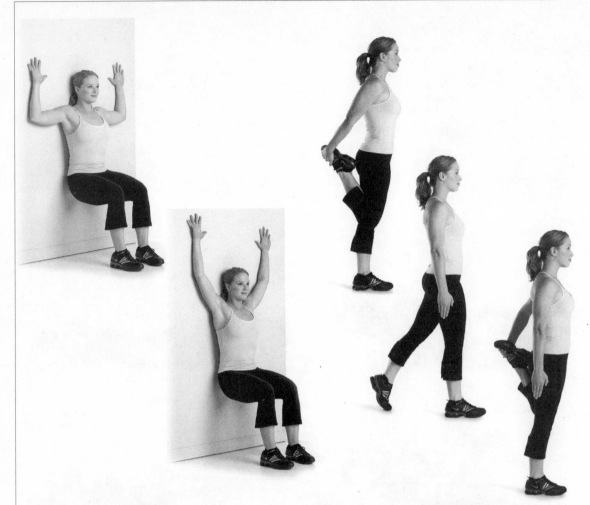

Wall Arm Slide

1 Standing with your back up against a wall and your shoulder blades squeezed in tight, raise your arms so your hands are overhead and your elbows are bent at 90-degree angles. Your shoulder blades, elbows, and wrists should be touching the wall.

2 Without losing contact with the wall at those three points, attempt to slide your arms up until they're straight (or as far as you can go without losing contact). Return to the starting position. Do 15 reps.

Walking Quad Stretch

1 Standing with your feet together, take one step while grabbing your other foot and pulling that heel in toward your butt, as shown, simultaneously pushing your hips forward.

2 Repeat on the other side, and keep traveling forward with each step/stretch until you've done 10 reps with each leg.

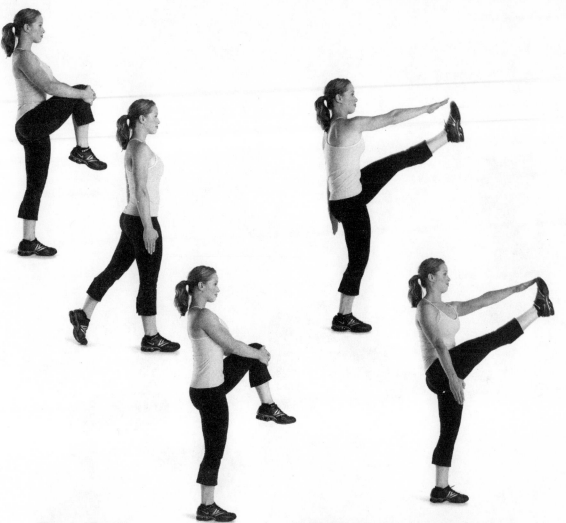

Knee Grab

❶ Standing with your feet together, take one step while grabbing your other knee up in front of you, as shown, and pulling it as high as you can while extending the rest of your body. Think about staying tall.

❷ Repeat on the other side, and keep traveling forward with each stretch until you've done 10 reps with each leg.

Walking Straight-Leg Kick

❶ Standing with your feet together, take one step while swinging the other leg straight up in front of you, keeping that knee straight and reaching for your toes with your opposite hand. Think about staying tall, and avoid bending at the waist.

❷ Repeat on the other side, and keep traveling forward with each stretch until you've done 8 reps with each leg.

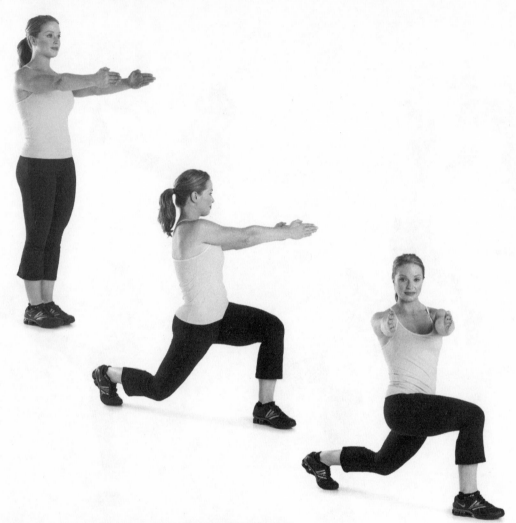

Forward Lunge with Outside Twist

1 Stand with your feet shoulder-width apart and your arms extended straight out in front of you.

2 Step forward into a lunge with your left leg, keeping your thigh parallel to the floor. With your arms straight, twist your torso toward your left leg, and then return your torso to a central position. While traveling forward, keep your arms extended, and return your body to a standing position.

3 Immediately from this position, step forward into a lunge with your right leg and twist your torso to the right. Return to a central position and keeping walking/lunging forward until you have performed 8 twists on each side.

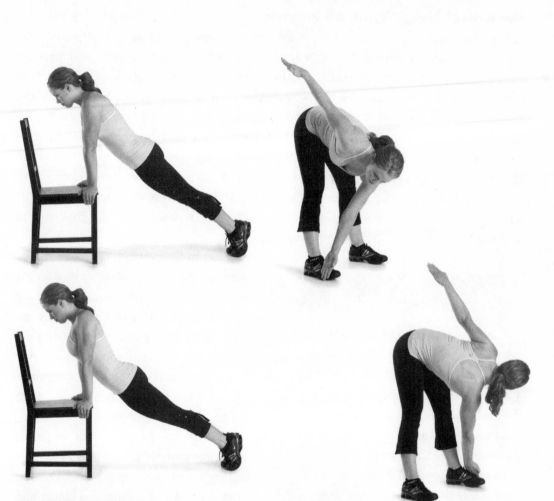

Scapular Pushup

❶ Assume a pushup position with your hands shoulder-width apart on either the floor or a chair (the floor is more difficult).

❷ Keeping your elbows locked, squeeze your shoulder blades together as if you were squeezing a penny between them, and then push them apart as far as you can. Try to avoid shrugging your shoulders and bending your elbows. Do 10 to 15 reps.

Windmill

❶ Stand with your legs more than shoulder-width apart and bend forward 90 degrees at the waist. Reach one hand to the opposite foot while the other arm swings back behind you.

❷ Then, quickly swing your other arm in front of your body and reach for the opposite foot. Do this back and forth, touching each foot 12 times. The purpose of this movement is to open up your hips and loosen your arms.

The Perfect Weight-Training Program

In the weight-training program, when exercises are grouped together as a "superset," you perform one exercise immediately after another, without resting in between, and then you rest for about 1 minute after all exercises in the grouping have been completed. The purpose of doing these back-to-back exercises with higher reps is to challenge your stamina and endurance. Once your rest is over, do another superset again, until you've completed 1 or 2 more supersets, as prescribed. Then move on to the next superset grouping of exercises.

On the days when the exercises are not grouped as supersets, you'll complete an entire circuit, performing a set of every exercise with little to no rest between sets. When you've completed the last exercise, rest for 2 to 3 minutes and then begin the circuit again. This aerobic-type circuit will burn as much fat as possible while still providing a challenge to your muscles.

Later in the program (Weeks 7 and 8), you will start your workouts with a single exercise. This exercise is alone because we want you to lift as much weight as you possibly can for 4 to 6 reps. It will help you to gain strength in places you never knew you had it. Rest for 2 to 3 minutes after this exercise, and then repeat 3 more times.

To make this program work, you must challenge yourself. Lifting heavier weights will not bulk you up; it will make you stronger, it will make you feel better, and it will sculpt your body into its perfect shape. When the guideline is to do 8 to 10 reps, it is absolutely imperative that you choose a weight with which you can do no more than 10 reps. The last 2 reps of each set should be extremely challenging, but you should be able to complete them with proper form and without help from someone else.

Short and Sweet

Can't squeeze a sumo-size gym session into your exercise schedule for the Perfect Body workout program? Not to worry. Short periods of exercise throughout the day may be better for your heart than one long workout, according to a study in the *Journal of Strength and Conditioning Research*. Scientists assigned 37 men and women to either one daily 30-minute treadmill walking session or two 15-minute sessions. Both groups showed cardiovascular improvements, but the twice-a-day walkers improved their blood pressure and heart rate more than the others. The researchers conclude, "Intermittent exercise may allow you to exercise at a greater intensity since you're working out in shorter bouts."

Here are all the resistance exercises you'll perform in your workout program. These moves will be put together in different combinations in the following chapters, based on the best workout for your body type. Chapter 13 outlines the workouts for Apples, Chapter 14 offers the prescription for Pears, and Chapter 15 gives the details for Avocados and Bananas.

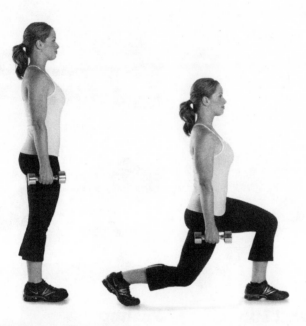

Dumbbell Reverse Lunge

1 Stand with both feet together, holding a dumbbell in each hand.

2 Step back with one foot behind you until both knees are bent at a 90-degree angle and you are in a split squat or lunge position. Now step forward, using your front leg to drive the action, until both feet are back together. Make sure that your toes are facing forward and your front knee is lined up directly over your heel throughout the movement.

3 Repeat on the same side until you've completed the prescribed number of repetitions, then switch sides.

» VARIATION: Perform this exercise without weights (not pictured).

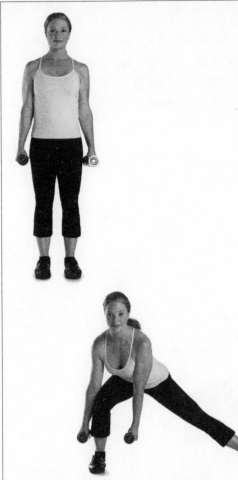

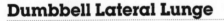

Dumbbell Lateral Lunge

1 Stand with your feet together, holding a dumbbell at each side.

2 Step out to the side, keeping the toes of both feet facing forward and your stationary leg straight with its foot flat on the floor. Position the weights so that they are on either side of your lunged leg. Be sure that your body weight falls to the heel of your outside leg and that your foot is flat on the floor once you step out. Return to the starting position. Repeat to the other side. Do the prescribed number of reps with each leg, continuing to alternate legs.

Pushup

1 Place your hands on the floor, slightly wider than shoulder-width apart, and extend your legs behind you, your toes on the floor. Lower your body by bending your elbows until your body is 2 inches off the floor.

2 Press up until your arms are straight. Return to the starting position.

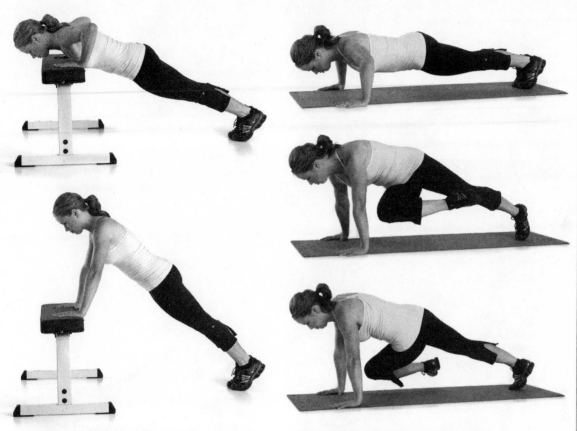

Bench Pushup

1 Facing the widest side of a bench, place both hands on the edge with your arms extended, and extend your feet behind you with your toes on the floor.

2 Lower your upper body until your chest touches the bench. Then push back up to the starting position.

Pushup with Leg Twist

1 Place your hands on the floor, slightly wider than shoulder-width apart, and extend your legs behind you, your toes on the floor. Lower your body by bending your elbows until your body is 2 inches off the floor.

2 Press up until your arms are straight, then draw in your belly button and raise one knee toward the opposite elbow while keeping your hips forward and your butt down. Return to the starting position.

3 Repeat this action with the opposite leg to complete one rep. Alternate legs until you've completed the prescribed number of reps.

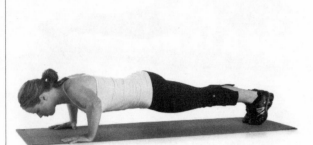

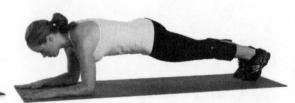

T-Pushup

① Place your hands on the floor, slightly wider than shoulder-width apart, and extend your legs behind you, your toes on the floor. Lower your body by bending your elbows until your body is 2 inches off the floor.

② Push up with your arms and, once they're straight, lift your left hand and roll onto the outside of your feet, keeping your body aligned. Extend your left arm toward the ceiling. Hold for 1 second before returning to the starting position. Repeat on the other side.

Front Plank

Assume a modified pushup position on your elbows and toes. Your body will form a straight line from your shoulders to your ankles. Pull your abs in, but don't stick out your butt. Hold this position with a straight body for the prescribed amount of time.

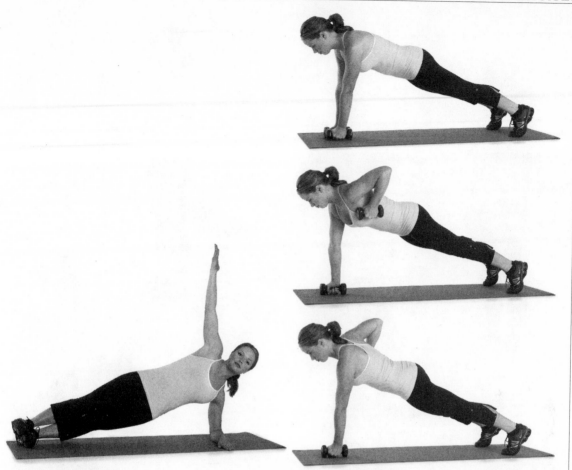

Side Plank

Lie on your side. Lift your body while facing forward, and support your weight with that forearm and the outside edge of your foot. Extend your other arm toward the ceiling. Your body will form a straight line from your shoulders to your ankles. Pull in your abs and keep your body in a straight line. Hold this position for at least 20 seconds, or the prescribed amount of time.

Plank Row

❶ Assume a pushup position with dumbbells in your hands on the floor. Place your hands right beside each other, extend your arms, and spread your feet a little wider than shoulder-width apart to increase stability.

❷ Without shifting your hips, and keeping your entire body as still as possible, pull one weight toward your chest. Lower it with control back to the floor.

❸ Alternate arms until you've completed the prescribed number of repetitions.

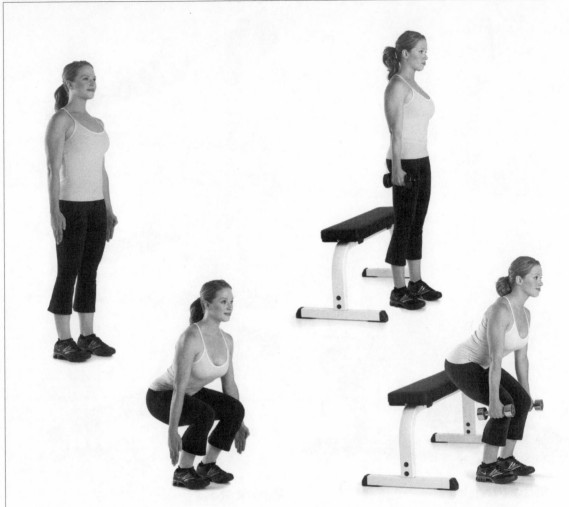

Body-Weight Squat

1 Stand with your feet hip-width apart, toes facing forward, abs tight, and arms at your sides.

2 Bend your knees and lower your body as if you were sitting back into a chair. Stop when your thighs are parallel to the floor. Return to the starting position.

Dumbbell Bench Squat

1 Holding a dumbbell in each hand, stand with your back to a bench.

2 Lower yourself onto the bench, keeping the weight of your body on your heels, the natural curve in your back, your arms relaxed, and the weights lined up with your heels. Very lightly touch the bench without releasing your weight completely. Then stand back up, driving up through your heels and squeezing your glutes and quads.

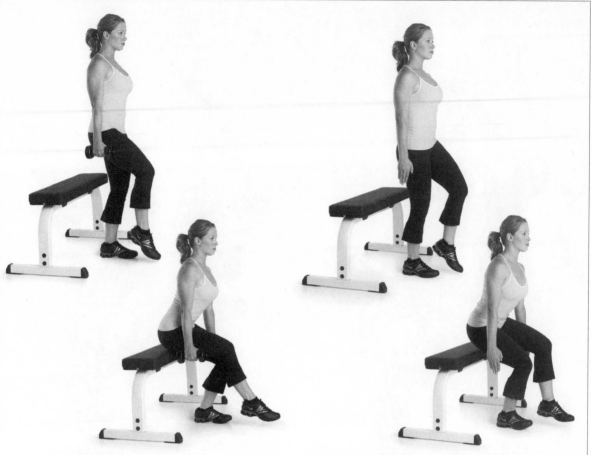

Dumbbell Single-Leg Bench Squat

1 Holding a dumbbell in each hand, stand on one leg with your back to a bench.

2 Lower yourself onto the bench, keeping the weight of your body on your supporting heel, the natural curve in your back, your arms relaxed, and the weights lined up with your heels. Very lightly touch the bench without releasing your weight completely. Then stand back up, driving up through your heel and squeezing your glutes and quads. Repeat for the prescribed number of reps, then repeat with your other leg.

Body-Weight Single-Leg Bench Squat

1 Stand on one leg with your back to a bench.

2 Lower yourself onto the bench, keeping the weight of your body on your supporting heel, the natural curve in your back, your arms relaxed, and the weights lined up with your heels. Very lightly touch the bench without releasing your weight completely. Then stand back up, driving up through your heel and squeezing your glutes and quads.

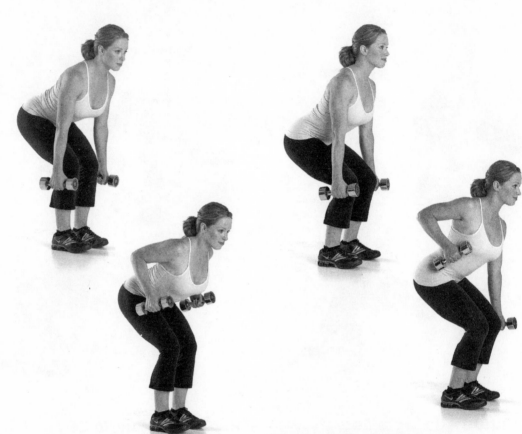

Bent-Over Dumbbell Row

1 Stand with your feet shoulder-width apart or slightly narrower and your knees bent, holding a dumbbell in each hand. Hinge yourself at the hips without losing the natural curve in your back. Your back should be at a 45-degree angle to the floor.

2 Bring the weights toward your chest by bending your elbows and squeezing your shoulder blades together without shrugging your shoulders. Return to the starting position.

Single-Arm Bent-Over Dumbbell Row

1 Stand with your feet shoulder-width apart or slightly narrower with your knees bent, holding a dumbbell in each hand. Hinge yourself at the hips without losing the natural curve in your back. Your back should be at a 45-degree angle to the floor.

2 Bring one of the weights toward your chest by bending your elbow and squeezing your shoulder blade up without shrugging your shoulder. Return to the starting position. Repeat for the prescribed number of reps, then repeat with the other arm.

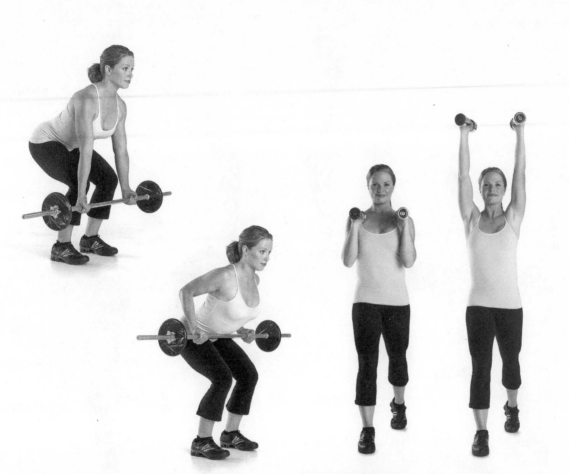

Bent-Over Barbell Row

❶ Stand with your feet shoulder-width apart or slightly narrower with your knees bent, holding a barbell with your palms facing up. Hinge yourself at the hips without losing the natural curve in your back. Your back should be at a 45-degree angle to the floor.

❷ Bring the bar toward your chest by bending your elbows and squeezing your shoulder blades together without shrugging your shoulders. Return to the starting position.

Lunge-Stance Dumbbell Shoulder Press

❶ Stand with one foot about 2 feet behind the other, its heel off the floor. Your toes should face forward. Hold a dumbbell in each hand at shoulder height, your palms facing your shoulders.

❷ Raise the weights directly overhead until your arms are fully extended. Then return to the starting position.

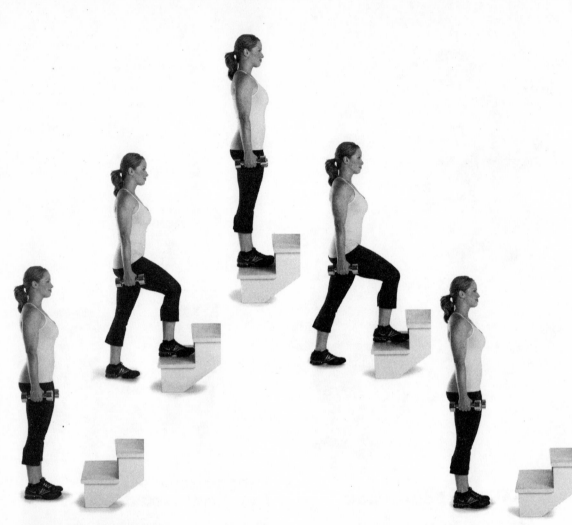

Dumbbell Stepup

❶ Stand facing a step, bench, or box, holding a dumbbell in each hand.

❷ Place your right foot on the step.

❸ Driving the weight of your body through your right heel, stand up on the step.

❹ Then lower yourself, with control, back to the floor, left foot first, and step off completely. Repeat on the other side (i.e., first right leg leads up, then left leg leads down; left leg leads up, right leg leads down). Complete the prescribed number of reps for each leg.

» VARIATION: Perform this exercise without weights (not pictured).

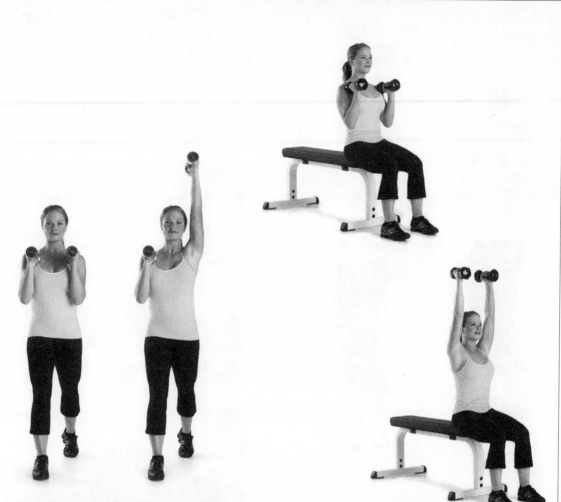

Lunge-Stance Single-Arm Dumbbell Shoulder Press

1 Stand with your left foot about 2 feet behind the other, its heel off the floor. Your toes should face forward. Hold a dumbbell in each hand at shoulder height, your palms facing your shoulders.

2 Raise the weight in your left hand directly overhead until your arm is fully extended. Complete the prescribed number of reps, then stagger your left foot in front of your right and repeat with your right arm.

Seated Shoulder Press

1 Sitting on the end of a bench, hold a dumbbell in each hand at shoulder height, your palms facing your shoulders.

2 Press the weights directly overhead until your arms are fully extended. Then return to the starting position.

» **VARIATION:** Perform this exercise while seated on a stability ball (not pictured).

Standing Alternating Shoulder Press

1 Standing with your feet shoulder-width apart, hold a dumbbell in each hand at shoulder height, your palms facing your shoulders.

2 Raise the weight in one hand directly overhead until your arm is fully extended. Lower to the starting position and repeat with the opposite arm. Alternate arms until the prescribed number of reps is completed.

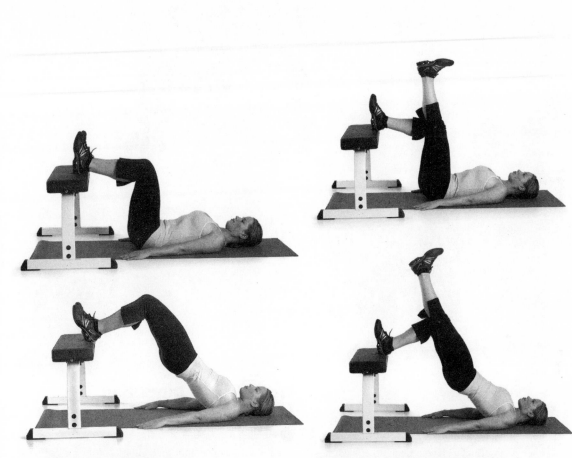

Bench or Stability Ball Hip-Pop

❶ Lie on the floor and place both heels on a bench or ball with your knees bent at about 90 degrees and your toes completely off the object.

❷ Keeping your head, shoulders, and arms on the floor, lift your hips until a straight line is formed from your shoulders to your knees.

Single-Leg Bench or Stability Ball Hip-Pop

❶ Lie on the floor and place one heel on a bench or ball with your knee bent at about 90 degrees and your toes off the device completely. Extend your other leg toward the ceiling.

❷ Keeping your head, shoulders, and arms on the floor, lift your hips until a straight line is formed from your shoulders to your knees. Do all reps with one leg and then switch to the other.

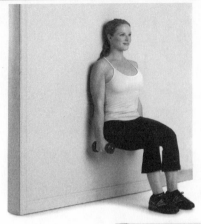

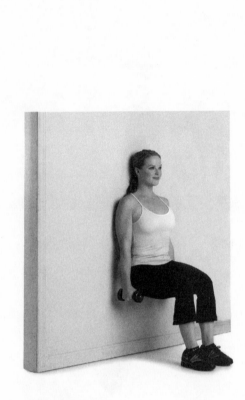

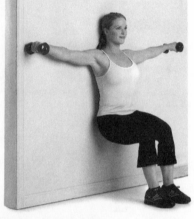

Wall Sit

Holding a dumbbell in each hand with your arms at your sides, stand with your back up against a wall, your shoulders pressed down and back. Bend your knees to 90 degrees, with your heels under your knees and the weight of your body on your heels. Keep your back and shoulders pressed against the wall while you remain in the squat position for the allotted time.

Wall Sit with Dumbbell Lateral Shoulder Raise

❶ Holding a dumbbell in each hand with your arms at your sides, stand with your back up against a wall and your shoulders pressed down and back. Bend your knees to 90 degrees, with your heels under your knees and the weight of your body on your heels.

❷ Keeping your back and shoulder blades against the wall, raise your arms out to your sides, lifting them no farther than shoulder height. Lower to the starting position.

》 VARIATION: Perform the dumbbell lateral shoulder raise in a standing position (not pictured).

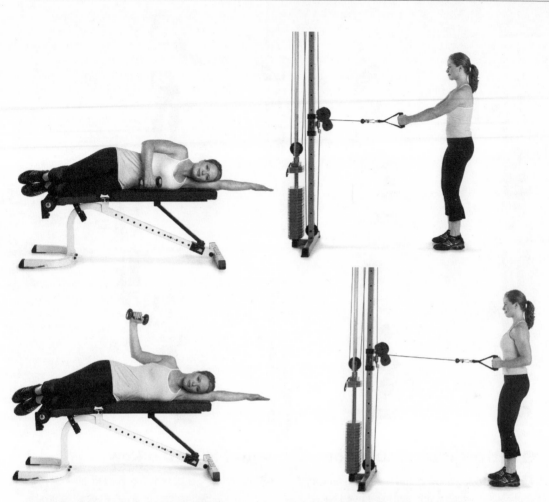

Lying External Rotation

❶ Lying on your side on a bench with a dumbbell in your outside hand, bend your elbow to 90 degrees with your palm facing the floor.

❷ Rotate your arm backward by squeezing your shoulder blade and keeping your elbow tight to your side until the back of your hand faces directly behind you. Return to the starting position and repeat for the prescribed number of reps. Then lie on your other side and repeat with the opposite arm.

Standing Cable Row

❶ Stand at a cable pulley station with movable pulleys, with your feet shoulder-width apart and your knees slightly bent. Set the cable handles so they are level with your belly button. Hold the handles with your arms straight and the weight stack slightly off the rack.

❷ Squeezing your shoulder blades together without shrugging your shoulders, pull back with both arms to bring the handle to your abs. Keep your chest out. Return to the starting position.

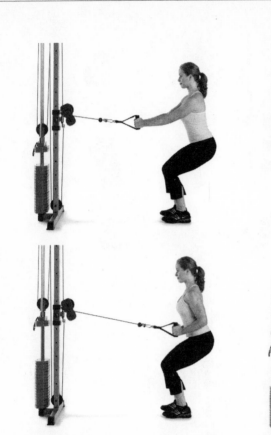

Quarter-Squat Cable Row

❶ Stand facing a low-cable pulley station with your feet shoulder-width apart and bend your knees, keeping your weight on your heels, until you reach a quarter-squat position. Set the cable handles so they are level with your belly button. Hold the handles with your arms straight and the weight stack slightly off the rack.

❷ Squeezing your shoulder blades together without shrugging your shoulders, pull back with both arms to bring the handle to your abs. Keep your chest out. Return to the starting position.

Squat to Cable Row

❶ Stand facing a low-cable pulley station with your feet shoulder-width apart and your knees slightly bent, Set the cable handles so they are level with your belly button. Hold the handles with your arms straight and the weight stack slightly off the rack.

❷ Bend your knees and lower your body as if you were sitting back into a chair. Stop when your thighs are parallel to the floor.

❸ As you stand back up, squeeze your shoulder blades together without shrugging your shoulders, pulling back with both arms to bring the handle to your abs. Keep your chest out. Return to the starting position.

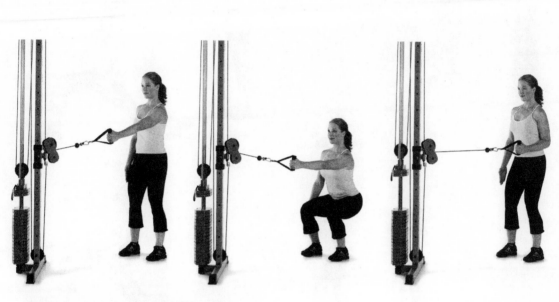

Squat to Single-Arm Cable Row

1 Stand facing a low-cable pulley station with your feet shoulder-width apart and your knees slightly bent. Set one D-shaped cable handle so it's level with your belly button. Hold the handle with one hand, keeping that arm straight and the weight stack slightly off the rack. Allow your other arm to hang at your side.

2 Bend your knees and lower your body as if you were sitting back into a chair. Stop when your thighs are parallel to the floor.

3 As you stand back up, pull back with your working arm to bring the handle to your abs. Keep your chest out. Return to the starting position. Do the prescribed number of reps with that arm, then repeat with the opposite arm, using the same cable that you were just using.

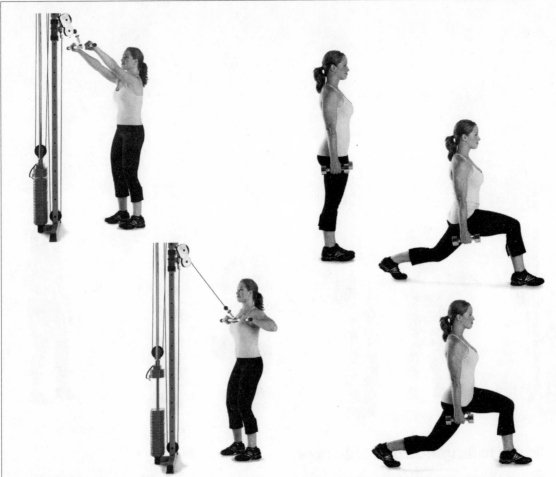

Cable Lat Pulldown

1 Attach a short straight bar to the high pulley of a cable machine and hold it with your palms facing away from your body a little bit wider than shoulder-width apart. Stand with your arms extended.

2 Keeping your shoulder blades down and back, pull the bar down to your chest. Slowly and with control, return to the starting position. Do not let your shoulders shrug on the way up.

Walking Dumbbell Lunge

1 Stand with your feet together and a challenging dumbbell in each hand.

2 Take a big step forward and lower yourself toward the floor until your forward thigh is parallel to the floor. Keep your knees and toes facing forward and the weight of your front foot on your heel.

3 Drive off your front foot to bring your feet back together as you move forward.

4 Then lunge forward with your other leg.

5 One rep counts as one lunge with one leg.

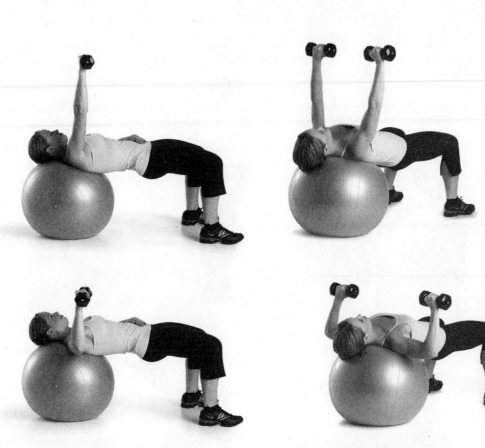

Single-Arm Dumbbell Chest Press on Ball

❶ With your shoulders and head on a stability ball, your feet on the floor, and your hips bridged up, hold a dumbbell in one hand with that arm extended straight up above you, your palm facing your feet. Rest your other hand on your belly.

❷ Lower the weight until your elbow reaches 90 degrees. Keep your hips level and your abs and glutes engaged throughout the entire movement. Press back up to the starting position. Do the prescribed number of reps with that arm, then repeat with the other arm.

Dumbbell Chest Press on Ball

❶ With your shoulders and head on a stability ball, your feet on the floor, and your hips bridged up, hold a dumbbell in each hand with your arms extended straight up above you, your palms facing your feet.

❷ Lower the weights until your elbows reach 90 degrees. Press back up to the starting position. Keep your hips level and your abs and glutes engaged throughout the entire movement.

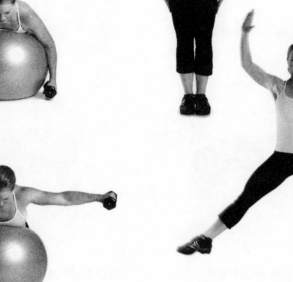

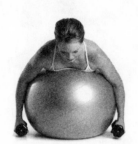

Reverse Dumbbell Fly on Ball

❶ Holding a dumbbell in each hand, lie with your chest on a stability ball, letting your arms hang down toward the floor, palms facing each other.

❷ Pinch your shoulder blades together as you raise your arms in a wide, arcing motion out to your sides, keeping your legs as straight as possible. Hold the weights at the top for a second or two, the lower back to the starting position with control. Don't rest the weights on the floor.

Jumping Jack

❶ Stand with your feet together and your arms at your sides.

❷ Jump up, kicking your legs out to your sides and bringing your arms together above your head. Return to the starting position.

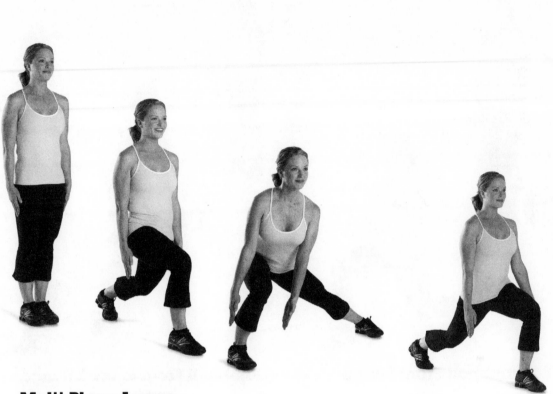

Multi-Plane Lunge

❶ Stand with your feet together.

❷ Take a big step forward and lower yourself toward the floor until your forward thigh is parallel to the floor. Keep your knees and toes facing forward and the weight of your front foot on your heel.

❸ Return to the starting position.

❹ Next, step out to the side with the same leg until that thigh is parallel to the floor, keeping the toes of both feet facing forward and your stationary leg straight with its foot flat on the floor. Be sure that your weight falls to the heel of your outside leg and that your foot is flat on the floor once you step out.

❺ Return to the starting position.

❻ Immediately step back with the same leg until your forward thigh is parallel to the floor.

❼ Return to the starting position.

❽ Do the prescribed number of reps with one leg, then repeat with the opposite leg.

》 VARIATION: Perform this exercise using dumbbells.

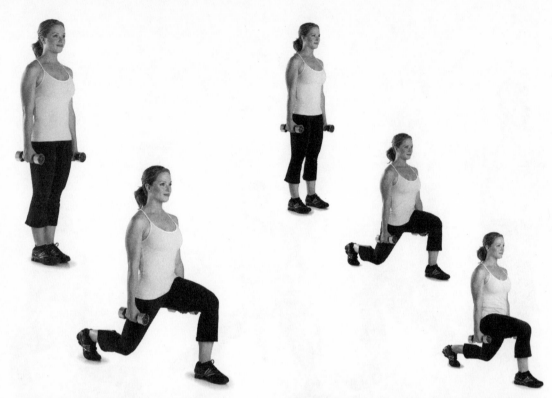

Dumbbell Front Lunge

1 Stand with your feet hip-width apart and hold a dumbbell in each hand, with your arms at your sides.

2 Step forward with one leg and lower yourself until that thigh is parallel to the floor. Return to the starting position.

3 Repeat with your opposite leg.

》 VARIATION: Perform this exercise without weights

Dumbbell Front to Back Lunge

1 Stand with your feet hip-width apart and hold a dumbbell in each hand with your arms at your sides.

2 With your left foot, step forward into a front lunge until your front thigh is parallel to the floor and your knee is aligned over your heel.

3 Immediately step back into a reverse lunge, placing the ball of your left foot on the floor 2 to 3 feet behind you and lowering your left knee to 2 to 3 inches above the floor. Your front leg should end up bent about 90 degrees, with that knee over the heel. This exercise can be a balance challenge, so make sure you focus and keep your toes facing forward and your knee aligned over the heel of your foot.

》 VARIATION: Perform this exercise without weights (not pictured).

Front Lunge with Biceps Curl

❶ Stand with your feet hip-width apart and hold a dumbbell in each hand with your arms at your sides, your palms facing forward.

❷ Step forward with one leg and then lower yourself until that thigh is parallel to the floor. Simultaneously curl the weights up to your shoulders. Return to the starting position.

❸ Repeat with your opposite leg.

Single-Arm Overhead Dumbbell Squat

❶ Standing with your feet shoulder-width apart, hold one dumbbell by your side and another half its weight overhead, your palm facing forward (e.g., 10 pounds by your side and 5 pounds overhead).

❷ Without letting the overhead dumbbell sway back or forth, bend your knees and lower your body until your thighs are parallel to the floor, keeping your hips square. The movement path for the dumbbell overhead should be straight up and down, and you should try to keep your chest out, a natural curve in your back, and your weight on your heels. Return to the starting position. Do the prescribed number of reps with that arm, then switch the weights into your opposite hands and repeat with the other arm.

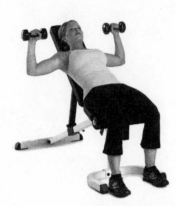

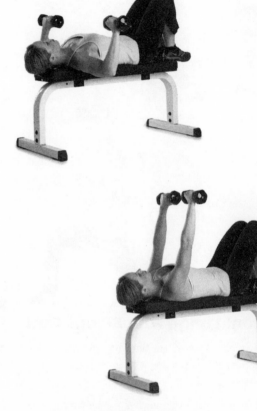

Dumbbell Incline Chest Press

1 Lie faceup on an incline bench with a dumbbell in each hand, palms facing forward. Extend your arms out to your sides and bend your elbows to 90 degrees.

2 Push the dumbbells straight up until your arms are fully extended. Return to the starting position.

Dumbbell Chest Press

1 Lie faceup on a flat bench, letting your elbows and shoulders drop. Hold a dumbbell in each hand on either side of your chest, with your elbows bent to 90 degrees.

2 Push both weights straight up at the same pace until your arms are fully extended. Hold them there for 1 second, then return to the starting position.

Triple Hamstring Series

This stability ball exercise is a combination of double-leg hip-pops with your heels on the ball immediately followed by leg curls (no rest in between), immediately followed by single-leg hip-pops with your toes on the ball. Keep a slight bend in your knees throughout this exercise.

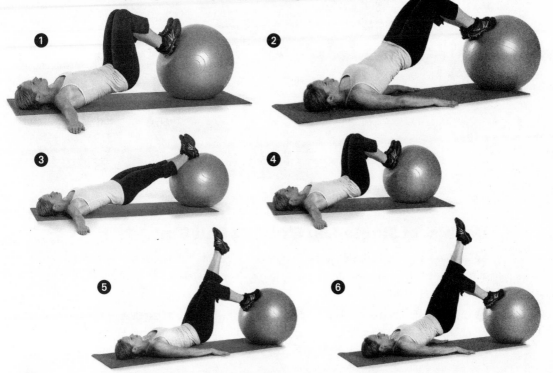

1 Lie faceup on the floor and place the heels of both feet on the ball, with your knees bent at about 90 degrees and the balls of your feet off the stability ball.

2 Keeping your head, shoulders, and arms on the floor, lift your hips until a straight line is formed from your shoulders to your knees.

3 Place just your heels on the ball, knees slightly bent and arms out to your sides. Push down on the ball with your feet, extending from your hips so your butt is 2 to 3 inches off the floor.

4 Curl the ball toward your body by bending your knees toward your chest as far as you can, keeping your hips off the floor.

5 Place the toes of one foot onto the ball with your knee bent at about 90 degrees and your heel off the device. Extend your other leg toward the ceiling.

6 Keeping your head, shoulders, and arms on the floor, lift your hips until a straight line is formed from your shoulders to your knees. Do the prescribed number of reps with that leg, then repeat with the other leg.

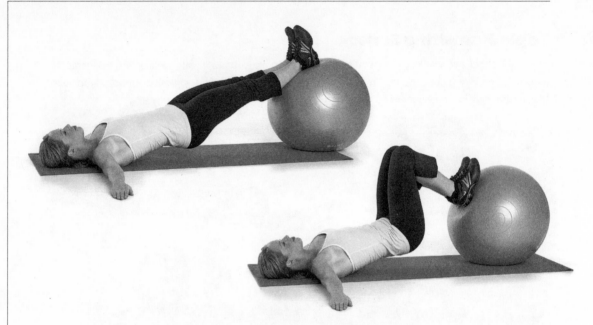

Double- or Single-Leg Stability Ball Curl

1 Lie faceup on the floor with just your heels on a stability ball, knees slightly bent and arms out to your sides. Push down on the ball with your feet, extending from your hips so that your butt is raised high off the floor.

2 Curl the ball with your heels placed on top toward your body by bending your knees toward your chest as far as you can, keeping your hips off the floor. Push the ball back out to the starting position, leaving a slight bend in your knees at the end of the movement. Keep your hips elevated throughout the repetitions.

» **VARIATION:** For added difficulty, attempt this exercise with one leg on the ball and one leg extended, heel pointed toward the ceiling and knee relatively straight.

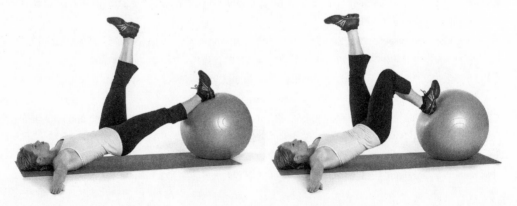

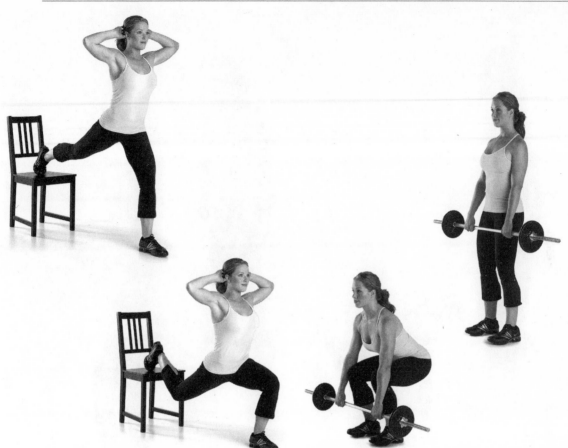

Balance Squat

1 Stand and place the instep of one foot on a chair or bench 2 to 3 feet behind you. Hold your hands behind your ears.

2 Balancing on your front foot, bend both knees to lower your body straight down until your back knee is a few inches from the floor and your front knee is at a 90-degree angle, the thigh parallel to the floor and the calf perpendicular to the floor. Your torso and rear thigh should form a straight line. Return to the starting position. Do the prescribed number of reps, then switch your front and back legs and repeat.

Deadlift

1 Standing with your feet shoulder-width apart and a 9- to 12-pound barbell in front of you, squat until your thighs are parallel to the floor and grasp the bar with an overhand grip, your hands just to the outside of your knees. Keep your back flat and do not let it round.

2 Push with your heels and pull the weight to your body as you stand up. Hold for 1 second, then return to the starting position.

Straight-Leg Dumbbell Deadlift

1 Standing with your knees slightly bent and aligned over your middle toes, hold a dumbbell in each hand with an overhand grip, your palms facing the front of your thighs.

2 Keeping your arms straight and your knees in place, slowly bend at your waist and lower the weights as far as possible toward the floor without rounding your back. Squeeze your glutes to pull yourself up.

Dumbbell Front Shoulder Raise

1 Standing with your feet shoulder-width apart and your knees slightly bent, hold a dumbbell in each hand with your palms facing your thighs, and lean forward very slightly at the hips.

2 Raise the weights out in front of you until your arms are parallel to the floor. Pause, then lower the weights to the starting position.

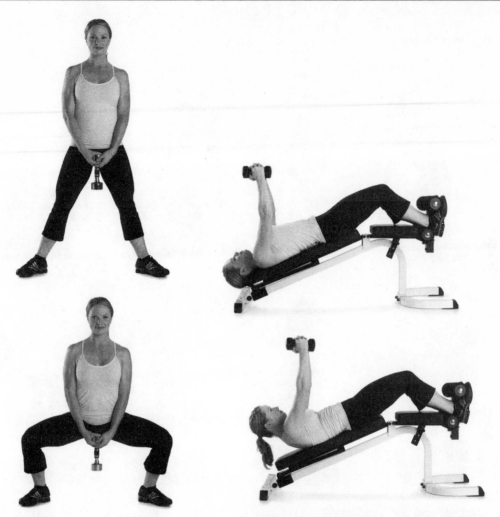

Dumbbell Plié Squat

❶ Grab a 5- to 8-pound dumbbell with both hands, stand with your feet slightly wider than your shoulders, and turn your toes out 45 degrees. Hold the weight between your thighs and keep your back straight and your shoulder blades squeezed tight.

❷ Keeping your butt as far back as possible, lower your tailbone until your thighs are parallel to the floor. Press back up to the starting position.

Weighted Decline Crunch

❶ Lie faceup on a decline bench and hook your feet under the holds. (If you don't have access to a decline bench, use a flat bench or lie on the floor.) Holding a single dumbbell in your hands, extend your arms straight above your shoulders.

❷ Push the weight directly toward the ceiling by lifting your shoulders. Return to the starting position.

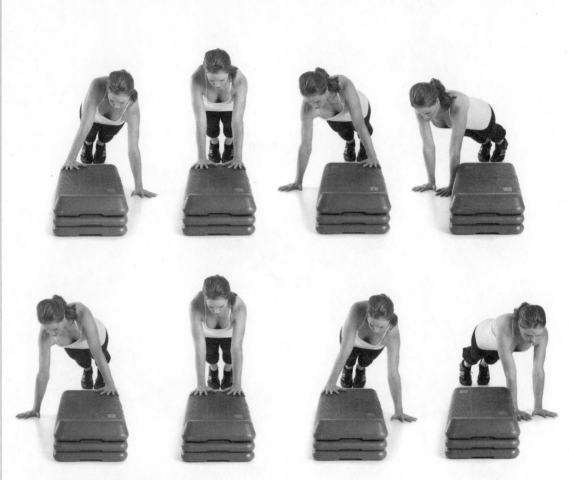

Upper-Body Stepover

❶ Using an aerobics step, get into a pushup position with your right hand on the step and the left on the floor, both arms extended and your legs extended behind you.

❷ Move your left hand up onto the step.

❸ Then move your right hand down onto the floor.

❹ Move your left hand down onto the floor.

❺ Then move your left and then right hands back onto the step and then back down off the other side.

❻ The entire sequence counts as one rep.

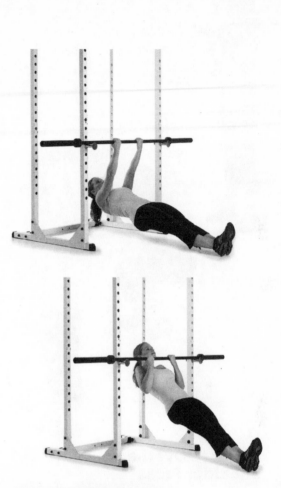

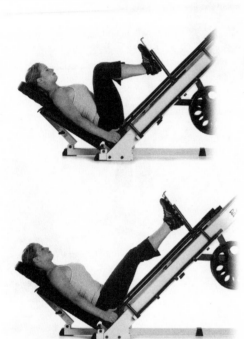

Leg Press

❶ Place your feet shoulder-width apart on the platform of a leg press machine, turning them slightly outward. Unlock any safety devices and allow the weight to lower toward your chest.

❷ Drive up, pressing through your heels and keeping your feet flat on the platform until your knees are almost fully extended. Try not to lock any joints while performing this exercise. Return to the starting position.

Inverted Body Row

❶ Set a chinning bar 3 to 4 feet from the floor (in a doorway or squat rack). Lie on your back with your chest directly below the bar. Reach up and grab the bar with a shoulder-width, underhand grip so that you're hanging from the bar and your body forms a straight diagonal line from your heels to your shoulders.

❷ Keeping your core tight, pull yourself up until your chest meets the bar. Lower yourself to the starting position.

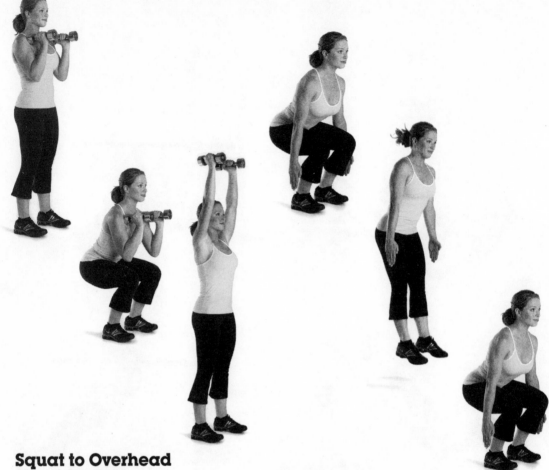

Squat to Overhead Shoulder Press

1 Standing with your feet shoulder-width apart, hold a dumbbell in each hand at shoulder level, palms facing each other.

2 Bend your knees and lower your body as if you were sitting back into a chair. Stop when your thighs are parallel to the floor.

3 Press back up and, as you do so, press the weights overhead until your arms are fully extended. Lower the weights as you descend into the next squat. Keep your chest out and the weight of your body on your heels.

Squat Jump

1 Stand with your feet shoulder-width apart. Keep your back straight, contract your abs, and lower your hips while pushing your glutes out until you're in a seated position with your thighs parallel to the floor and your knees aligned over your toes.

2 Press through your legs to jump up.

3 Land in the squat position. Then immediately jump straight up again.

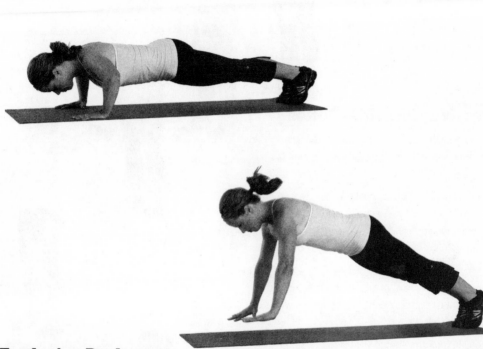

Explosive Pushup

❶ Place your hands on the floor, slightly wider than shoulder-width apart, and extend your legs behind you, your toes on the floor. Lower your body by bending your elbows until your body is 2 inches off the floor.

❷ Push up as fast as you can, catching a bit of air at the top.

Three-Way Shoulder Series

1 Standing with your feet shoulder-width apart, hold a light dumbbell in each hand with your palms facing the fronts of your thighs.

2 Complete a front shoulder raise, raising the weights out in front of you until your arms are parallel to the floor (keep your shoulder blades pulled down and back—no shrugging). Return to the starting position. Complete the prescribed number of reps.

3 Immediately do a set of lateral shoulder raises: First, hold the weights in front of your thighs with your palms facing each other.

4 Then lift your arms out to your sides, raising them no farther than shoulder height. Return to the starting position. Complete the prescribed number of reps.

5 Immediately do a set of bent-over reverse flies: Bend your knees and bend over at the hips until your torso is at a 45-degree angle to the floor, letting your arms hang straight down.

6 Pinch your shoulder blades together as you raise your arms in a wide, arcing motion out to your sides. Return to the starting position. Complete the prescribed number of reps. For example, if your designated number of reps is 10, do 10 front raises, 10 lateral raises, and then 10 bent-over reverse flies all in a row.

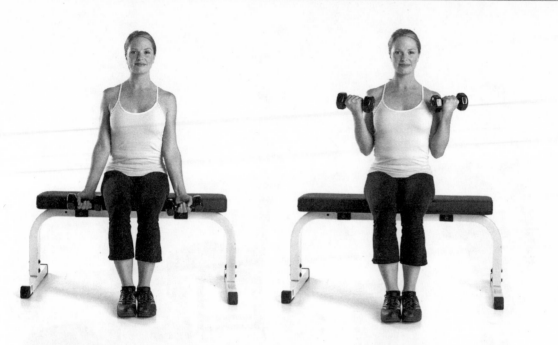

Biceps/Triceps Dumbbell Combo on Bench/Ball

❶ While sitting on a bench or ball, hold dumbbells at your sides with your palms facing forward. Curl the weights up to your shoulders and then lower them slowly to the starting position. Repeat for the prescribed number of reps.

❷ Now lie faceup on the bench or ball and do lying triceps crushers: Hold the dumbbells next to your ears, palms facing your face. Straighten your elbows until your arms are extended. Return to the starting position, then repeat for the prescribed number of reps.

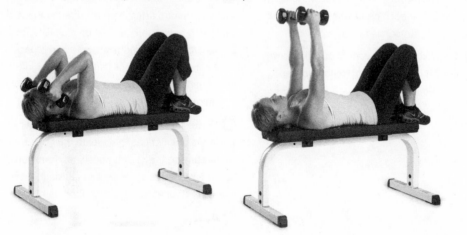

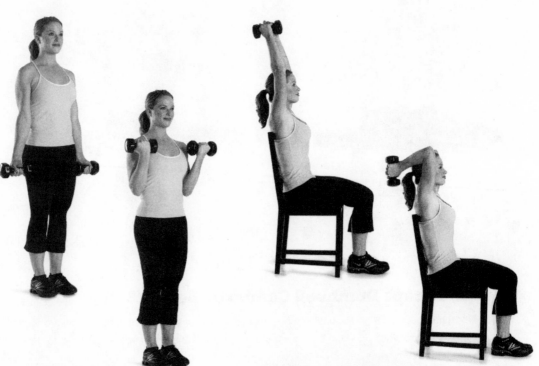

Standing Biceps Curl

❶ Standing with your feet shoulder-width apart, hold a dumbbell in each hand with your arms at your sides and your palms facing forward.

❷ Curl the weights up to your shoulders. Slowly return to the starting position. Repeat for the prescribed number of reps.

Seated Overhead Triceps Extension

❶ Grab the end of a dumbbell, heavy enough so that you fatigue after the prescribed amount of reps, with both hands and sit on a chair. With your palms around the weight's handle and pressing up on the inside of the upper end, lift the weight over your head and hold it there with your elbows close to your ears.

❷ Lower the weight behind your head until your forearms are just past parallel to the floor. Pause, then return to the starting position. Keep your upper arms in the same position throughout the exercise. Repeat for the prescribed number of reps.

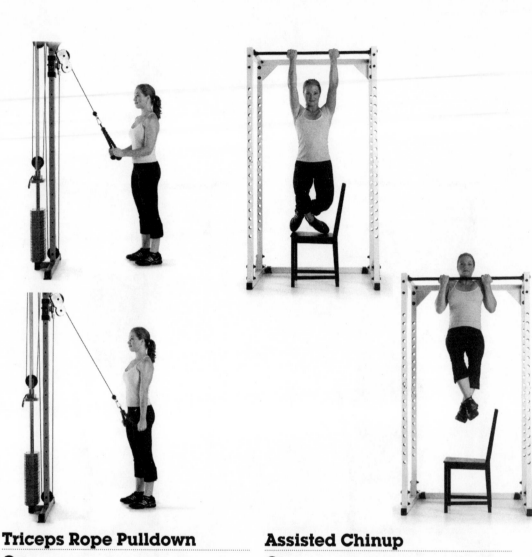

Triceps Rope Pulldown

1 Stand facing a cable machine with a rope handle on the high pulley. Grab an end of the rope in each hand and pull the handle down until your elbows are bent 90 degrees.

2 Straighten your arms until they're fully extended at your sides. Return to the starting position, then repeat for the prescribed number of reps.

Assisted Chinup

1 With a chair beneath you, grab a chinning bar with an underhand, shoulder-width grip and hang with your elbows slightly bent.

2 Keeping your chest out and your body straight beneath you, pull yourself straight up over the bar, pushing off the chair a bit with your legs. Return to the starting position.

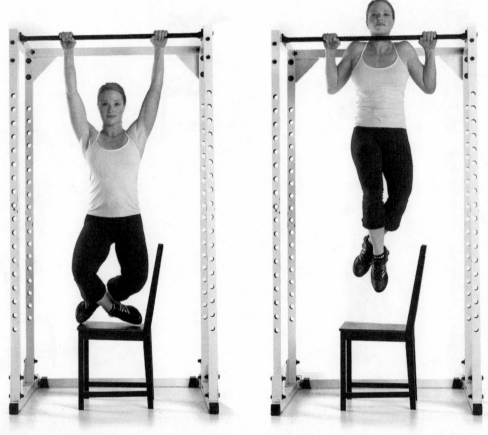

Assisted Pullup

1 With a chair beneath you, grab a chinning bar with an overhand grip that's slightly wider than shoulder-width and hang with your elbows slightly bent.

2 Keeping your chest out and your body straight beneath you, pull yourself straight up over the bar, pushing off the chair a bit with your legs. Return to the starting position.

The Perfect Cardio Plan

Including cardiovascular workouts in your exercise program will help you get to your perfect body goals faster. Although weight training is effective for fat loss, cardio will give you a day off from lifting while still keeping you exercising.

Regardless of your body type, you'll perform one of the following six cardio options on 3 of your days "off" from weight lifting. Any of the workouts can be done in your home or outdoors. You don't necessarily have to go to a gym. All of the options can be performed using any type of cardio machine or activity that you prefer, such as running, swimming, cycling, using an elliptical machine or a rowing machine, or stairclimbing. However, you should take your body type into account when you pick a cardio modality. Apples should focus on activities that engage the abdominal muscles to help make the tummy tight, so they should avoid bikes and holding on to the railings of a stairclimber.

Pears should focus on aerobic activities that really challenge the leg muscles and butt for the maximum possible fat burning in those areas. Pears will do well with incline treadmill or hill running or those grueling 1-hour Spinning classes.

Avocado and Banana bods can do whatever activities they like, but Bananas should do cardio one less day per week because they don't need to jeopardize their chances of adding extra muscle.

Choose whichever one of the six cardio workouts you feel is best for your body based on how you feel at workout time. If you're tired, do the lower-intensity options, #1 or 5. To gauge the intensity of your workouts, you can use either the *target heart rate* method or the *rating of perceived exertion*.

THE TARGET HEART RATE METHOD

Measure your *resting heart rate* (RHR) first thing when you wake up in the morning or after you've been reclining for at least 30 minutes. To measure your heart rate, you can either use a heart rate monitor or check your pulse at your wrist, using your index and middle fingers, not your thumb. When counting your pulse, count the pulses up to 10 seconds and then multiply that number by 6 to get your heart rate. Then, calculate your target heart rate with the following table.

RHR = _____
(measured with a heart rate monitor or counting your pulse at your wrist)

Maximum heart rate (MHR): 220 − your age = _____

Now, find your maximal *training heart rate* (THR) by subtracting your maximum heart rate from your resting heart rate.

MHR _____ – RHR _____ = _____ THR

Determine the percentages of your training heart rate with the following equations.

THR _____ × 60–70% (0.60–0.70) + RHR _____ = _____ target rate for Zone 1

THR _____ × 70–80% (0.70–0.80) + RHR _____ = _____ target rate for Zone 2

THR _____ × 80–90% (0.80–0.90) + RHR _____ = _____ target rate for Zone 3

THR _____ × 90–95% (0.90–0.95) + RHR _____ = _____ target rate for Zone 4

THE RATING OF PERCEIVED EXERTION METHOD

These zones describe how you feel during a cardiovascular workout. See if you can recognize each one. A good way to test this out is on a treadmill or elliptical machine, so you can see the differences between the zones.

Zone 1 = Conversation/warmup/recovery pace—you're sweating but can still talk in full sentences.

Zone 2 = You can feel that you're working harder now and can only answer questions in short sentences; you cannot talk continuously but still feel fresh and strong.

Zone 3 = You're really starting to feel short of breath and can hold this intensity for only 3 to 5 minutes.

Zone 4 = You're working just about as hard as you can and can answer questions only in one-word breaths; you can only hold this intensity for about 1 minute.

Your Seven Cardio Workouts

OPTION #1: LOWER-INTENSITY, LONGER WORKOUT

Warm up in Zone 1 (60–70% of your THR) for 5 minutes.

Gradually increase to the top of Zone 2 (70–80% of your THR) for 10 minutes.

Switch activities and hold the top of Zone 2 (70–80% of your THR) for 15 minutes.

Switch activities and hold the top of Zone 2 (70–80% of your THR) for 10 to 15 minutes.

Cool down at or below Zone 1 for 5 minutes.

Total Time = 45 to 50 minutes

OPTION #2: MODERATE-INTENSITY VARIABLE INTERVAL WORKOUT

Warm up in Zone 1 (60–70% of your THR) for 5 minutes.

Gradually increase to the top of Zone 2 (70–80% of your THR) over the next 2 minutes.

Increase to the middle-top of Zone 3 (80–90% of your THR) for 3 minutes.

Recover in Zone 1 (60–70% of your THR) for 2 minutes.

Increase to the middle-top of Zone 3 (80–90% of your THR) for 3 minutes.

Recover in Zone 1 (60–70% of your THR) for 2 minutes.

Increase to the middle-top of Zone 3 (80–90% of your THR) for 3 minutes.

Recover in Zone 1 (60–70% of your THR) for 2 minutes.

Increase to the middle-top of Zone 3 (80–90% of your THR) for 3 minutes.

Recover in Zone 1 (60–70% of your THR) for 2 minutes.

Increase to the middle-top of Zone 3 (80–90% of your THR) for 3 minutes.

Cool down in Zone 1 (60–70% of your THR) for 5 to 7 minutes.

Total Time = 35 to 37 minutes

OPTION #3: SHORTER-DURATION, VERY HIGH INTENSITY WORKOUT

Warm up in Zone 1 (60–70% of your THR) for 5 minutes.

Gradually increase to the top of Zone 2 (70–80% of your THR) over the next 2 minutes.

Increase 1 level each minute until you are at the top of Zone 4.

Recover in Zone 1 (60–70% of your THR) for 2 to 3 minutes.

Repeat the above instructions 2 or 3 times.

Cool down in Zone 1 (60–70% of your THR) for 5 to 7 minutes.

Total Time = 27 to 43 minutes

OPTION #4: HIGH-INTENSITY VARIABLE INTERVAL WORKOUT

Warm up in Zone 1 (60–70% of your THR) for 5 minutes.

Gradually increase to the top of Zone 1 (60–70% of your THR) over next 2 minutes.

Ramp up to Zone 4 (90–95% of your THR) for 30 seconds.

Recover in Zone 2 (70–80% of your THR) for 1 minute.

Ramp up to Zone 4 (90–95% of your THR) for 1 minute.

Recover in Zone 2 (70–80% of your THR) for 1 minute.

Ramp up to the top of Zone 3/bottom of Zone 4 (90% of your THR) for 1.5 minutes.

Recover in Zone 2 (70–80% of your THR) for 1 minute.

Ramp up to Zone 4 (90–95% of your THR) for 1 minute.

Recover in Zone 2 (70–80% of your THR) for 1 minute.

Ramp up to Zone 4 (90–95% of your THR) for 30 seconds

Recover in Zone 2 (70–80% of your THR) for 3 minutes.

Perform the above instructions 1 or 2 more times.

Cool down in Zone 1 (60–70% of your THR) for 5 to 7 minutes.

Total Time = 21.5 to 40 minutes

OPTION #5: RECOVERY WORKOUT

Warm up in Zone 1 (60–70% of your THR) for 5 minutes.

Increase to the top of Zone 1/bottom of Zone 2 (70% of your THR) over the next 2 minutes.

Gradually increase to the top of Zone 2 (80% of your THR) for 5 minutes.

Stay in Zone 2 (70–80% of your THR; fluctuate from bottom to top however you want) for 15 more minutes.

Cool down at Zone 1 (60–70% of your THR) for 5 minutes.

Total Time = 32 minutes

OPTION #6: AT-HOME CARDIO/STRENGTH-TRAINING WORKOUT

Complete the Active Dynamic Warmup (see page 243) to get your heart ready.

Perform the following exercises at a fast pace with no rest in between:

Body-Weight Squat (page 260): 20 reps

Jumping Jack (page 274): 15 reps

Dumbbell Front Lunge (page 276): 20 reps each leg

Dumbbell Reverse Lunge (page 255): 20 reps each leg

Dumbbell Lateral Lunge (page 256): 20 reps each leg

Pushup (page 256): as many as you can for 30 seconds

Lunge-Stance Dumbbell Shoulder Press (page 263): 30 reps

Straight-Leg Dumbbell Deadlift (page 282): 20 reps

Front Lunge with Biceps Curl (page 277): 15 reps each leg

Rest for 2 to 3 minutes and repeat the circuit again.

Cool down with your choice of an abdominal workout.

OPTION #7: AT-HOME CARDIO/STRENGTH-TRAINING WORKOUT

Complete one entire Active Dynamic Warmup (see page 243).

Perform the following exercises at a fast pace with no rest in between:

Squat Jump (page 286): 20 reps

Single-Arm Bent-Over Dumbbell Row (page 262): 10 reps each side

Dumbbell Reverse Lunge (page 255): 20 reps each leg

Bent-Over Dumbbell Row (page 262): 20 reps

Dumbbell Lateral Lunge (page 256): 20 reps each leg

Pushup (page 256): as many as you can for 30 seconds

Wall Sit with Dumbbell Lateral Shoulder Raise (page 268): 12–15 reps

Standing Biceps Curl (page 290): 15 reps

Pushup (page 256): as many as you can for 30 seconds

Front Plank (page 307): 30 seconds

Side Plank (page 307): 30 seconds each side

Rest for 2 to 3 minutes and repeat the circuit again.

Cool down with your choice of an abdominal workout.

The Perfect Abs Workout

In addition to your resistance training and cardio workouts, you'll do abs workouts three times a week, on the same days as your cardio workouts (that is, on days when you don't do resistance training). Abs workouts designed specifically for Apples are laid out in Chapter 13. Pears will find their custom-made programs in Chapter 14. Avocados and Bananas can choose any of the routines in the book; you'll find all six abs options in Chapter 15.

On the following pages are the abs exercises you'll need to know.

Countdown to Abs-olute Perfection

When you have a high-profile deadline just a few days away, use these four ab-sculpting tricks to look even more svelte.

THREE DAYS BEFORE

Cut the carbs (except fruits and nonstarchy veggies). You'll shed any extra water you may have been holding on to, which can knock the scale down a notch or two. Skip excess salt, too (it has the same water-retaining effect). Limit your daily sodium intake to 2,300 milligrams.

TWO DAYS BEFORE

Hit snooze. The amount of sleep you get affects the function of ghrelin and leptin—hormones that regulate your appetite and metabolism. Skimping on shut-eye can cause the hormone levels to fluctuate, which makes you hungry (especially for sugary, carb-heavy foods) and less able to tell when you're full. Aim for at least 7 hours of sleep a night and you won't be as likely to give in to that hot-dog hankering.

Pass on the gas. Steer clear of cruciferous vegetables like broccoli, cabbage, and Brussels sprouts—they're high in fiber and hard to digest, which means they make you bloated and, well, flatulent. They also contain sulfur, so when you let one rip, it's stinkier than a port-o-potty at Lollapalooza.

ONE DAY BEFORE

Say sayonara to soda. When you drink carbonated beverages, you consume extra air, which makes your paunch puff up right after you've finished that Diet Dr Pepper. So ditch the soda and seltzer and down water instead.

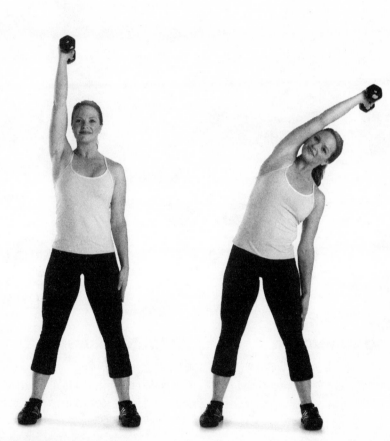

Weighted Side Bend

1 Standing tall with your feet slightly wider than shoulder-width apart, hold a 5- to 10-pound dumbbell straight above your head with your right arm. Let your left arm hang at your side.

2 Bend to your left side. Return to the starting position. Do the prescribed number of reps to the left, then switch sides and repeat.

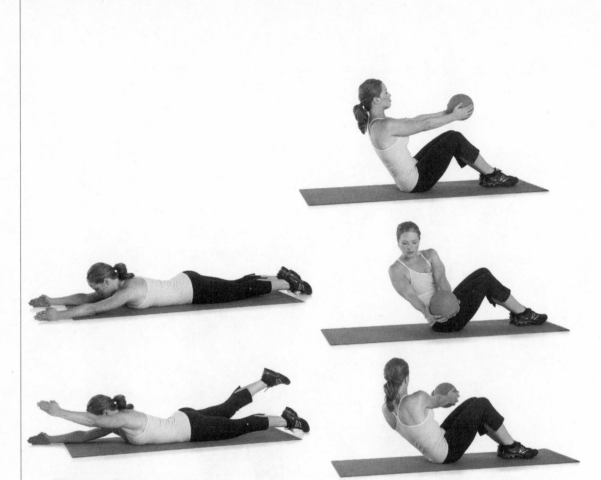

Single-Arm, Single-Leg Superman

1 Lie facedown on the floor with your arms extended in front of you, palms facing in and thumbs toward the ceiling.

2 Keeping your eyes looking straight at the floor in front of you, simultaneously raise your left arm and right leg, keeping your knees straight and your hips square to the floor. Return to the starting position. Do 10 reps on one side before switching to the other.

Weighted Russian Twist

1 Sit on the floor with your knees bent and your feet flat on the floor or lifted a few inches above the floor. Hold a medicine ball with both arms extended straight out in front of you. Lean back until your torso is at a 60- to 75-degree angle from the floor.

2 Twist your torso to one side, reaching with the ball toward the floor behind you. Return to the starting position.

3 Twist to the other side. That's one rep.

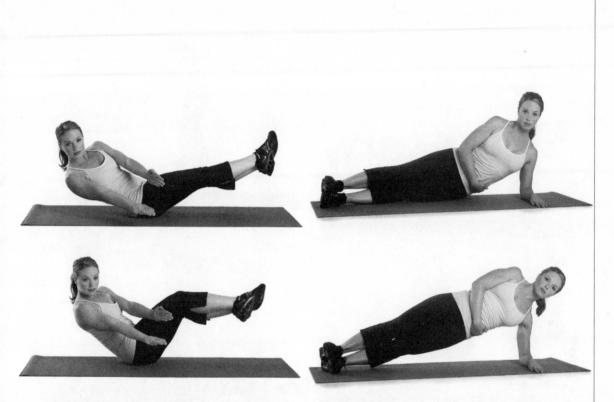

Knee Double Crunch

1 Sit on the floor balanced on your right buttock, with your legs raised off the floor and straightened (but not locked) and your arms extended out over your right hip, palms up.

2 Simultaneously crunch your legs and torso together, bending your knees toward your chest while still balancing on your right buttock. Return to the starting position. Do the prescribed number of reps, then switch sides.

Side Hip-Pop

1 Lie on your side with your forearm on the floor under your shoulder to prop you up and your feet stacked.

2 Contract your core, squeeze your butt, and press your forearm against the floor to raise your hips until your body is a straight diagonal from ankles to shoulders. Return to the starting position. Do the prescribed number of reps, then repeat on your other side.

》 VARIATION: Hold a dumbbell on your top hip (not pictured).

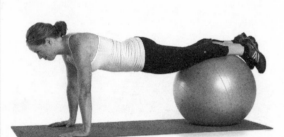

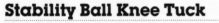

Stability Ball Knee Tuck

1 Assume the pushup position with your shins resting on a stability ball, hands slightly more than shoulder-width apart. With your arms straight and your back flat, your body should form a straight line from your shoulders to your ankles.

2 Keeping your abs tight, draw your knees toward your chest until your toes are on top of the ball. Slowly straighten your legs so the ball rolls back to the starting position.

Single-Leg Lowering

1 Lie faceup on the floor with your legs extended straight up toward the ceiling and your arms at your sides.

2 Keeping your legs straight, your core contracted, and your lower back pressed to the floor, lower one leg toward the floor until your foot is 2 to 3 inches off the ground. Return to the starting position and then repeat with your other leg. Think about keeping your pelvis absolutely still and "sucking in" your belly button toward your spine.

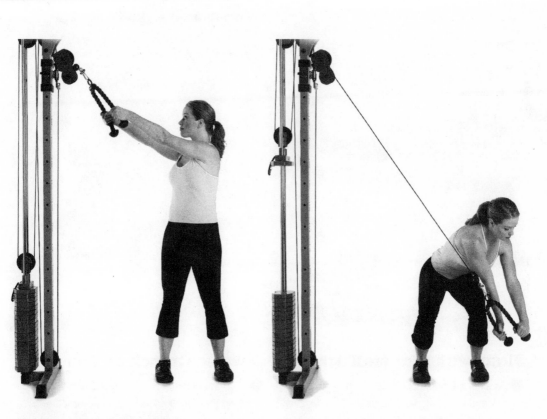

Cable Wood Chop

1 At a high-cable pulley station, grab an end of rope with each hand. Standing with your feet shoulder-width apart and your knees slightly bent, turn your body so your arms are reaching the cable rope at one side (your feet should be perpendicular to the cable).

2 Keeping your arms straight, pull the cable down and across your body to the outside of your opposite knee, shifting your weight to the outside leg. Return to the starting position with control, shifting your weight back to the inside leg. Do the prescribed number of reps, then repeat on the other side.

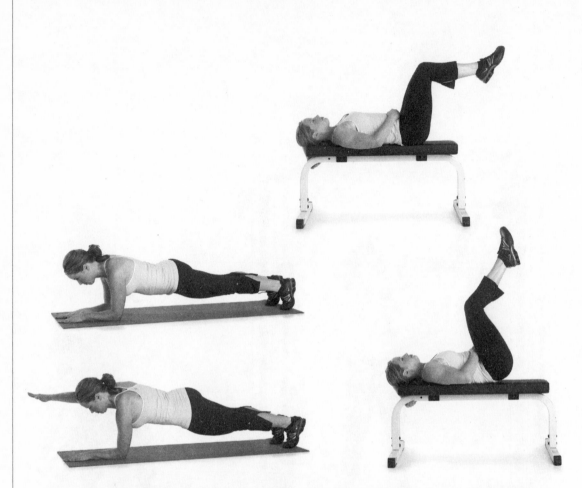

Plank with Diagonal Arm Lift

1 Assume a modified pushup position on your elbows and toes, with your feet slightly wider than shoulder-width apart and your elbows only a few inches apart.

2 Raise one arm forward and out to the side and hold for 2 seconds. Make a strong effort to keep your entire body steady by tightening and focusing on your torso. Return to the starting position. Do the prescribed number of reps with that arm, then repeat with the other arm.

Reverse Crunch on Bench

1 Lie faceup on a bench with one arm lightly gripping the bench underneath and the other resting on your abdomen. Bring your knees to a 90-degree angle.

2 Squeeze your glutes and abs to raise your lower body off the bench with control. This is a small movement where your knees and feet go straight up toward the ceiling, not toward your chest. Return to the starting position.

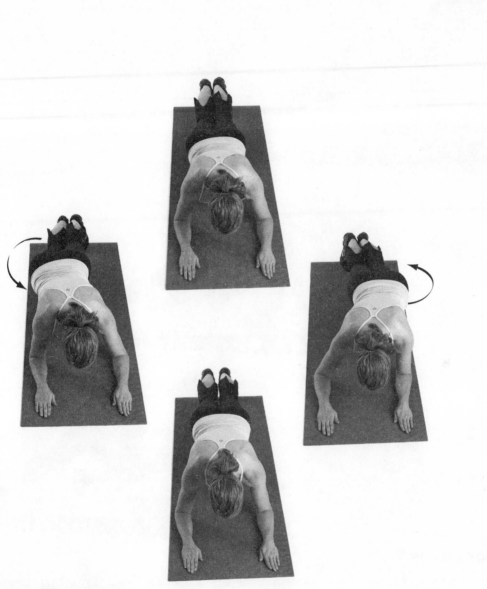

Plank Hip Circle

❶ Assume a modified pushup position on your elbows and toes.

❷ Keeping your shoulders lined up over your elbows, draw a circle with your hips to the right and then to the left, as if swinging a hula hoop around your waist. Repeat in the other direction.

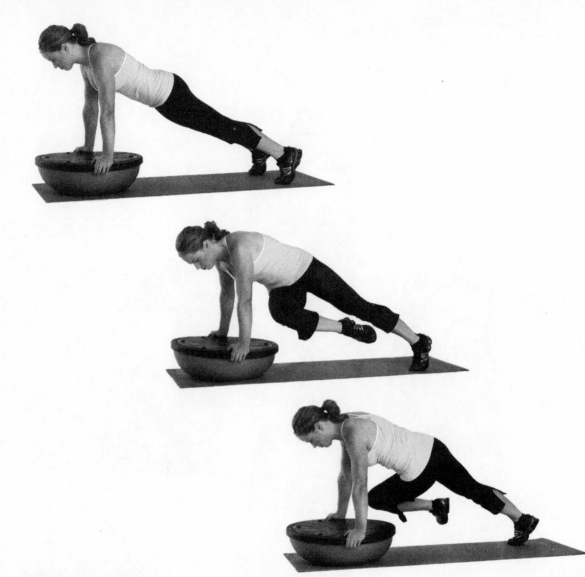

Bosu Knee Twist

1 Assume a pushup position with your hands on the flat side of a Bosu (blue side down), your arms extended, and your legs extended behind you, your toes on the floor.

2 Draw in your belly button and bring one knee toward your opposite elbow, keeping your hips forward and butt down. Return your foot to the floor.

3 Perform the movement with the opposite leg.

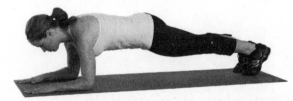

Front Plank

Assume a modified pushup position, on your elbows and toes. Your body will form a straight line from your shoulders to your ankles. Pull your abs in but don't stick out your butt. Hold this position with a straight body for the prescribed amount of time.

Side Plank

Lie on your side. Lift your body while facing forward, and support your weight with that forearm and the outside edge of your foot. Extend your other arm toward the ceiling. Your body will form a straight line from your shoulders to your ankles. Pull in your abs and keep your body in a straight line. Hold this position for at least 20 seconds, or the prescribed amount of time.

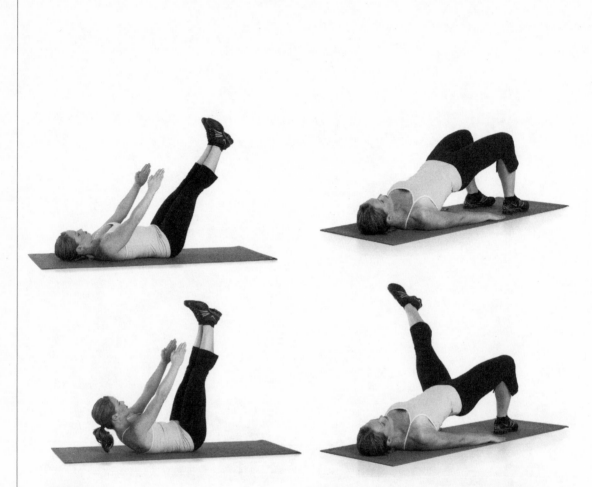

V-Up

1 Lie faceup on the floor with your legs and arms extended at 45-degree angles.

2 Reach toward your legs, simultaneously raising them to bring them in line with your hips. Return to the starting position.

Single-Leg Hip-Pop Hold

1 Lying faceup on the floor with your knees bent and feet flat, press your hips up into a bridge, creating a 90-degree angle with your knees.

2 Holding the position, pick up your left foot and extend your left leg out to the side. Keep your hips up. Hold for 30 seconds. If your hips start to dip to the side or fold, stop and rest for a few seconds. Return to the starting position, then repeat with your right leg.

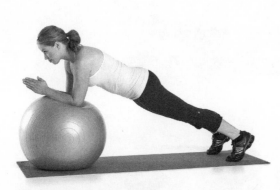

Stability Ball Plank

Assume a modified pushup position with your elbows on a ball and your toes on the floor. Hold this position for 30 to 60 seconds.

Medicine Ball Twisting Lunge

1 Stand with your feet shoulder-width apart and hold a medicine ball straight out in front of you. Step your right leg forward into a lunge, keeping your thigh parallel to the floor. With your arms straight, twist from your torso over your right leg with the ball. Return to the starting position.

2 Repeat to the other side.

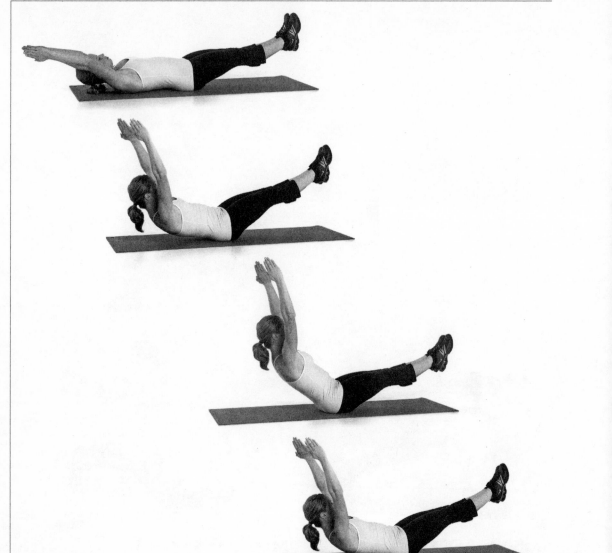

Banana Boat

Lie faceup on the floor and contract your abdominal muscles together while bringing your arms and feet slightly off the ground to form a banana shape. Rock your body up and down like a boat while keeping your abs as tight as possible. Do 20 rocks total.

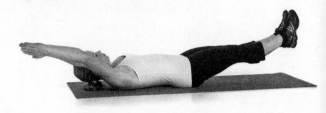

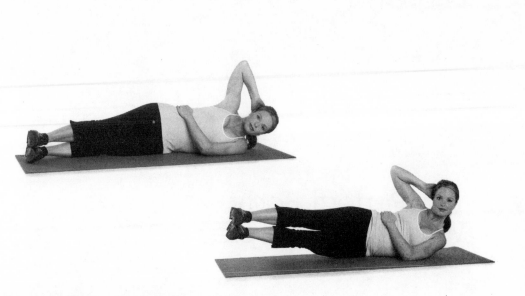

Double-Side Jackknife

1 Lie on your left side with your legs stacked and straight. Wrap your left arm in front of your torso, placing it on your right hip, and put your right hand behind your head.

2 Simultaneously raise your torso and legs, bringing your head toward your hips. Return to the starting position in a controlled motion. Do 20 reps. Repeat on your other side.

» VARIATION: Too hard? Start by lifting just your legs (not pictured).

Take the First Step

For your body-type specific workout plan, read on. Apples will find their workout programs, complete with logs to track the amount of weight used and the numbers of sets and reps completed, in Chapter 13. Chapter 14 lays out the plan for Pears. And Avocados (and Bananas) should turn right to Chapter 15. So let's get moving!

The Perfect Body Workout for Apples

Okay, Apple, get ready to get a literal leg up on sculpting your perfect body.

Your goal: You're going to flatten and tone your belly and upper body, where most of your body fat resides, and develop your leg musculature to balance your top and bottom halves.

Your strength workouts: Your legs are made up of some of the largest muscles in your body, so working them burns lots of calories, helping to speed up your weight loss. Your Perfect Body workout program therefore focuses most of your muscle-building efforts on your legs. For your belly, you'll focus on non-weighted abdominal work to tone those muscles without bulking them up to create a blocky waist.

Remember to always do the Active Dynamic Warmup from Chapter 12 (page 243) before your weight workout as a warmup.

Your cardio workouts: Rotate through machines and activities that activate your abdominals at all times, such as running or fast walking (either outside or on a treadmill) or using an elliptical machine. Other great cardio choices include swimming and running or walking steps at a stadium or on your gym's stairclimber. Stay away from activities where you might forget to engage your abs. For example, avoid bikes—both inside and outside, standard and recumbent. Choose any of the seven cardio options on pages 294 to 297.

Your ab workouts: After your cardio workout, do one of the abs-specific workouts on pages 328, 345, and 363 to 364. These focus on nonweighted abs exercises such as several types of planks to strengthen your middle without adding mass.

Week 1

The game plan: For Week 1, you will do strength training only twice to ease into your new workout program. Break up your lifting days with at least 1 day of cardiovascular activity in between.

Complete the following exercises individually for 2 to 3 sets before moving on to the next exercise. For example, do 2 or 3 sets of the first exercise with 30 seconds to 1 minute of rest between each set, then rest for 2 minutes before moving on to the next exercise for 2 or 3 more sets. Use a weight that allows you to complete all repetitions with perfect form but is heavy enough to be challenging. Use the following logs to record the amount of weight you use for each appropriate exercise.

Follow each workout with 10 to 15 minutes of light cardiovascular exercise, such as walking on a flat treadmill or taking the dog around the block a few times.

APPLE PERFECT BODY WORKOUT

DAY 1	2 OR 3 SETS	WEIGHT	SET 1 REPS	SET 2 REPS	SET 3 REPS
Dumbbell Reverse Lunge (page 255)	6–8 reps each leg				
Bench Pushup (page 257)	12–15 reps	N/A			
Plank Row (page 259)	10 reps each arm				
Dumbbell Bench Squat (page 260)	12–15 reps				
Bent-Over Dumbbell Row (page 262)	12–15 reps				
Dumbbell Stepup (page 264)	6–8 reps each leg				
Lunge-Stance Dumbbell Shoulder Press (page 263)	12–15 reps				
Bench or Stability Ball Hip-Pop (page 267)	12–15 reps	N/A			
Wall Sit (page 268)	30 sec hold				

DAY 2	2 OR 3 SETS	WEIGHT	SET 1 REPS	SET 2 REPS	SET 3 REPS
Dumbbell Reverse Lunge (page 255)	6–8 reps each leg				
Bench Pushup (page 257)	12–15 reps	N/A			
Plank Row (page 259)	6–8 reps each arm				
Dumbbell Bench Squat (page 260)	12–15 reps				
Bent-Over Dumbbell Row (page 262)	12–15 reps				
Dumbbell Stepup (page 264)	6–8 reps each leg				
Lunge-Stance Dumbbell Shoulder Press (page 263)	12–15 reps				
Bench or Stability Ball Hip-Pop (page 267)	12–15 reps	N/A			
Wall Sit (page 268)	30-sec hold				

Week 2

The game plan: Week 2 starts the 3-day weight-lifting program. Exercises grouped together as supersets should be performed back-to-back with no rest in between. After each superset, rest for 1 to 2 minutes, then repeat the same superset once or twice more. After 2 or 3 sets of a superset, rest for 3 to 4 minutes before moving on to the next superset.

DAY 1	2 OR 3 SETS	WEIGHT	SET 1 REPS	SET 2 REPS	SET 3 REPS
Superset A					
Dumbbell Reverse Lunge (page 255)	10–12 reps each leg				
Pushup with Leg Twist (page 257)	Max*	N/A			
Side Plank (page 259)	30-sec hold each side	N/A			
Superset B					
Dumbbell Bench Squat (page 260)	10–12 reps				
Standing Cable Row (page 269)	12–15 reps				
Superset C					
Dumbbell Stepup (page 264)	10–12 reps each leg				
Lunge-Stance Dumbbell Shoulder Press (page 263)	12–15 reps				
Single-Leg Bench or Stability Ball Hip-Pop (page 267)	15 reps each leg	N/A			

*Max = as many reps as possible

APPLE PERFECT BODY WORKOUT

DAY 2	2 OR 3 SETS	WEIGHT	SET 1 REPS	SET 2 REPS	SET 3 REPS
Superset A					
Cable Lat Pulldown (page 272)	12–15 reps				
Front to Back Dumbbell Lunge (page 276)	8–10 reps each leg				
Superset B					
Standing Cable Row (page 269)	12–15 reps				
Lunge-Stance Dumbbell Shoulder Press (page 263)	8–10 reps				
Wall Sit with Dumbbell Lateral Shoulder Raise (page 268)	12–15 reps				
Superset C					
Single-Arm Dumbbell Chest Press on Ball (page 273)	12–15 reps each arm				
Dumbbell Bench Squat (page 260)	8–10 reps				
Reverse Dumbbell Fly on Ball (page 274)	8–10 reps each arm				

For Day 3, there are 2 supersets containing 4 exercises each. Rest 1 to 2 minutes after each superset, then repeat the same superset once or twice. After 2 or 3 sets of a superset, rest for 3 to 4 minutes before moving on. Remember, exercises grouped together will be performed back-to-back with no rest in between, so bring all your weights and situate yourself near the equipment you need to use so you can move through the exercises without missing a beat.

DAY 3	2 OR 3 SETS	WEIGHT	SET 1 REPS	SET 2 REPS	SET 3 REPS
Superset A					
Lunge-Stance Dumbbell Shoulder Press (page 263)	12–15 reps				
Dumbbell Bench Squat (page 260)	12–15 reps				
Bent-Over Dumbbell Row (page 262)	12–15 reps				
Pushup with Leg Twist (page 257)	Max*	N/A			
Superset B					
Dumbbell Stepup (page 264)	12–15 reps each leg				
Wall Sit (page 268)	45-sec hold				
Dumbbell Reverse Lunge (page 255)	6–8 reps each leg				
Single-Leg Bench or Stability Ball Hip-Pop (page 267)	12–15 reps each leg	N/A			

*Max = as many reps as possible

Week 3

The game plan: As in Week 2, exercises grouped together as a superset will be performed back-to-back without rest. After each superset, rest for 1 to 2 minutes. Then repeat the same superset once or twice. After 2 or 3 sets of a superset, rest for 3 to 4 minutes before moving on to the next superset.

DAY 1	2 OR 3 SETS	WEIGHT	SET 1 REPS	SET 2 REPS	SET 3 REPS
Superset A					
Dumbbell Front Lunge (page 276)	10–12 reps each leg				
Pushup with Leg Twist (page 257)	Max*	N/A			
Superset B					
Single-Arm Overheard Dumbbell Squat (page 277)	10 reps each arm				
Quarter-Squat Cable Row (page 270)	12–15 reps each arm				
Superset C					
Dumbbell Stepup (page 264)	8–10 reps each leg				
Dumbbell Incline Chest Press (page 278)	12–15 reps				
Double-Leg Stability Ball Curl (page 280)	12–15 reps	N/A			

*Max = as many reps as possible

APPLE PERFECT BODY WORKOUT

DAY 2	2 OR 3 SETS	WEIGHT	SET 1 REPS	SET 2 REPS	SET 3 REPS
Superset A					
Balance Squat (page 281)	8–10 reps each leg	N/A			
Dumbbell Chest Press (page 278)	12–15 reps				
Deadlift (page 281)	8–10 reps				
Superset B					
Squat to Single-Arm Cable Row (page 271)	10 reps each arm				
Upper-Body Stepover (page 284)	Max*	N/A			
Lunge-Stance Single-Arm Dumbbell Shoulder Press (page 265)	10–12 reps each arm				
Superset C					
Dumbbell Front Shoulder Raise (page 282)	12–15 reps				
Dumbbell Front to Back Lunge (page 276)	8–10 reps each leg				
Front Plank (page 307)	30 sec hold	N/A			

*Max = as many reps as possible

Week 3, Day 3 is structured like Week 2, Day 3: There are 2 supersets containing 4 exercises each. Rest 1 to 2 minutes after each superset, then repeat the same superset twice. After 3 sets of a superset, rest for 3 to 4 minutes before moving on to the next superset. Remember, exercises grouped together will be performed back-to-back with no rest in between, so bring all your weights and situate yourself near the equipment you need to use so you can move through the exercises without missing a beat.

DAY 3	3 SETS	WEIGHT	SET 1 REPS	SET 2 REPS	SET 3 REPS
Superset A					
Dumbbell Bench Squat (page 260)	12–15 reps				
Bent-Over Dumbbell Row (page 262)	12–15 reps				
Pushup with Leg Twist (page 257)	Max*	N/A			
Dumbbell Stepup (page 264)	10–12 reps each leg				
Superset B					
Cable Lat Pulldown (page 272)	12–15 reps				
Wall Sit (page 268)	45 sec hold				
Dumbbell Reverse Lunge (page 255)	6–8 reps each leg				
Single-Leg Bench or Stability Ball Hip-Pop (page 267)	12–15 reps each leg				

*Max = as many reps as possible

Week 4

The game plan: This is a recovery week. You'll take an extra day off this week, doing only two resistance workouts, to prevent overtraining that could lead to injury.

DAY 1	2 SETS	WEIGHT	SET 1 REPS	SET 2 REPS
Superset A				
Dumbbell Front Lunge (page 276)	12–15 reps each leg			
Pushup (page 256)	Max*	N/A		
Superset B				
Single-Arm Overhead Dumbbell Squat (page 277)	10 reps each arm			
Quarter-Squat Cable Row (page 270)	12–15 reps			
Superset C				
Dumbbell Stepup (page 264)	12–15 reps each leg			
Dumbbell Incline Chest Press (page 278)	12–15 reps			
Superset D				
Double-Leg Stability Ball Curl (page 280)	12–15 reps	N/A		
Front Plank (page 307)	30-sec hold			

*Max = as many reps as possible

DAY 2	2 SETS	WEIGHT	SET 1 REPS	SET 2 REPS
Superset A				
Balance Squat (page 281)	12–15 reps each leg	N/A		
Dumbbell Chest Press (page 278)	12–15 reps			
Straight-Leg Dumbbell Deadlift (page 282)	12–15 reps			
Superset B				
Squat to Single-Arm Cable Row (page 271)	12–15 reps each arm			
Dumbbell Plié Squat (page 283)	12–15 reps	N/A		
Superset C				
Dumbbell Front Shoulder Raise (page 282)	12–15 reps			
Dumbbell Front to Back Lunge (page 276)	8–10 reps each leg			
Reverse Dumbbell Fly on Ball (page 274)	12–15 reps			

Week 5

The game plan: Now you're back in action! Day 1 features 3 supersets, the first combining three exercises, the second pairing two exercises, and the third consisting of another three exercises.

DAY 1	2 OR 3 SETS	WEIGHT	SET 1 REPS	SET 2 REPS	SET 3 REPS
Superset A					
Leg Press (page 285)	10–12 reps				
Dumbbell Chest Press on Ball (page 273)	10–12 reps				
Lunge-Stance Dumbbell Shoulder Press (page 263)	10–12 reps				
Superset B					
Deadlift (page 281)	10–12 reps				
Inverted Body Row (page 285)	10–12 reps	N/A			
Superset C					
Triple Hamstring Series (page 279)	10–12 each	N/A			
Standing Biceps Curl (page 290)	10–12 reps				
Dumbbell Lateral Lunge (page 256)	6–8 reps each leg				

Day 2 features 2 supersets of four exercises each.

DAY 2	3 SETS	WEIGHT	SET 1 REPS	SET 2 REPS	SET 3 REPS
Superset A					
Single-Arm Overhead Dumbbell Squat (page 277)	10 reps each arm				
Single-Arm Dumbbell Chest Press on Ball (page 273)	12–15 reps each arm				
Squat Jump (page 286)	15–20 reps	N/A			
Single-Arm Bent-Over Dumbbell Row (page 262)	12–15 reps each arm				
Superset B					
Dumbbell Plié Squat (page 283)	12–15 reps	N/A			
Single-Leg Bench or Stability Ball Hip-Pop (page 267)	15 reps each leg	N/A			
Three-Way Shoulder Series (page 288)	10 each way				
Straight-Leg Dumbbell Deadlift (page 282)	12–15 reps				

On Day 3, you'll do 2 supersets of three exercises each and a third superset of two exercises.

DAY 3	2 OR 3 SETS	WEIGHT	SET 1 REPS	SET 2 REPS	SET 3 REPS
Superset A					
Balance Squat (page 281)	10–12 reps each leg	N/A			
Dumbbell Incline Chest Press (page 278)	10–12 reps				
Straight-Leg Dumbbell Deadlift (page 282)	10–12 reps				
Superset B					
Squat to Single-Arm Cable Row (page 271)	10–12 reps each arm				
Dumbbell Single-Leg Bench Squat (page 261)	10–12 reps each leg				
Lunge-Stance Single-Arm Dumbbell Shoulder Press (page 265)	10–12 reps each arm				
Superset C					
Side Plank (page 307)	30-sec hold each side	N/A			
Triceps Rope Pulldown (page 291)	10–12 reps				

Week 6

The game plan: Choose heavier weights this week to meet the goal of 6 to 8 reps for the specified exercises. Opt for a weight that lets you barely eke out the 6th rep with perfect form.

DAY 1	3 SETS	WEIGHT	SET 1 REPS	SET 2 REPS	SET 3 REPS
Superset A					
Leg Press (page 285)	6–8 reps				
Dumbbell Chest Press (page 278)	10–12 reps				
Superset B					
Inverted Body Row (page 285)	10–12 reps	N/A			
Deadlift (page 281)	6–8 reps				
Superset C					
Single-Arm Bent-Over Dumbbell Row (page 262)	10–12 reps each arm				
Triple Hamstring Series (page 279)	10–12 each	N/A			
Standing Biceps Curl (page 290)	6–8 reps				

DAY 2	3 SETS	WEIGHT	SET 1 REPS	SET 2 REPS	SET 3 REPS
Superset A					
Dumbbell Bench Squat (page 260)	10–12 reps				
Single-Arm Dumbbell Chest Press on Ball (page 273)	12–15 reps each arm				
Squat Jump (page 286)	10–12 reps	N/A			
Plank Row (page 259)	10 reps each arm	N/A			
Superset B					
Explosive Pushup (page 287)	Max*	N/A			
Single-Leg Bench or Stability Ball Hip-Pop (page 267)	12–15 reps each leg	N/A			
Biceps/Triceps Dumbbell Combo on Bench/Ball (page 289)	12 each				

*Max = as many reps as possible

DAY 3	3 SETS	WEIGHT	SET 1 REPS	SET 2 REPS	SET 3 REPS
Superset A					
Cable Lat Pulldown (page 272)	10–12 reps				
Dumbbell Incline Chest Press (page 278)	10–12 reps				
Superset B					
Straight-Leg Dumbbell Deadlift (page 282)	6–8 reps				
Squat to Single-Arm Cable Row (page 271)	8–10 reps each arm				
Superset C					
Front Plank (page 307)	30-sec hold	N/A			
Lunge-Stance Single-Arm Dumbbell Shoulder Press (page 265)	10–12 reps each arm				
Superset D					
Triceps Rope Pulldown (page 291)	10–12 reps				
Wall Sit (page 268)	45-sec hold				

Week 7

The game plan: On Days 1 and 3, your heaviest exercise is the first one in each day of the workouts. Give yourself a 2- or 3-minute rest after each set of these first exercises to allow you to lift just as heavy a weight for all 4 sets. Opt for a weight that lets you barely eke out the 6th rep with perfect form.

On Day 2, you'll do supersets of four exercises each.

DAY 1	4 SETS	WEIGHT	SET 1 REPS	SET 2 REPS	SET 3 REPS	SET 4 REPS
Dumbbell Chest Press (page 278)	4–6 reps					
Superset A	3 Sets	Weight	Set 1 Reps	Set 2 Reps	Set 3 Reps	N/A
Dumbbell Front to Back Lunge (page 276)	6–8 reps each leg					–
Assisted Chinup (page 291) or Cable Lat Pulldown (page 272)	10–12 reps					–
Superset B	3 Sets	Weight	Set 1 Reps	Set 2 Reps	Set 3 Reps	N/A
Bent-Over Dumbbell Row (page 262)	10–12 reps					–
Dumbbell Single-Leg Bench Squat (page 261)	6–8 reps each leg					–
Superset C	3 Sets	Weight	Set 1 Reps	Set 2 Reps	Set 3 Reps	N/A
Leg Press (page 285)	6–8 reps					–
Plank Row (page 259)	10 reps each arm					–

DAY 2	3 SETS	WEIGHT	SET 1 REPS	SET 2 REPS	SET 3 REPS
Superset A					
Single-Arm Overhead Dumbbell Squat (page 277)	12–15 reps each arm				
Plank Row (page 259)	12–15 reps each arm				
Squat Jump (page 286)	12 reps	N/A			
Single-Arm Bent-Over Dumbbell Row (page 262)	12–15 reps each arm				
Superset B					
Pushup (page 256)	Max*	N/A			
Single-Leg Bench or Stability Ball Hip-Pop (page 267)	12–15 reps each leg	N/A			
Three-Way Shoulder Series (page 288)	10 each way				
Biceps/Triceps Dumbbell Combo on Bench/Ball (page 289)	12 each				

*Max = as many reps as possible

DAY 3	4 SETS	WEIGHT	SET 1 REPS	SET 2 REPS	SET 3 REPS	SET 4 REPS
Balance Squat (page 281)	4–6 reps each leg	N/A				
Superset A	3 Sets	Weight	Set 1 Reps	Set 2 Reps	Set 3 Reps	N/A
T-Pushup (page 258)	Max*	N/A				–
Walking Dumbbell Lunge (page 272)	6–8 reps each leg					–
Superset B	3 Sets	Weight	Set 1 Reps	Set 2 Reps	Set 3 Reps	N/A
Straight-Leg Dumbbell Deadlift (page 282)	6–8 reps					–
Front Plank (page 307)	45 sec hold	N/A				–
Seated Overhead Triceps Extension (page 290)	6–8 reps					–

*Max = as many reps as possible

Week 8

The game plan: Just as in Week 7, on Days 1 and 3 your heaviest exercise is the first one in each workout. Give yourself a 2- or 3-minute rest after each set to allow you to lift just as heavy a weight for all 4 sets. Opt for a weight that lets you barely eke out the 6th rep with perfect form.

This week brings everything together so that you can really see your Perfect Body taking shape.

DAY 1	4 SETS	WEIGHT	SET 1 REPS	SET 2 REPS	SET 3 REPS	SET 4 REPS
Dumbbell Chest Press (page 278)	4–6 reps					
Superset A	**3 Sets**	**Weight**	**Set 1 Reps**	**Set 2 Reps**	**Set 3 Reps**	**N/A**
Dumbbell Reverse Lunge (page 255)	6–8 reps each leg					–
Assisted Chinup (page 291)	10–12 reps	N/A				–
Bent-Over Dumbbell Row (page 262)	10–12 reps					–
Superset B	**3 Sets**	**Weight**	**Set 1 Reps**	**Set 2 Reps**	**Set 3 Reps**	**N/A**
Dumbbell Single-Leg Bench Squat (page 261)	6–8 reps each leg					–
Side Plank (page 307)	30-sec hold each side	N/A				–
Plank Row (page 259)	10 reps each arm					–

DAY 2	3 SETS	WEIGHT	SET 1 REPS	SET 2 REPS	SET 3 REPS
Superset A					
Single-Arm Overhead Dumbbell Squat (page 277)	12–15 reps each arm				
Pushup (page 256)	Max*	N/A			
Squat Jump (page 286)	12 reps	N/A			
Single-Arm Bent-Over Dumbbell Row (page 262)	12–15 reps each arm				
Superset B					
Body-Weight Squat (page 260)	20 reps	N/A			
Pushup (page 256)	Max*	N/A			
Single-Leg Bench or Stability Ball Hip-Pop (page 267)	12–15 reps each leg	N/A			
Three-Way Shoulder Series (page 288)	10 each way				
Biceps/Triceps Dumbbell Combo on Bench/Ball (page 289)	12 each				

*Max = as many reps as possible

DAY 3	4 SETS	WEIGHT	SET 1 REPS	SET 2 REPS	SET 3 REPS	SET 4 REPS
Balance Squat (page 281)	4–6 reps each leg	N/A				
Superset A	3 Sets	Weight	Set 1 Reps	Set 2 Reps	Set 3 Reps	N/A
T-Pushup (page 258)	Max*	N/A				–
Walking Dumbbell Lunge (page 272)	6–8 reps each leg					–
Superset B	3 Sets	Weight	Set 1 Reps	Set 2 Reps	Set 3 Reps	N/A
Straight-Leg Dumbbell Deadlift (page 282)	6–8 reps					–
Quarter-Squat Cable Row (page 270)	12–15 reps					–
Reverse Dumbbell Fly on Ball (page 274)	6–8 reps					–

*Max = as many reps as possible

Ab Workouts

After your cardio workouts, on your days off from weight training, perform one of the following abdominal routines. Mix it up throughout the week. Perform the exercises back to back or do 2 sets of each individual exercise and then move on to the next.

AB #1	2 SETS	SET 1 REPS	SET 2 REPS
Bosu Knee Twist (page 306)	8–10 reps each leg		
Plank Hip Circle (page 305)	5 each way		
V-Up (page 308)	15–20 reps		
Single-Leg Hip-Pop Hold (page 308)	30-sec hold each leg		

AB #2	2 SETS	SET 1 REPS	SET 2 REPS
Stability Ball Plank (page 309)	30–60-sec hold		
Side Plank (page 307)	30-sec hold each side		
Reverse Crunch on Bench (page 304)	15–20 reps		
Medicine Ball Twisting Lunge (page 309)	10 reps each side		

AB #3	2 SETS	SET 1 REPS	SET 2 REPS
Double-Side Jackknife (page 311)	20 reps each side		
Plank with Diagonal Arm Lift (page 304)	10 reps each arm		
Stability Ball Knee Tuck (page 302)	12–15 reps		
Banana Boat (page 310)	20 total rocks		

CHAPTER 14

The Perfect Body Workout for Pears

Get ready to top off your existing assets to build your perfect body: the classic hourglass shape.

Your goal: Your Perfect Body workout program will build muscle and strength in your upper body while slimming your legs and butt.

Your strength workouts: You'll tone your legs and bump up the fat-loss process by working your body's largest muscles, but you won't give them as much resistance or attention as you will your upper half. As a result, you will often do exercises that are shown as weighted in the photographs, but you will do them using only your body weight.

Remember to always do the Active Dynamic Workout from Chapter 12 before your weight workout as a warmup.

Your cardio workouts: Pick an activity that really challenges your butt and legs. Put the treadmill at a slight incline, or do sprint intervals on the bike or track. Pears can really benefit from a Spinning class, cycling or running, climbing stairs, and hiking long distances. Whatever you choose, any of the seven cardio workouts on pages 294 to 297 will be an effective challenge.

Your ab workouts: After your cardio workout, do one of the abs-specific workouts on page 345.

Week 1

The game plan: For Week 1 you will strength train only twice to ease into the program. Separate your lifting days with at least 1 day of cardiovascular activity.

For this week you will complete 2 or 3 sets of an individual exercise before moving on to the next exercise. The structure is known as doing straight sets and is used here to get you accustomed to weight training—after this first week, you will incorporate supersets. For straight sets here, you will, for example, do 2 or 3 sets of the Body Weight Reverse Lunge with 30 seconds to 1 minute of rest between each set of that exercise, then rest for 2 minutes before moving on to the Bench Pushup for 2 or 3 more sets. Use a weight (if specified) that allows you to complete all repetitions with perfect form but is heavy enough to be challenging. Do not use weight if the exercise is to be done with just your body weight. In the charts that follow, record the amount of weight you use for each exercise that uses weights.

Follow each workout with 10 to 15 minutes of light cardiovascular exercise, such as walking on a flat treadmill or taking the dog around the block a few times.

DAY 1	2 OR 3 SETS	WEIGHT	SET 1 REPS	SET 2 REPS	SET 3 REPS
Dumbbell Reverse Lunge, No-Weight Variation (not pictured, page 255)	12–15 reps each leg	N/A			
Bench Pushup (page 257)	Max*	N/A			
Cable Lat Pulldown (page 272)	12–15 reps				
Body-Weight Squat (page 260)	12–15 reps	N/A			
Standing Cable Row (page 269)	12–15 reps				
Dumbbell Stepup, No-Weight Variation (not pictured, page 264)	6–8 reps each leg	N/A			
Lunge-Stance Dumbbell Shoulder Press (page 263)	12–15 reps				
Bench or Stability Ball Hip-Pop (page 267)	12–15 reps	N/A			

*Max = as many reps as possible

DAY 2	2 OR 3 SETS	WEIGHT	SET 1 REPS	SET 2 REPS	SET 3 REPS
Dumbbell Reverse Lunge, No-Weight Variation (not pictured, page 255)	12–15 reps each leg	N/A			
Bench Pushup (page 257)	12–15 reps	N/A			
Cable Lat Pulldown (page 272)	12–15 reps				
Body-Weight Squat (page 260)	12–15 reps	N/A			
Standing Cable Row (page 269)	12–15 reps				
Dumbbell Stepup, No-Weight Variation (not pictured, page 264)	6–8 reps each leg	N/A			
Lunge-Stance Dumbbell Shoulder Press (page 263)	12–15 reps				
Single-Leg Bench or Stability Ball Hip-Pop (page 267)	12–15 reps each leg	N/A			

Week 2

The game plan: Week 2 starts the 3-day weight-lifting program. Instead of doing straight sets, you will perform your exercises as supersets, as indicated. Supersets increase the amount of calories you burn with your workout. Exercises grouped together as supersets should be performed back-to-back with no rest in between. After each superset, rest for 1 to 2 minutes, then repeat the same superset once or twice more. After 2 or 3 sets of a super-set, rest for 3 to 4 minutes before moving on to the next superset.

DAY 1	2 OR 3 SETS	WEIGHT	SET 1 REPS	SET 2 REPS	SET 3 REPS
Superset A					
Dumbbell Front to Back Lunge, No-Weight Variation (not pictured, page 276)	6–8 reps each leg	N/A			
Pushup (page 256)	Max*	N/A			
Cable Lat Pulldown (page 272)	8–10 reps				
Superset B					
Single-Arm Bent-Over Dumbbell Row (page 262)	8–10 reps each arm				
Body-Weight Single-Leg Bench Squat (page 261)	8–10 reps each leg	N/A			
Superset C					
Seated Shoulder Press (page 265)	8–10 reps				
Reverse Dumbbell Fly on Ball (page 274)	8–10 reps				
Cable Wood Chop (page 303)	15–20 reps each side				

*Max = as many reps as possible

DAY 2	2 OR 3 SETS	WEIGHT	SET 1 REPS	SET 2 REPS	SET 3 REPS
Superset A					
Pushup (page 256)	Max*	N/A			
Standing Cable Row (page 269)	8–10 reps				
Seated Shoulder Press (page 265)	8–10 reps				
Superset B					
Dumbbell Chest Press (page 278)	8–10 reps				
Lying External Rotation (page 269)	8–10 reps each side				
Superset C					
Biceps/Triceps Dumbbell Combo on Bench/Ball (page 289)	10–12 each				
Reverse Dumbbell Fly on Ball (page 274)	10–12 reps				

*Max = as many reps as possible

For Day 3, there are 2 supersets containing 4 exercises each. Rest 1 to 2 minutes after each superset, then repeat the same superset once or twice. After 2 or 3 sets of a superset, rest for 3 to 4 minutes before moving on. Remember, exercises grouped together will be performed back-to-back with no rest in between, so bring all your weights and situate yourself near the equipment you need to use so you can move through the exercises without missing a beat.

DAY 3	2 OR 3 SETS	WEIGHT	SET 1 REPS	SET 2 REPS	SET 3 REPS
Superset A					
Seated Shoulder Press (page 265)	12–15 reps				
Squat Jump (page 286)	12–15 reps	N/A			
Bent-Over Dumbbell Row (page 262)	12–15 reps				
Pushup with Leg Twist (page 257)	12–15 reps each leg	N/A			
Superset B					
Dumbbell Stepup, No-Weight Variation (not pictured, page 264)	12–15 reps each leg	N/A			
Cable Lat Pulldown (page 272)	12–15 reps				
Dumbbell Front Shoulder Raise (page 282)	12–15 reps				
Single-Leg Bench or Stability Ball Hip-Pop (page 267)	12–15 reps each leg	N/A			

Week 3

The game plan: As in Week 2, exercises grouped together as a superset will be performed back-to-back without rest. After each superset, rest for 1 to 2 minutes. Then repeat the same superset once or twice. After 2 or 3 sets of a superset, rest for 3 to 4 minutes before moving on to the next superset.

DAY 1	2 OR 3 SETS	WEIGHT	SET 1 REPS	SET 2 REPS	SET 3 REPS
Superset A					
Dumbbell Front Lunge, No-Weight Variation (page 276)	12–15 reps each leg	N/A			
Pushup (page 256)	Max*	N/A			
Assisted Chinup (page 291)	8–10 reps	N/A			
Superset B					
Body-Weight Single-Leg Bench Squat variation (page 261)	10–12 reps each leg	N/A			
Standing Cable Row (page 269)	8–10 reps				
Superset C					
Single-Arm Bent-Over Dumbbell Row (page 262)	8–10 reps each arm				
Double- or Single-Leg Stability Ball Curl (page 280)	12–15 reps	N/A			
Lying External Rotation (page 269)	8–10 reps each side				

*Max = as many reps as possible

DAY 2	2 OR 3 SETS	WEIGHT	SET 1 REPS	SET 2 REPS	SET 3 REPS
Superset A					
Cable Lat Pulldown (page 272)	8–10 reps				
Dumbbell Chest Press (page 278)	8–10 reps				
Straight-Leg Dumbbell Deadlift (page 282)	12–15 reps				
Superset B					
Squat to Single-Arm Cable Row (page 271)	10 reps each arm				
Upper-Body Stepover (page 284)	12 reps	N/A			
Lunge-Stance Single-Arm Dumbbell Shoulder Press (page 265)	8–10 reps each arm				
Superset C					
Inverted Body Row (page 285)	8–10 reps	N/A			
Weighted Decline Crunch (page 283)	15–20 reps				
Side Plank (page 307)	30 sec hold each side	N/A			

For Day 3, there are 2 supersets containing 4 exercises each. Rest 1 to 2 minutes after each superset, then repeat the same superset twice. After 3 sets of a superset, rest for 3 to 4 minutes before moving on to the next superset. Remember, exercises grouped together will be performed back-to-back with no rest in between, so bring all your weights and situate yourself near the equipment you need to use so you can move through the exercises without missing a beat.

DAY 3	3 SETS	WEIGHT	SET 1 REPS	SET 2 REPS	SET 3 REPS
Superset A					
Lunge-Stance Dumbbell Shoulder Press (page 263)	12–15 reps				
Bent-Over Barbell Row (page 263)	12–15 reps				
Pushup (page 256)	Max*	N/A			
Weighted Russian Twist (page 300)	12–15 reps				
Superset B					
Assisted Chinup (page 291)	8–10 reps	N/A			
Multi-Plane Lunge (page 275)	6 reps each leg each way	N/A			
Single-Leg Bench or Stability Ball Hip-Pop (page 267)	12–15 reps each leg	N/A			
Front Plank (page 307)	30 sec hold	N/A			

*Max = as many reps as possible

Week 4

The game plan: This is a recovery week. You'll take an extra day off this week, doing only two resistance workouts, to prevent overtraining that could lead to injury.

DAY 1	2 SETS	WEIGHT	SET 1 REPS	SET 2 REPS
Superset A				
Dumbbell Front Lunge, No-Weight Variation (page 276)	12–15 reps each leg	N/A		
Pushup with Leg Twist (page 257)	Max*	N/A		
Cable Lat Pulldown (page 272)	12–15 reps			
Superset B				
Cable Wood Chop (page 303)	12–15 reps			
Quarter-Squat Cable Row (page 270)	12–15 reps			
Superset C				
Dumbbell Incline Chest Press (page 278)	12–15 reps			
Bent-Over Barbell Row (page 263)	12–15 reps			
Superset D				
Double- or Single-Leg Stability Ball Curl (page 280)	12–15 reps	N/A		
Wall Sit with Dumbbell Lateral Shoulder Raise, Standing Variation (not pictured, page 268)	12–15 reps			

*Max = as many reps as possible

DAY 2	2 SETS	WEIGHT	SET 1 REPS	SET 2 REPS
Superset A				
Balance Squat (page 281)	12–15 reps each leg	N/A		
Dumbbell Chest Press (page 278)	12–15 reps			
Straight-Leg Dumbbell Deadlift (page 282)	12–15 reps			
Superset B				
Standing Cable Row (page 269)	12–15 reps			
Cable Wood Chop (page 303)	12–15 reps each side			
Lunge-Stance Dumbbell Shoulder Press (page 263)	12–15 reps			
Superset C				
Dumbbell Front Shoulder Raise (page 282)	12–15 reps			
Dumbbell Front to Back Lunge, No-Weight Variation (not pictured, page 276)	8–10 reps each leg	N/A		
Reverse Dumbbell Fly on Ball (page 274)	12–15 reps			

Week 5

The game plan: Now you're back in action, working out 3 days this week.

DAY 1	2 OR 3 SETS	WEIGHT	SET 1 REPS	SET 2 REPS	SET 3 REPS
Superset A					
Dumbbell Chest Press (page 278)	10–12 reps				
Lying External Rotation (page 269)	10 reps each side				
Inverted Body Row (page 285)	10–12 reps	N/A			
Superset B					
Straight-Leg Dumbbell Deadlift (page 282)	10–12 reps				
Single-Arm Bent-Over Dumbbell Row (page 262)	10–12 reps each arm				
Assisted Pullup (page 292)	10–12 reps	N/A			
Superset C					
Triple Hamstring Series (page 279)	10–12 each	N/A			
Reverse Dumbbell Fly on Ball (page 274)	10–12 reps				

DAY 2	3 SETS	WEIGHT	SET 1 REPS	SET 2 REPS	SET 3 REPS
Superset A					
Seated Shoulder Press on Stability Ball (not pictured, page 265)	12–15 reps				
Single-Arm Dumbbell Chest Press on Ball (page 273)	12–15 reps each arm				
Squat Jump (page 286)	10–12 reps	N/A			
Single-Arm Bent-Over Dumbbell Row (page 262)	12–15 reps each arm				
Superset B					
Plank Hip Circle (page 305)	5 each way	N/A			
Explosive Pushup (page 287)	Max*	N/A			
Single-Leg Bench or Stability Ball Hip-Pop (page 267)	12–15 reps each leg	N/A			
Three-Way Shoulder Series (page 288)	8 each way				
Biceps/Triceps Dumbbell Combo on Bench/Ball (page 289)	12 each				

*Max = as many reps as possible

PEAR PERFECT BODY WORKOUT

DAY 3	2 OR 3 SETS	WEIGHT	SET 1 REPS	SET 2 REPS	SET 3 REPS
Superset A					
Dumbbell Incline Chest Press (page 278)	10–12 reps				
Straight-Leg Dumbbell Deadlift (page 282)	10–12 reps				
Superset B					
Squat to Single-Arm Cable Row (page 271)	10–12 reps each arm				
Cable Wood Chop (page 303)	10–12 reps each side				
Lunge-Stance Single-Arm Dumbbell Shoulder Press (page 265)	10–12 reps each arm				
Superset C					
Standing Biceps Curl (page 290)	10–12 reps				
Triceps Rope Pulldown (page 291)	10–12 reps				

Week 6

The game plan: Choose heavier weights this week to meet the goal of 6 to 8 reps for the specified exercises. Opt for a weight that lets you barely eke out the 6th rep with perfect form.

DAY 1	3 SETS	WEIGHT	SET 1 REPS	SET 2 REPS	SET 3 REPS
Superset A					
Multi-Plane Lunge (page 275)	10 reps each leg each way	N/A			
Single-Arm Dumbbell Chest Press on Ball (page 273)	6–8 reps each arm				
Superset B					
Inverted Body Row (page 285)	Max*	N/A			
Single-Arm Bent-Over Dumbbell Row (page 262)	6–8 reps each arm				
Biceps/Triceps Dumbbell Combo on Bench/Ball (page 289)	12 reps each				
Superset C					
Triple Hamstring Series (page 279)	15 reps each	N/A			
Reverse Dumbbell Fly on Ball (page 274)	6–8 reps				

*Max = as many reps as possible

DAY 2	3 SETS	WEIGHT	SET 1 REPS	SET 2 REPS	SET 3 REPS
Superset A					
Lunge-Stance Single-Arm Dumbbell Shoulder Press (page 265)	12–15 reps each arm				
Dumbbell Chest Press on Ball (page 273)	12–15 reps				
Single-Leg Bench or Stability Ball Hip-Pop (page 267)	12–15 reps each leg	N/A			
Weighted Decline Crunch (page 283)	12–15 reps				
Superset B					
Body-Weight Squat (page 260)	20 reps	N/A			
Explosive Pushup (page 287)	Max*	N/A			
Three-Way Shoulder Series (page 288)	5 reps each way				
Standing Biceps Curl (page 290)	12 reps				

*Max = as many reps as possible

PEAR PERFECT BODY WORKOUT

DAY 3	3 SETS	WEIGHT	SET 1 REPS	SET 2 REPS	SET 3 REPS
Superset A					
Balance Squat (page 281)	8–10 reps each leg	N/A			
Assisted Chinup (page 291)	6–8 reps	N/A			
Superset B					
Straight-Leg Dumbbell Deadlift (page 282)	12–15 reps				
Squat to Cable Row (page 270)	6–8 reps				
Superset C					
Dumbbell Single-Leg Bench Squat, with light weights (page 261)	10 reps each leg				
Lunge-Stance Single-Arm Dumbbell Shoulder Press (page 265)	12–15 reps each arm				
Superset D					
Dumbbell Front Shoulder Raise (page 282)	12–15 reps				
Triceps Rope Pulldown (page 291)	10–12 reps				

Week 7

The game plan: On Days 1 and 3, your heaviest exercise is the first one on each day of the workouts. Give yourself a 2- or 3-minute rest after each set of these first exercises to allow you to lift just as heavy a weight for all 4 sets. Opt for a weight that lets you barely eke out the 6th rep with perfect form.

On Day 2, you'll do supersets of four exercises each.

DAY 1	4 SETS	WEIGHT	SET 1 REPS	SET 2 REPS	SET 3 REPS	SET 4 REPS
Dumbbell Chest Press (page 278)	4–6 reps					
Superset A	3 Sets	Weight	Set 1 Reps	Set 2 Reps	Set 3 Reps	N/A
Dumbbell Front to Back Lunge, No-Weight Variation (not pictured, page 276)	12–15 reps each leg	N/A				–
Assisted Chinup (page 291)	6–8 reps	N/A				–
Superset B	3 Sets	Weight	Set 1 Reps	Set 2 Reps	Set 3 Reps	N/A
Bent-Over Dumbbell Row (page 262)	6–8 reps					–
Pushup (page 256)	Max*	N/A				–
Superset C	3 Sets	Weight	Set 1 Reps	Set 2 Reps	Set 3 Reps	N/A
Straight-Leg Dumbbell Deadlift (page 282)	10–12 reps					–
Single-Leg Bench or Stability Ball Hip-Pop (page 267)	12–15 reps each leg	N/A				–

*Max = as many reps as possible

PEAR PERFECT BODY WORKOUT

DAY 2	3 SETS	WEIGHT	SET 1 REPS	SET 2 REPS	SET 3 REPS
Superset A					
Squat to Overhead Shoulder Press (page 286)	12–15 reps				
Single-Arm Dumbbell Chest Press on Ball (page 273)	12–15 reps				
Single-Arm Bent-Over Dumbbell Row (page 262)	12–15 reps each arm				
Body-Weight Squat (page 260)	20 reps	N/A			
Superset B					
Explosive Pushup (page 287)	Max*	N/A			
Single-Leg Bench or Stability Ball Hip-Pop (page 267)	12–15 reps each leg	N/A			
Three-Way Shoulder Series (page 288)	5 each way				
Biceps/Triceps Dumbbell Combo on Bench/Ball (page 289)	10 each				

*Max = as many reps as possible

DAY 3	4 SETS	WEIGHT	SET 1 REPS	SET 2 REPS	SET 3 REPS	SET 4 REPS
Balance Squat (page 281)	4–6 reps each leg	N/A				
Superset A	3 sets	Weight	Set 1 Reps	Set 2 Reps	Set 3 Reps	N/A
Pushup (page 256)	Max*	N/A				–
Weighted Decline Crunch (page 283)	6–8 reps					–
Superset B	3 Sets	Weight	Set 1 Reps	Set 2 Reps	Set 3 Reps	N/A
Straight-Leg Dumbbell Deadlift (page 282)	6–8 reps					–
Squat to Cable Row (page 270)	10 reps					–
Superset C	3 Sets	Weight	Set 1 Reps	Set 2 Reps	Set 3 Reps	N/A
Lying External Rotation (page 269)	10 reps each side					–
Reverse Dumbbell Fly on Ball (page 274)	6–8 reps					–

*Max = as many reps as possible

Week 8

The game plan: Just as in Week 7, on Days 1 and 3 your heaviest exercise is the first one in each workout. Give yourself a 2- or 3-minute rest after each set to allow you to lift just as heavy a weight for all 4 sets. Opt for a weight that lets you barely eke out the 6th rep with perfect form.

This week brings everything together so you really see your perfect body taking shape.

DAY 1	4 SETS	WEIGHT	SET 1 REPS	SET 2 REPS	SET 3 REPS	SET 4 REPS
Dumbbell Chest Press (page 278)	4–6 reps					
Superset A	**3 Sets**	**Weight**	**Set 1 Reps**	**Set 2 Reps**	**Set 3 Reps**	**N/A**
Dumbbell Front to Back Lunge (page 276)	6–8 reps each leg					–
Assisted Chinup (page 291)	6–8 reps	N/A				–
Superset B	**3 Sets**	**Weight**	**Set 1 Reps**	**Set 2 Reps**	**Set 3 Reps**	**N/A**
Bent-Over Dumbbell Row (page 262)	6–8 reps					–
Pushup (page 256)	Max*	N/A				–
Superset C	**3 Sets**	**Weight**	**Set 1 Reps**	**Set 2 Reps**	**Set 3 Reps**	**N/A**
Side Plank (page 307)	30-sec hold each side	N/A				–
Plank Row (page 259)	10 reps each arm	N/A				–

*Max = as many reps as possible

DAY 2	3 SETS	WEIGHT	SET 1 REPS	SET 2 REPS	SET 3 REPS
Superset A					
Squat to Overhead Shoulder Press (page 286)	12–15 reps				
Single-Arm Dumbbell Chest Press on Ball (page 273)	12–15 reps				
Single-Arm Bent-Over Dumbbell Row (page 262)	12–15 reps each arm				
Body-Weight Squat (page 260)	20 reps	N/A			
Superset B					
Explosive Pushup (page 287)	Max*	N/A			
Single-Leg Bench Hip-Pop (page 267)	12–15 reps each leg	N/A			
Three-Way Shoulder Series (page 288)	8 each way				
Biceps/Triceps Dumbbell Combo on Bench/Ball (page 289)	12 each				

*Max = as many reps as possible

PEAR PERFECT BODY WORKOUT

DAY 3	4 SETS	WEIGHT	SET 1 REPS	SET 2 REPS	SET 3 REPS	SET 4 REPS
Balance Squat (page 281)	4–6 reps each leg	N/A				
Superset A	**3 Sets**	**Weight**	**Set 1 Reps**	**Set 2 Reps**	**Set 3 Reps**	**N/A**
Pushup (page 256)	Max	N/A				–
Weighted Decline Crunch (page 283)	6–8 reps					–
Superset B	**3 Sets**	**Weight**	**Set 1 Reps**	**Set 2 Reps**	**Set 3 Reps**	**N/A**
Straight-Leg Dumbbell Deadlift (page 282)	6–8 reps					–
Squat to Cable Row (page 270)	10 reps					–
Superset C	**3 Sets**	**Weight**	**Set 1 Reps**	**Set 2 Reps**	**Set 3 Reps**	**N/A**
Cable Wood Chop (page 303)	10 reps each side					–
Reverse Dumbbell Fly on Ball (page 274)	6–8 reps					–

Ab Workout

After your cardio workouts, on your days off from weight training, perform one of the following abdominal routines. Mix it up throughout the week. Perform the exercises back-to-back, or do 2 sets of each individual exercise and then move on to the next.

AB #1	2 SETS	SET 1 REPS	SET 2 REPS
Weighted Side Bend (page 299)	12 reps each side		
Single-Arm, Single-Leg Superman (page 300)	12 reps each side		
Weighted Russian Twist (page 300)	10 reps each side		
V-Up (page 308)	15–20 reps		

AB #2	2 SETS	SET 1 REPS	SET 2 REPS
Knee Double Crunch (page 301)	12–15 reps each side		
Side Hip-Pop, Weighted Variation (not pictured, page 301)	12 reps each side		
Stability Ball Knee Tuck (page 302)	12–15 reps		
Single-Leg Lowering (page 302)	10 reps each side		

AB #3	2 SETS	SET 1 REPS	SET 2 REPS
Cable Wood Chop (page 303)	15 reps each side		
Weighted Side Bend (page 299)	12 reps each side		
Plank with Diagonal Arm Lift (page 304)	10 reps each arm		
Reverse Crunch on Bench (page 304)	15–20 reps		

CHAPTER 15

The Perfect Body Workout for Avocados and Bananas

Here's an all-around program for both Avocado and Banana body types that will earn you a perfect 10 in your quest for a perfect body.

Your goal: Your ideal strength-training program focuses on building muscle and burning fat evenly, without focusing on a specific body part.

Your strength workouts: Your plan includes full-body workouts 3 days a week. Remember to always do the Active Dynamic Warmup from Chapter 12 (page 243) before your weight workout as a warmup.

Your cardio workouts: Pick the type of cardio activity that you enjoy doing most, and rotate through a variety every once in a while to prevent weight-loss plateaus. Whatever you choose, any of the seven cardio workouts on pages 294 to 297 will be an effective fat burner.

Banana bods are the exception; they will do less cardio than Avocados. This means they will choose the recovery options more often, which are less intense, or take a day off from gym cardio and do another lighter activity such as cleaning, yoga, or washing the car.

Your ab workouts: After your cardio workout, both bods can do one of the six abs-specific workouts starting on page 363. The choice is yours.

Week 1

The game plan: For Week 1 you will do strength training only twice to ease into your new program. Separate your lifting days with at least 1 day of cardiovascular activity in between.

For this week you will complete 2 or 3 sets of an individual exercise before moving on to the next exercise. The structure is known as doing straight sets and is used here to get you accustomed to weight training—after this first week, you will incorporate supersets. For straight sets here, you will, for example, do 2 or 3 sets of Dumbbell Reverse Lunges with 30 seconds to 1 minute of rest between each set of that exercise, then rest for 2 minutes before moving on to Bench Pushups for 2 or 3 sets. Use a weight that allows you to complete all repetitions but is heavy enough to be challenging. Write down here the amount of weight you use for each appropriate exercise, if specified.

Follow this workout with 10 to 15 minutes of light cardiovascular exercise, such as walking on a flat treadmill or taking the dog around the block a few times.

AVOCADO AND BANANA PERFECT BODY WORKOUT

DAY 1	2 OR 3 SETS	WEIGHT	SET 1 REPS	SET 2 REPS	SET 3 REPS
Dumbbell Reverse Lunge (page 255)	8–10 reps each leg				
Bench Pushup (page 257)	12–15 reps	N/A			
Cable Lat Pulldown (page 272)	12–15 reps				
Dumbbell Bench Squat (page 260)	12–15 reps				
Squat to Cable Row (page 270)	12–15 reps				
Dumbbell Stepup (page 264)	12–15 reps each leg				
Lunge-Stance Dumbbell Shoulder Press (page 263)	12–15 reps				
Bench or Stability Ball Hip-Pop (page 267)	12–15 reps	N/A			
Wall Sit with Dumbbell Lateral Shoulder Raise (page 268)	12–15 reps				

DAY 2	2 OR 3 SETS	WEIGHT	SET 1 REPS	SET 2 REPS	SET 3 REPS
Dumbbell Reverse Lunge (page 255)	12–15 reps				
Pushup (page 256)	Max*	N/A			
Cable Lat Pulldown (page 272)	12–15 reps				
Dumbbell Bench Squat (page 260)	12–15 reps				
Standing Cable Row (page 269)	12–15 reps				
Dumbbell Stepup (page 264)	12–15 reps each leg				
Lunge-Stance Dumbbell Shoulder Press (page 263)	12–15 reps				
Single-Leg Bench or Stability Ball Hip-Pop (page 267)	12–15 reps each leg	N/A			
Wall Sit with Dumbbell Lateral Shoulder Raise, Standing Variation (not pictured, page 268)	12–15 reps				

*Max = as many reps as possible

Week 2

The game plan: Week 2 starts the 3-day weight-lifting program. Exercises grouped together as supersets should be performed back-to-back with no rest in between. After each superset, rest for 1 to 2 minutes, then repeat the same superset once or twice more. After 2 or 3 sets of a superset, rest for 3 to 4 minutes before moving on to the next superset.

DAY 1	2 OR 3 SETS	WEIGHT	SET 1 REPS	SET 2 REPS	SET 3 REPS
Superset A					
Dumbbell Reverse Lunge (page 255)	10–12 reps each leg				
Pushup (page 256)	10–12 reps	N/A			
Cable Lat Pulldown (page 272)	10–12 reps				
Superset B					
Dumbbell Bench Squat (page 260)	10–12 reps				
Squat to Cable Row (page 270)	10–12 reps				
Superset C					
Dumbbell Stepup (page 264)	10–12 reps each leg				
Lunge-Stance Dumbbell Shoulder Press (page 263)	10–12 reps				
Bench or Stability Ball Hip-Pop (page 267)	10–12 reps	N/A			
Wall Sit with Dumbbell Lateral Shoulder Raise (page 268)	10–12 reps				

AVOCADO AND BANANA PERFECT BODY WORKOUT

DAY 2	2 OR 3 SETS	WEIGHT	SET 1 REPS	SET 2 REPS	SET 3 REPS
Superset A					
Cable Lat Pulldown (page 272)	10–12 reps				
Pushup (page 256)	Max*	N/A			
Superset B					
Standing Cable Row (page 269)	10–12 reps				
Lunge-Stance Dumbbell Shoulder Press (page 263)	10–12 reps				
Dumbbell Stepup (page 264)	12–15 reps each leg				
Superset C					
Dumbbell Chest Press (page 278)	10–12 reps				
Biceps/Triceps Dumbbell Combo on Bench/Ball (page 289)	10–12 each				
Reverse Dumbbell Fly on Ball (page 274)	10–12 reps				

*Max = as many reps as possible

For Day 3, there are 2 supersets containing 4 exercises each. Rest 1 to 2 minutes after each superset, then repeat the same superset once or twice. After 2 or 3 sets of a superset, rest for 3 to 4 minutes before moving on. Remember, exercises grouped together will be performed back to back with no rest in between, so bring all your weights and situate yourself near the equipment you need to use so you can move through the exercises without missing a beat.

DAY 3	2 OR 3 SETS	WEIGHT	SET 1 REPS	SET 2 REPS	SET 3 REPS
Superset A					
Plank Row (page 259)	8–10 reps				
Dumbbell Bench Squat (page 260)	12–15 reps				
Bent-Over Dumbbell Row (page 262)	12–15 reps				
Pushup (page 256)	Max*	N/A			
Superset B					
Front Plank (page 258)	30 sec hold	N/A			
Three-Way Shoulder Series (page 288)	5 each way				
Dumbbell Reverse Lunge (page 255)	10–12 reps each leg				
Single-Leg Bench or Stability Ball Hip-Pop (page 267)	12–15 reps each leg	N/A			

*Max = as many reps as possible

Week 3

The game plan: As in Week 2, exercises grouped together as a superset will be performed back-to-back without rest. After each superset, rest for 1 to 2 minutes. Then repeat the same superset once or twice. After 2 or 3 sets of a superset, rest for 3 to 4 minutes before moving on to the next superset.

DAY 1	2 OR 3 SETS	WEIGHT	SET 1 REPS	SET 2 REPS	SET 3 REPS
Superset A					
Dumbbell Front Lunge (page 276)	10–12 reps each leg				
Pushup with Leg Twist (page 257)	Max*	N/A			
Superset B					
Dumbbell Bench Squat (page 260)	8–10 reps				
Standing Cable Row (page 269)	8–10 reps				
Superset C					
Dumbbell Stepup (page 264)	8–10 reps each leg				
Wall Sit with Dumbbell Lateral Shoulder Raise, Standing Variation (not pictured, page 268)	12–15 reps				
Double-Leg Stability Ball Curl (page 280)	8–10 reps	N/A			

*Max = as many reps as possible

DAY 2	2 OR 3 SETS	WEIGHT	SET 1 REPS	SET 2 REPS	SET 3 REPS
Superset A					
Cable Lat Pulldown (page 272)	8–10 reps				
Pushup (page 256)	Max*	N/A			
Superset B					
Squat to Single-Arm Cable Row (page 271)	8–10 reps each arm				
Dumbbell Chest Press (page 278)	8–10 reps				
Lunge-Stance Single-Arm Dumbbell Shoulder Press (page 265)	8–10 reps				
Superset C					
Dumbbell Front Shoulder Raise (page 282)	8–10 reps				
Dumbbell Front to Back Lunge (page 276)	8–10 reps each leg				
Reverse Dumbbell Fly on Ball (page 274)	8–10 reps				

*Max = as many reps as possible

AVOCADO AND BANANA PERFECT BODY WORKOUT

For Day 3, there are 2 supersets containing 4 exercises each. Rest 1 to 2 minutes after each superset, then repeat the same superset twice. After 3 sets of a superset, rest for 3 to 4 minutes before moving on to the next superset. Remember, exercises grouped together will be performed back-to-back with no rest in between, so bring all your weights and situate yourself near the equipment you need to use so you can move through the exercises without missing a beat.

DAY 3	2 OR 3 SETS	WEIGHT	SET 1 REPS	SET 2 REPS	SET 3 REPS
Superset A					
Seated Shoulder Press (page 265)	12–15 reps				
Dumbbell Bench Squat (page 260)	12–15 reps				
Bent-Over Dumbbell Row (page 262)	12–15 reps				
Front Plank (page 258)	30 sec hold	N/A			
Superset B					
Dumbbell Stepup (page 264)	10–12 reps each leg				
Cable Lat Pulldown (page 272)	12–15 reps				
Wall Sit with Dumbbell Lateral Shoulder Raise (page 268)	12–15 reps				
Single-Leg Bench or Stability Ball Hip-Pop (page 267)	12–15 reps each leg	N/A			

Week 4

The game plan: This is a recovery week. You'll take an extra day off this week, doing only two resistance workouts to prevent overtraining that could lead to injury.

DAY 1	2 SETS	WEIGHT	SET 1 REPS	SET 2 REPS
Superset A				
Dumbbell Front Lunge (page 276)	12–15 reps each leg			
Pushup (page 256)	Max*	N/A		
Cable Lat Pulldown (page 272)	12–15 reps			
Superset B				
Single-Arm Overhead Dumbbell Squat (page 277)	10 reps each arm			
Standing Cable Row (page 269)	12–15 reps			
Superset C				
Dumbbell Stepup (page 264)	12–15 reps each leg			
Dumbbell Incline Chest Press (page 278)	12–15 reps			
Superset D				
Double-Leg Stability Ball Curl (page 280)	12–15 reps	N/A		
Wall Sit with Dumbbell Lateral Shoulder Raise (page 268)	12–15 reps			

*Max = as many reps as possible

AVOCADO AND BANANA PERFECT BODY WORKOUT

DAY 2	2 SETS	WEIGHT	SET 1 REPS	SET 2 REPS
Superset A				
Balance Squat (page 281)	12–15 reps each leg	N/A		
Single-Arm Dumbbell Chest Press on Ball (page 273)	8–12 reps each arm			
Straight-Leg Dumbbell Deadlift (page 282)	12–15 reps			
Superset B				
Squat to Single-Arm Cable Row (page 271)	12–15 reps each arm			
Wall Sit (page 268)	30 sec hold			
Lunge-Stance Single-Arm Dumbbell Shoulder Press (page 265)	12–15 reps each arm			
Superset C				
Single-Leg Bench or Stability Ball Hip-Pop (page 267)	12–15 reps each leg	N/A		
Dumbbell Reverse Lunge (page 255)	8–10 reps each leg			
Reverse Dumbbell Fly on Ball (page 274)	12–15 reps			

Week 5

The game plan: Now you're back in action, working out 3 days this week.

DAY 1	2 OR 3 SETS	WEIGHT	SET 1 REPS	SET 2 REPS	SET 3 REPS
Superset A					
Multi-Plane Lunge, Dumbbell Variation (not pictured, page 275)	6 reps each leg each way				
Dumbbell Chest Press on Ball (page 273)	10–12 reps				
Superset B					
Deadlift (page 281)	10–12 reps				
Front Plank (page 258)	30 sec hold	N/A			
Single-Arm Bent-Over Dumbbell Row (page 262)	10–12 reps each arm				
Superset C					
Triple Hamstring Series (page 279)	10–12 each	N/A			
Three-Way Shoulder Series (page 288)	5 each way				

DAY 2	2 OR 3 SETS	WEIGHT	SET 1 REPS	SET 2 REPS	SET 3 REPS
Superset A					
Seated Shoulder Press, Variation on Stability Ball (not pictured, page 265)	12–15 reps				
Single-Arm Dumbbell Chest Press on Ball (page 273)	12–15 reps each arm				
Squat Jump (page 286)	20 reps	N/A			
Single-Arm Bent-Over Dumbbell Row (page 262)	12–15 reps each arm				
Superset B					
Explosive Pushup (page 287)	Max*	N/A			
Single-Leg Bench or Stability Ball Hip-Pop (page 267)	15 reps each leg	N/A			
Three-Way Shoulder Series (page 288)	8 reps each way				
Biceps/Triceps Dumbbell Combo on Bench/Ball (page 289)	12 reps each				

*Max = as many reps as possible

AVOCADO AND BANANA PERFECT BODY WORKOUT

DAY 3	2 OR 3 SETS	WEIGHT	SET 1 REPS	SET 2 REPS	SET 3 REPS
Superset A					
Balance Squat (page 281)	10–12 reps each leg	N/A			
Dumbbell Incline Chest Press (page 278)	10–12 reps				
Straight-Leg Dumbbell Deadlift (page 282)	10–12 reps				
Superset B					
Squat to Single-Arm Cable Row (page 271)	10–12 reps each arm				
Dumbbell Pliè Squat (page 271)	10–12 reps				
Lunge-Stance Single-Arm Dumbbell Shoulder Press (page 265)	10–12 reps each arm				
Superset C					
Standing Biceps Curl (page 290)	10–12 reps				
Triceps Rope Pulldown (page 291)	10–12 reps				

Week 6

The game plan: Choose heavier weights this week to meet the goal of 6 to 8 reps for the specified exercises. Opt for a weight that lets you barely eke out the 6th rep with perfect form.

DAY 1	3 SETS	WEIGHT	SET 1 REPS	SET 2 REPS	SET 3 REPS
Superset A					
Walking Dumbbell Lunge (page 272)	6–8 reps each leg				
Dumbbell Chest Press (page 278)	6–8 reps				
Superset B					
Inverted Body Row (page 285)	6–8 reps	N/A			
Deadlift (page 281)	6–8 reps				
Single-Leg Bench or Stability Ball Hip-Pop (page 267)	12–15 reps each leg	N/A			
Superset C					
Triple Hamstring Series (page 279)	6–8 each				
Reverse Dumbbell Fly on Ball (page 274)	6–8 reps				

DAY 2	3 SETS	WEIGHT	SET 1 REPS	SET 2 REPS	SET 3 REPS
Superset A					
Squat to Overhead Shoulder Press (page 286)	12–15 reps				
Dumbbell Chest Press on Ball (page 273)	12–15 reps				
Squat Jump (page 286)	15–20 reps	N/A			
Plank Row (page 259)	10 reps each arm				
Superset B					
Body-Weight Squat (page 260)	20 reps	N/A			
Explosive Pushup (page 287)	Max*	N/A			
Single-Leg Bench or Stability Ball Hip-Pop (page 267)	10 reps each leg	N/A			
Biceps/Triceps Dumbbell Combo on Bench/Ball (page 289)	12 each				

*Max = as many reps as possible

DAY 3	3 SETS	WEIGHT	SET 1 REPS	SET 2 REPS	SET 3 REPS
Superset A					
Balance Squat (page 281)	6–8 reps each leg	N/A			
Dumbbell Incline Chest Press (page 278)	6–8 reps				
Superset B					
Straight-Leg Dumbbell Deadlift (page 282)	6–8 reps				
Squat to Cable Row (page 270)	6–8 reps				
Superset C					
Dumbbell Single-Leg Bench Squat (page 261)	6–8 reps each leg				
Standing Alternating Shoulder Press (page 266)	6–8 reps each arm				
Superset D					
Wall Sit with Dumbbell Lateral Shoulder Raise (page 268)	6–8 reps				
Triceps Rope Pulldown (page 291)	10–12 reps				

Week 7

The game plan: On Days 1 and 3, your heaviest exercise is the first one in each day of the workouts. Give yourself a 2- or 3-minute rest after each set of these first exercises to allow you to lift just as heavy a weight for all 4 sets. Opt for a weight that lets you barely eke out the 6th rep with perfect form.

On Day 2, you'll do supersets of four exercises each.

DAY 1	4 SETS	WEIGHT	SET 1 REPS	SET 2 REPS	SET 3 REPS	SET 4 REPS
Dumbbell Chest Press (page 278)	4–6 reps					
Superset A	**3 Sets**	**Weight**	**Set 1 Reps**	**Set 2 Reps**	**Set 3 Reps**	**N/A**
Dumbbell Front to Back Lunge (page 276)	6–8 reps each leg					–
Assisted Chinup (page 291)	6–8 reps	N/A				–
Superset B	**3 Sets**	**Weight**	**Set 1 Reps**	**Set 2 Reps**	**Set 3 Reps**	**N/A**
Bent-Over Dumbbell Row (page 262)	6–8 reps					–
Pushup (page 256)	Max*	N/A				–
Superset C	**3 Sets**	**Weight**	**Set 1 Reps**	**Set 2 Reps**	**Set 3 Reps**	**N/A**
Straight-Leg Dumbbell Deadlift (page 282)	10–12 reps					–
Single-Leg Bench or Stability Ball Hip-Pop (page 267)	12–15 reps each leg	N/A				–

*Max = as many reps as possible

DAY 2	3 SETS	WEIGHT	SET 1 REPS	SET 2 REPS	SET 3 REPS
Superset A					
Squat to Overhead Shoulder Press (page 286)	12–15 reps				
Plank Row (page 259)	12–15 reps each arm				
Squat Jump (page 286)	20 reps	N/A			
Front Plank (page 307)	30 sec hold	N/A			
Superset B					
Explosive Pushup (page 287)	Max*	N/A			
Single-Leg Bench or Stability Ball Hip-Pop (page 267)	12–15 reps each leg	N/A			
Three-Way Shoulder Series (page 288)	10 each way				
Biceps/Triceps Dumbbell Combo on Bench/Ball (page 289)	12 each				

*Max = as many reps as possible

AVOCADO AND BANANA PERFECT BODY WORKOUT

DAY 3	4 SETS	WEIGHT	SET 1 REPS	SET 2 REPS	SET 3 REPS	SET 4 REPS
Balance Squat (page 281)	4–6 reps each leg	N/A				
Superset A	**3 Sets**	**Weight**	**Set 1 Reps**	**Set 2 Reps**	**Set 3 Reps**	**N/A**
T-Pushup (page 258)	Max*	N/A				–
Weighted Decline Crunch (page 283)	6–8 reps					–
Superset B	**3 Sets**	**Weight**	**Set 1 Reps**	**Set 2 Reps**	**Set 3 Reps**	**N/A**
Straight-Leg Dumbbell Deadlift (page 282)	6–8 reps					–
Squat to Single-Arm Cable Row (page 271)	6–8 reps each arm					–
Superset C	**3 Sets**	**Weight**	**Set 1 Reps**	**Set 2 Reps**	**Set 3 Reps**	**N/A**
Lying External Rotation (page 269)	10 reps each side					–
Reverse Dumbbell Fly on Ball (page 274)	6–8 reps	N/A				–

*Max = as many reps as possible

Week 8

The game plan: Just as in Week 7, on Days 1 and 3 your heaviest exercise is the first one in each workout. Give yourself a 2- or 3-minute rest after each set to allow you to lift just as heavy a weight for all 4 sets. Opt for a weight that lets you barely eke out the 6th rep with perfect form.

This week brings everything together so that you can really see your perfect body taking shape.

DAY 1	4 SETS	WEIGHT	SET 1 REPS	SET 2 REPS	SET 3 REPS	SET 4 REPS
Dumbbell Chest Press (page 278)	4–6 reps					
Superset A	**3 Sets**	**Weight**	**Set 1 Reps**	**Set 2 Reps**	**Set 3 Reps**	**N/A**
Dumbbell Front to Back Lunge (page 276)	12–15 reps each leg					–
Assisted Chinup (page 291)	6–8 reps	N/A				–
Superset B	**3 Sets**	**Weight**	**Set 1 Reps**	**Set 2 Reps**	**Set 3 Reps**	**N/A**
Bent-Over Dumbbell Row (page 262)	8–10 reps					–
Dumbbell Single-Leg Bench Squat (page 261)	Max*					–
Superset C	**3 Sets**	**Weight**	**Set 1 Reps**	**Set 2 Reps**	**Set 3 Reps**	**N/A**
Side Plank (page 259)	30-sec hold each side	N/A				–
Front Plank (page 258)	30-sec hold	N/A				–
Plank Row (page 259)	10 reps each arm	N/A				–

*Max = as many reps as possible

AVOCADO AND BANANA PERFECT BODY WORKOUT

DAY 2	3 SETS	WEIGHT	SET 1 REPS	SET 2 REPS	SET 3 REPS
Superset A					
Squat to Overhead Shoulder Press (page 286)	12–15 reps				
Single-Arm Dumbbell Chest Press on Ball (page 273)	12–15 reps each arm				
Squat Jump (page 286)	10 reps	N/A			
Three-Way Shoulder Series (page 288)	8 reps each way				
Superset B					
Body-Weight Squat (page 260)	20 reps	N/A			
Explosive Pushup (page 287)	Max*	N/A			
Single-Leg Bench or Stability Ball Hip-Pop (page 267)	12–15 reps each leg	N/A			
Biceps/Triceps Dumbbell Combo on Bench/Ball (page 289)	12 each				

*Max = as many reps as possible

DAY 3	4 SETS	WEIGHT	SET 1 REPS	SET 2 REPS	SET 3 REPS	SET 4 REPS
Balance Squat (page 281)	4–6 reps each leg	N/A				
Superset A	3 Sets	Weight	Set 1 Reps	Set 2 Reps	Set 3 Reps	N/A
Pushup (page 256)	Max*	N/A				–
Walking Dumbbell Lunge (page 272)	8–10 reps each leg					–
Superset B	3 Sets	Weight	Set 1 Reps	Set 2 Reps	Set 3 Reps	N/A
Straight-Leg Dumbbell Deadlift (page 282)	8–10 reps					–
Plank Row (page 259)	8–10 reps					–
Superset C	3 Sets	Weight	Set 1 Reps	Set 2 Reps	Set 3 Reps	N/A
Lying External Rotation (page 269)	10 reps each side					–
Standing Biceps Curl (page 290)	8–10 reps					–

*Max = as many reps as possible

Ab Workout

The game plan: After your cardio workouts, on your days off from weight training, perform one of the following abdominal routines. Mix it up throughout the week. Perform the exercises back-to-back or do 2 sets of each individual exercise and then move on to the next.

AB #1	2 SETS OR HOLD	SET 1 REPS	SET 2 REPS OR HOLD
Bosu Knee Twist (page 306)	8–10 reps each leg		
Plank Hip Circle (page 305)	5 each way		
V-Up (page 308)	15–20 reps		
Single-Leg Hip-Pop Hold (page 308)	30-sec hold each leg		

AB #2	2 SETS	SET 1 REPS	SET 2 REPS OR HOLD
Stability Ball Plank (page 309)	30–60-sec hold		
Side Plank (page 307)	30-sec hold each side		
Reverse Crunch on Bench (page 304)	15–20 reps		
Medicine Ball Twisting Lunge (page 309)	10 reps each side		

AB #3	2 SETS	SET 1 REPS	SET 2 REPS
Double-Side Jackknife (page 311)	20 reps each side		
Plank with Diagonal Arm Lift (page 304)	10 reps each arm		
Stability Ball Knee Tuck (page 302)	12–15 reps		
Banana Boat (page 310)	20 total rocks		

(continued)

AB #4	2 SETS	SET 1 REPS	SET 2 REPS
Weighted Side Bend (page 299)	15 reps each side		
Single-Arm, Single-Leg Superman (page 300)	12 reps each side		
Weighted Russian Twist (page 300)	10 reps each side		
V-Up (page 308)	15–20 reps		

AB #5	2 SETS	SET 1 REPS	SET 2 REPS
Knee Double Crunch (page 301)	12–15 reps each side		
Side Hip-Pop, Weighted Variation (not pictured, page 301)	12 reps each side		
Stability Ball Knee Tuck (page 302)	12–15 reps		
Single-Leg Lowering (page 302)	10 reps each side		

AB #6	2 SETS	SET 1 REPS	SET 2 REPS
Cable Wood Chop (page 303)	15 reps each side		
Weighted Side Bend (page 299)	12 reps each side		
Plank with Diagonal Arm Lift (page 304)	10 reps each arm		
Reverse Crunch on Bench (page 304)	15–20 reps		

CHAPTER 16

Perfect Made Permanent

Are we there yet? Well, yeah, in a lot of ways we are. When you follow the diet and exercise advice we've laid out in previous chapters, you *will* reach your goal: a shape that makes you look great in the mirror and a level of health and fitness that makes you feel great (and feel great about yourself)—in short, a body that's perfect for you.

From here on out, your job is simply to hold on to that perfect body. Now don't get us wrong: That doesn't mean you should simply slide back into your old eating and (non)exercise habits. Too many women do that, which is why 80 percent of the people who lose weight end up slowly gaining it back once they go off their diets. But this is where the *Women's Health Perfect Body Diet* is different. Because you tailored a plan to your individual shape and body tendencies, you'll be able to follow it long after the initial 8 weeks are up. You'll still see benefits and weight loss without the usual weight regain. You haven't just changed your body, you've changed your lifestyle—and your new lifestyle is going to keep your old body a thing of the past.

There are a few things to focus on as you go forward. For starters, stick with your eating plan. You've determined what types of foods are best for your body, and you have the proof right in front of you: You look better, you feel better, and your health has improved. Don't stop eating according to the plan just because you've reached your weight-loss goal.

That means continuing to eat five or six meals per day and using glucomannan. Glucomannan will continue to help you stay full and satisfied and keep your blood sugars and subsequent hunger levels more controlled, even after you have achieved your perfect body. One of this book's contributors has been using it with her meals for the past 3 years, and she still experiences the benefits. She uses the same amount of glucomannan as she did when she was cutting calories to initially lose weight, and her weight has been stable now for years. She also continues to eat five or six small meals a day, so she hardly ever makes bad or rash food choices based on insane hunger.

Finally, sticking with the Perfect Body exercise plan, with its emphasis on weight lifting, will prevent your fat cells from growing. While eating the right foods is important for losing weight in the first place, exercise is really the more important element in terms of keeping your perfect body. Continue to exercise 5 or 6 days a week, and on days without planned and purposeful exercise, make sure that you are physically active for at least 30 minutes.

Eating for the New You

As you lost weight, your *resting energy expenditure* (REE)—the number of calories your body needs just to exist—got lower. That means you can't keep eating for your old weight; you have to adjust your caloric intake for your new Perfect Body weight. In Chapter 7, we helped you figure out how many calories you should eat each day to lose weight. Break out your calculator again, because we're going to crunch some new numbers: the number of calories you need to eat to stay at your perfect weight.

Step 1: Recalculate your resting energy expenditure (REE). This is the absolute minimum number of calories your new body needs just to keep functioning.

》 Multiply your body weight in pounds by 7.18.   _____

》 Divide that number by 2.2.   _____

》 Add 795.   _____

REE =   _____

Step 2: Now factor in your *physical activity level* (PAL).

》 Under 35 years old and less than 30 pounds over your ideal weight, use 1.5 for your PAL.

》 Under 35 and more than 30 pounds over your ideal weight, use 1.4 for your PAL.

» 35 years and over and less than 30 pounds over your ideal weight, use 1.4 for your PAL.

» 35 years and over and more than 30 pounds over your ideal weight, use 1.2 for your PAL.

REE (from Step 1) × PAL = _____

This is the number of calories you need to eat each day to *maintain* your current weight. We suggest playing it safe and following meal plans with slightly fewer calories (this allows for the occasional miscalculation or bout of cheating). On days when you're exercising, subtract 100 from the number you calculated in Step 2. On sedentary days, subtract 200. This formula will keep you on track—and keep your body perfect forever.

Why You Should Keep Weighing In

You've gotten into the habit of weighing yourself every day, so why stop now? A recent study in the *New England Journal of Medicine* found that among 314 dieters who had lost 10 percent of their body weight over 2 years, daily weigh-ins were associated with a decreased risk of regaining weight.

Stepping on the scale will let you know if it's time to change your behavior because your weight is starting to creep back up. You'll be able to squelch any problems before you gain all the weight back.

Even if you're doing everything perfectly, there are lots of reasons why the number on the scale could be up by a pound or two every now and again. Here are some of the usual suspects.

You were thirsty. Downing 16 ounces of any fluid can cause an immediate gain of 1 pound.

You're backed up. If it's been more than a couple of days since your bowels did their thing, constipation can tilt the scale by as much as 2 pounds.

When Weight Loss Flatlines

If, after 8 weeks, you've lost significant weight but are still not at your goal, keep going. If you've stalled, with no weight loss in more than 2 weeks, recalculate your caloric score again. As your weight goes down, so does the number of calories you need to keep your body running. And don't forget your "Take a Perfect Body Break" day, which will also boost your metabolism and give you that extra bit of energy to burn more calories going forward.

You're on vacation. The changes in air pressure during travel can make you retain water on flights longer than 4 hours, which can show up as an extra 1 to 3 pounds on the scale.

You ate the Kung Pao Chicken. Have a salty dinner and you could wake up 2 to 3 pounds heavier—your body retains water to dilute all that sodium.

Your period is on its way. Hormone fluctuations in the 3 days leading up to your period can make you retain up to 5 pounds of water.

If any of these are the culprits, don't sweat it. Your scale will readjust quickly. However, if you're getting heavier because you've suddenly developed an apple cider doughnut fetish, we think you know what to do. But don't get discouraged—you've already proved that you have the discipline it takes to get the body you want.

Exercise: Move More, Add More Variety

Physical activity and exercise seem to be more important than diet in preventing weight gain, according to James Hill, PhD, of the National Institutes of Health's Center for Human Nutrition. That's because your newly trim body may burn calories more efficiently, finding a way to work with less energy expended. As a result, you'll need to keep your exercise intensity high by creating new challenges in your workouts. Lift more weight, add an extra set, or do a few more interval cardio options. The good news is that as your body develops more muscle with consistent exercise, your metabolism will increase and it will be easier to maintain your perfect body.

The Importance of Recovery

Even though you've amped up your workout, you still have to give your body enough recovery time. The soreness that accompanies a workout is usually caused by torn muscle fiber. A rest day allows the muscle fiber to heal, so you'll find that you won't feel as sore the next time you work out. As the muscle is repairing itself, it will also drive up your metabolism, so you'll burn even more calories. You will need to eat a bit more during recovery to help your muscles repair themselves. So if you've been working out hard for the past 2 months, a whole week off is well deserved. When you do come back to the gym, you'll regain the vigor that you had when you first started training.

"For weight maintenance, it's the total amount of physical activity and exercise that counts, even if it's in small bouts throughout the day," says Dr. Hill. Remember, everything counts toward your exercise time: rigorous cleaning, brisk mall walking, hiking, biking, beach volleyball, mountain climbing, tennis, and even golf.

You also have to keep changing the routine so your body doesn't get bored. If your body becomes too used to any one type of exercise, no matter what your weight is, it'll stop making beneficial changes. So mix it up a bit.

Thankfully, the Perfect Body workout offers you lots of variety so you always have something new to choose. You can continue following the program as outlined for several more months, but try increasing the resistance by lifting heavier weights. You'll even find that you may be able to add another day of weight training to your exercise routine. These simple modifications will make this program one that will work for a long time.

To keep improving your aerobic fitness, explore the world beyond the cardio machines. Your gym may offer yoga, Pilates, kickboxing, or even samba lessons. It's now open season for those classes you were too intimidated to join. If you can get a perfect body in 8 weeks, you can definitely conquer Spinning class.

What to Do If the Weight Comes Back

As we've said time and again throughout this book, the beauty of the *Women's Health Perfect Body Diet* is that it's tailored to *you*. It's helped you figure out what's best for *your* body—not someone else's. So if putting on your favorite jeans ever starts to feel like an Olympic event again, the solution is simple: Just get back to basics.

Remember, the *Women's Health Perfect Body Diet* is really just six simple steps:

1. Determine what you should weigh.

2. Determine which of the two diets is best for you, and always select from the vast array of good foods prescribed by your plan.

3. Calculate your personal caloric score.

Set Aside Time to Eat

Most of us are so busy that it's almost impossible not to do two things at once, like eat and drive, or eat and work. But when you eat at the same time you're doing something else, you often eat too much, and those pounds you worked so hard to lose will bounce right back on. So stop. Slow down. And whenever you eat, make that your only task.

4. Add glucomannan to your foods.

5. Eat five or six meals a day.

6. Exercise 6 days a week, and be physically active for at least 30 minutes on the remaining day.

In a lot of ways, you should consider this book a friend—one who wants what's best for you and is always ready to help you get it. So put us up on your bookshelf. We're always here if you need us.

Moving Forward: The Power of a Perfect Body

The diet and exercise advice in this book have helped you reach your physical goals. You're leaner, stronger, and healthier than you were when you started. But it's a funny thing about physical changes: They have a way of spilling over into your entire life. If you look better, you feel better. And if you feel great about yourself, then there's hardly any limit to what you can do.

The Introduction to this book dealt with a simple question: *What does it mean to have a perfect body?* As we said then, every woman answers that question differently, and that's exactly as it should be. *Perfect* comes in all shapes and sizes. But what underlies all those versions of perfect is one simple idea: giving the world—and yourself—the very best version of you, the one who looks her best, feels her best, performs her best. So, yes, you've achieved a perfect body, but now the real fun starts: enjoying your perfect life.

INDEX

Underscored page references indicate boxed text and tables. **Boldface** references indicate photographs.

Bent-over dumbbell row, 262, **262**

Berries, 102. *See also specific berries*

Beverages
    alcoholic, 96, 97, <u>98</u>
    coffee, 80, <u>81</u>, 95, <u>95</u>
    meal-replacement, 86
    sports drinks, 95
    water, 90, 93, 95, 161

Biceps curl
    front lunge with, 277, **277**
    standing, 290, **290**

Biceps/triceps dumbbell combo on ball/bench, 289, **289**

Binge eating disorders, 23

Bingeing, cause of, 17

Bioelectrical impedance, for measuring body fat, 15

Bird dog, 247, **247**

Birth control pills, increasing estrogen levels in Pear shapes, 8

Blackberries
    Apple and Blackberry Fiber Crumble, 190

Blood glucose
    caffeine affecting, 95
    effect of low-fat diet on, xix–xx
    fiber steadying, 27
    glucomannan reducing, <u>35</u>
    normal vs. abnormal ranges of, 20–21
    stress depleting, 18
    testing levels of, 21

Blueberries
    Blueberry Beet Almond Smoothie, 224

BMI. *See* Body mass index

Body fat
    controlling distribution of, 4
    excess sugar causing, 47
    factors affecting distribution of, 3–6
    loss of
        dietary fats for, 57–59
        from problem areas, 4–5
    low-fat diets increasing, xx
    protein for burning, 67

Body fat percentage
    as indicator of healthy weight, 14–15
    methods of measuring, 15–16
    recommended, 14

Body shape(s). *See also* Apple shapes; Avocado shapes; Banana shapes; Pear shapes
    identifying, 6–7
    weight loss affecting, 5–6

Body-weight single-leg bench squat, 261, **261**

Body-weight squat, 260, **260**

Bone structure, for determining perfect weight, 13–14, <u>14</u>

Borage oil, for preventing weight regain, 59

Bosu knee twist, 306, **306**

Bowel regularity
    fiber for, 27
    glucomannan for, 92

Brain, fullness detected by, <u>24</u>, 24–25

Brain chemical response, hunger and, 21–22

Bran
    Bran Date Muffins, 228

Breads
    in Grains and Fruits Diet, 135, <u>135</u>
    poor-choice, 51–52
    sprouted grain, <u>135</u>
    Zucchini Bread, 226

Breakfasts
    guidelines for, 80–81, <u>81</u>
    for testing carbohydrate tolerance, 41, <u>41</u>

Breast cancer, soy foods and, 68

Broccoli
    Creamy Broccoli Soup, 200
    No-Crust Vegetable Quiche, 192
    Rainbow Broccoli Slaw, 177

Burgers
    Turkey and Bean Burgers, 167

Butter, 55, 64, 65

Buttermilk
    Whole Wheat Buttermilk Gluco-Pancakes, 180

»C

Cable lat pulldown, 272, **272**

Cable row
    quarter-squat, 270, **270**
    squat to, 270, **270**
    squat to single-arm, 271, **271**
    standing, 269, **269**

Cable wood chop, 303, **303**

Caffeine, 95

Cake
    Strawberry Cheesecake, 189

Calcium
  for lactose-intolerant
      women, 92
  for weight loss, 63
CALERIE study, results from,
      xviii
Calipers, for measuring body
      fat, 15–16
Calories
  fiber for reducing, 28
  glucomannan for reducing,
      35
  weight loss and, xviii, 77,
      366–67
Cancer
  good fats preventing, 54
  soy foods and, 68
Canola oil, 64
Carbohydrate enzymes, taken
      with glucomannan,
      92
Carbohydrate intolerance
  alcohol and, 96, 97
  in Apple shapes, 40, 48
  caffeine sensitivity with, 95
  indicators of, 39, 40
  testing for, 39–45
Carbohydrates. See also
      Low-carb diets
  Apple shape response to, 7
  caveats about, 52
  complex, 47
  cutting, for quick ab
      sculpting, 298
  determining daily intake of,
      100, 130
  in diet for Apple shapes, 7
  in diet for Avocado shapes, 8
  in diet for Pear shapes, 8

excess
  converted to fat, xx
  problems from, 39, 40
exercise and, 49
in frequent meals, 21
in Grains and Fruits Diet,
      49–51, 50, 129–37
in Greens and Berries Diet,
      48, 50, 99–104
insulin response and, 20
in low-fat diets, xix
100-calorie, 79
poor-choice, 51–53
in postworkout meal, 85
for reducing ghrelin levels,
      20
simple, 47–48
sources of, 46–47, 49–51
as sugar, starch, or fiber,
      47
weight loss and, xxii–xxiii
in *Your Perfect Body Plan*,
      xviii
Carbohydrate tolerance
  in Pear shapes, 40
  testing for, 39–45
Carbohydrate tolerance
      questionnaire, 42–43
Cardio exercise
  for Apple shapes, 7–8, 312
  for Avocado shapes, 8–9,
      346
  for Banana shapes, 9, 346
  for Pear shapes, 329
  in Your Perfect Body
      Workout, 238, 239,
      293–97
Carrot juice
  Carrot Cake Smoothie, 206

Casserole
  Turkey and Cauliflower
      Casserole, 198
Cauliflower
  Bangers and Cauliflower
      Mash, 200
  Milk-Free Creamed
      Cauliflower, 179
  Turkey and Cauliflower
      Casserole, 198
CCK. *See* Cholecystokinin
Cereals
  in Grains and Fruits Diet,
      135, 135, 136, 136
  in Greens and Berries Diet,
      104, 104
  high-fiber, 81
  poor-choice, 52
  Super Fiber Breakfast Bowl,
      201, 220
Cheese
  Balanced-Body Smoothie,
      185
  Chocolate Protein Pudding,
      208, 228
  Goat Cheese and Herb
      Gluco-Omelette, 193
  High-Fiber Cottage Cheese
      and Yogurt, 202
  Mixed Greens with
      Strawberries, Feta, and
      Walnuts, 178
  protein content of, 107, 140
  Ricotta Mango Breakfast,
      202, 222
  Scrambled Eggs with Feta
      Cheese and Salsa, 41
Cheesecake
  Strawberry Cheesecake, 189

No-Crust Vegetable Quiche, 192

Scrambled Eggs with Feta Cheese and Salsa, 41

Scrambled Egg Whites with Spinach, 162

Sweet Egg White Splendor, 209

Enova oil, 57–58, 64

Ephedra, 36

Estrogen

affecting body fat distribution, 4

controlling, in Pear shapes, 8

good fats producing, 54

Ethnic background, affecting body fat distribution, 3–4

Evening primrose oil, for preventing weight regain, 59

Exercise, xxiii–xxiv. *See also* Your Perfect Body Workout

affecting body fat, 4, 5

for Apple shapes, 7–8

for Avocado shapes, 8–9

for Banana shapes, 9

for burning off extra calories, 98

carbohydrates and, 49

eating to support, 84–85, 95–96

improving carbohydrate metabolism, 40

monounsaturated fats and, 55

for Pear shapes, 8

vs. physical activity, 238

protein needs with, 70

recovery from, 368

short periods of, 254

for weight loss, 237–38

for weight maintenance, 368–69

Explosive pushup, 287, **287**

External rotation, lying, 269, **269**

»F

Fast food, 86–88

Fat, body. *See* Body fat

Fat-burner supplements, 36

Fat burning, effect of frequent meals on, 78, 80

Fats, dietary

in animal protein, 67

in dairy products, 62–63

determining daily intake of, 100–101, 130–31

in diet for Apple shapes, 7

in diet for Avocado shapes, 8

in diet for Pear shapes, 8

for fat loss, 57–59, 66

in frequent meals, 21

ghrelin levels and, 20

in Grains and Fruits Diet, 65, 137–39

in Greens and Berries Diet, 65, 104–7

health benefits from, 53–54, 66

in nuts, 60–61

100-calorie, 79

oxidized, health risks from, 64

perfect ratios of, 64–65

for slowing carbohydrate breakdown, 47–48

types of (*see* Interesterified fats; Monounsaturated fats; Omega-3 fatty acids; Omega-6 fatty acids; Polyunsaturated fats; Saturated fats; Trans fats)

types to avoid, 66

in *Your Perfect Body Plan,* xviii

Feta cheese

Mixed Greens with Strawberries, Feta, and Walnuts, 178

Scrambled Eggs with Feta Cheese and Salsa, 41

Fiber

in beans and legumes, 103, 103, 134, 134

in carbohydrates, 47

depleted from foods, 30

enzyme for digesting, 92

for fullness, 27–28

gas from, 30

insoluble, 28, 30–31

recommended intake of, 30

for slowing carbohydrate breakdown, 47–48

soluble, 28, 30

sources of, 30–31, 31

for weight loss, 50

in whole wheat bread, 51

Fiber supplements, 32

Fish and shellfish

Brown Rice and Salmon Salad, 214

Coconut Curry Shrimp, 199

Mantra, for refusing food, 19
Maple syrup, as sweetener, 94
Mayonnaise
    Glorious Gluco-Mayo, 203
Meal frequency and size
    for avoiding low blood
        glucose, 21
    for cortisol control, 7
    for hunger control, 26
    for speeding metabolism,
        78, 80
Meal plans
    in Grains and Fruits Diet,
        75–76, 143, 143–56
    in Greens and Berries Diet,
        75–76, 111, 111–24
Meal-replacement drinks and
    bars, 86
Meats. *See also specific meats*
    fat content of, 105, 138
    protein content of, 107, 108,
        140, 141
Medicine ball twisting lunge,
    309, **309**
Menopause, soy foods and, 68
Metabolic Drive by Biotest, 68
Metabolism
    determining calorie intake, 77
    dieting lowering, 9, 223
    dopamine maintaining, 22
    factors increasing
        exercise, 237–38
        frequent meals, 78, 80
        good fats, 54
        muscle repair, 368
        protein, 66
        snacks, 84
        Your Perfect Body Break,
            98

Methylcellulose, as fiber
    supplement, 32
Mexican Americans, belly fat
    in, 3
Milk
    protein content of, 108, 141
    soy, 68
Mindless eating, 229–30
Monounsaturated fats, 55
    balancing intake of, 64–65
    frying with, 64
    in Grains and Fruits Diet,
        138
    in Greens and Berries Diet,
        105
    in nuts, 60–61
    for satiety, 55
    in steak, 67
Mood changes, from low-fat
    diet, xix–xx
Motivation, for Your Perfect
    Body Workout, 242
Muffins
    Bran Date Muffins, 228
    Pumpkin Protein Fiber
        Muffins, 191
Multi-plane lunge, 275, **275**
Multivitamin, 92–93
Muscle mass. *See also* Muscles
    depletion of, 84
    effect of dieting on, xxi
    protein for preserving, 66,
        70
Muscles. *See also* Muscle mass
    increasing, in
        Apple shapes, 7, 8
        Avocado shapes, 8
        Pear shapes, 8
    recovery time for, 368

Mushrooms
    Crab-Stuffed Mushroom
        Caps, 173
    Creamy Mushroom Soup,
        217
    No-Crust Vegetable Quiche,
        192
Mustard, Dijon
    Asparagus with Dill
        Mustard Sauce, 176
    Dijon Chicken Salad, 164

»N

NexGen Foods, 90
NSI Glucomannan, 90
Nut butters, 65
    Chicken Satay with Peanut
        Dipping Sauce, 195
    fat content of, 105, 138
    protein content of, 110,
        142
Nutrient information, Web
    sites on, 231
Nuts. *See also* Almonds; Nut
    butters; Walnuts
    benefits of, 60–62, 61
    fat content of, 105, 106, 138,
        139
    protein content of, 110, 142
    storing, 61
    uses for, 60

»O

Oats
    Gluco-Granola, 181
    Pumpkin-Spiced Oatmeal,
        221
    Simple Oats with Whey,
        220

Obesity, stomach size and, 22, 23

Oils. *See also specific oils*
  classification of, 54
  cooking, choosing, 64–65
  fat content of, 105, 106, 138, 139
  for fat loss, 57–59

Olive oil, 54, 64, 65

Omega-3 fatty acids, 55–56, 56, 57, 65, 67, 93

Omega-6 fatty acids, 56–57, 57, 65

Omelette
  Goat Cheese and Herb Gluco-Omelette, 193

100-calorie cheat sheet, 79

Onions
  No-Crust Vegetable Quiche, 192
  Vegetable-Stuffed Peppers, 218

Optimum Nutrition Whey, 68

Orzo
  Chicken Orzo Salad, 212
  Tasty Orzo Pilaf, 221

Osteoporosis, testing for, 16

Overeating
  contributors to, 24
  fiber preventing, 27, 28
  from low-fat diet, xx

» P

Pancakes
  Whole Wheat Buttermilk Gluco-Pancakes, 180

Peanut butter
  Chicken Satay with Peanut Dipping Sauce, 195

Peanuts, benefits of, 61

Pear shapes
  carbohydrate tolerance in, 40
  diet and exercise for, 8
  exercise goals for, 238
  fat distribution in, 5
  Grains and Fruits Diet for, 40
  insulin response in, 20
  waist-hip ratio of, 6
  Your Perfect Body Workout for, 329, 330–45

Peas
  Quick Turkey, Bean, and Pea Chili, 166
  Slow Cooker Split-Pea Soup, 175

Pecans, benefits of, 61

Peppers
  Stuffed Peppers with Tuna Salad, 169
  Vegetable-Stuffed Peppers, 218

"Perfect" body, individual views on, xv, 370

Perfect Body Break, xxiii, 97–98, 367

Perfect weight. *See* Weight, perfect

Periodization, in weight-training workouts, 238–39

Pesto
  Chicken with Pistachio Pesto, 196
  Sun-Dried Tomato Pesto, 204

Physical activity
  vs. exercise, 238
  for weight maintenance, 368–69

Physical activity level
  calculating, 77
  recalculating, after weight loss, 366–67

Phytoestrogens
  increasing estrogen levels in Pear shapes, 8
  in soy foods, 68

Pilaf
  Tasty Orzo Pilaf, 221

Pistachios
  benefits of, 61
  Chicken with Pistachio Pesto, 196

Plank
  front, 258, **258**, 307, **307**
  side, 259, **259**, 307, **307**
  stability ball, 309, **309**

Plank hip circle, 305, **305**

Plank row, 259, **259**

Plank with diagonal arm lift, 304, **304**

Plateaus, weight, reasons for, 237, 367

Plié squat, dumbbell, 283, **283**

Polyunsaturated fats, 55–57, 57
  balancing intake of, 64–65
  in Grains and Fruits Diet, 138–39
  in Greens and Berries Diet, 106
  in nuts, 60
  oxidation of, 64

Portion control, 87

Spot reduction, myth of, 4
Sprouted grain breads, 135
Squat
  balance, 281, **281**
  body-weight, 260, **260**
  body-weight single-leg
    bench, 261, **261**
  dumbbell bench, 260, **260**
  dumbbell plié, 283, **283**
  dumbbell single-leg bench,
    261, **261**
  to overhead shoulder press,
    286, **286**
  prisoner, 245, **245**
  single-arm overhead
    dumbbell, 277, **277**
  Y, 245, **245**
Squat jump, 286, **286**
Squat to cable row, 270, **270**
Squat to overhead shoulder
  press, 286, **286**
Squat to single-arm cable row,
  271, **271**
Stability ball curl, double- or
  single-leg, 280, **280**
Stability ball hip-pop
  bench or, 267, **267**
  single-leg bench or, 267, **267**
Stability ball knee tuck, 302,
  302
Stability ball plank, 309, **309**
Standing alternating shoulder
  press, 266, **266**
Standing biceps curl, 290, **290**
Standing cable row, 269, **269**
Starch, in carbohydrates, 47
Static stretch, problem with,
  240
Stepover, upper-body, 284, **284**

Stepup, dumbbell, 264, **264**
Stevia, 94, 133
Stew
  Curried Chickpea Stew, 174
Stomach size
  adjusting to smaller meals,
    23, 24
  hunger and, 22–23
Stool frequency, glucomannan
  increasing, 92
Straight-leg dumbbell deadlift,
  282, **282**
Straight-leg kick, walking, 251,
  251
Strawberries
  Gluco-Berry Protein Sorbet,
    191
  Mixed Greens with
    Strawberries, Feta, and
    Walnuts, 178
  Strawberry Cheesecake, 189
Strength exercises. *See also*
    Weight-training
    workouts
  for Apple shapes, 312,
    314–27
  assisted chinup, 291, **291**
  assisted pullup, 292, **292**
  for Avocado and Banana
    shapes, 346, 347,
    348–62
  balance squat, 281, **281**
  bench or stability ball
    hip-pop, 267, **267**
  bench pushup, 257, **257**
  bent-over barbell row, 263,
    263
  bent-over dumbbell row,
    262, **262**

biceps/triceps dumbbell
  combo on ball/bench,
  289, **289**
body-weight single-leg bench
  squat, 261, **261**
body-weight squat, 260, **260**
cable lat pulldown, 272, **272**
deadlift, 281, **281**
double- or single-leg stability
  ball curl, 280, **280**
dumbbell bench squat, 260,
  260
dumbbell chest press, 278,
  278
dumbbell chest press on
  ball, 273, **273**
dumbbell front lunge, 276,
  276
dumbbell front shoulder
  raise, 282, **282**
dumbbell front to back
  lunge, 276, **276**
dumbbell incline chest
  press, 278, **278**
dumbbell lateral lunge, 256,
  256
dumbbell plié squat, 283,
  283
dumbbell reverse lunge, 255,
  255
dumbbell single-leg bench
  squat, 261, **261**
dumbbell stepup, 264, **264**
explosive pushup, 287, **287**
front lunge with biceps curl,
  277, **277**
front plank, 258, **258**
inverted body row, 285, **285**
leg press, 285, **285**